LEGION
•XXII•

THE
CAPSARIUS

LEGION
•XXII•

THE
CAPSARIUS

SIMON TURNEY

HEAD
of
ZEUS

An Aries Book

First published in the UK in 2022 by Head of Zeus Ltd
This paperback edition first published in 2022 by Head of Zeus Ltd,
part of Bloomsbury Publishing Plc

9 7 5 3 1 2 4 6 8

A catalogue record for this book is available from
the British Library.

ISBN (PB): 9781801108942
ISBN (E): 9781801108911

Typeset by Divaddict Publishing Solutions Ltd

Map design by Michael Athanson

Printed and bound in Great Britain by
CPI Group (UK) Ltd, Croydon CR0 4YY

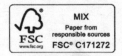

Head of Zeus Ltd
First Floor East
5–8 Hardwick Street
London EC1R 4RG

WWW.HEADOFZEUS.COM

*To the tireless and heroic staff of
the National Health Service*

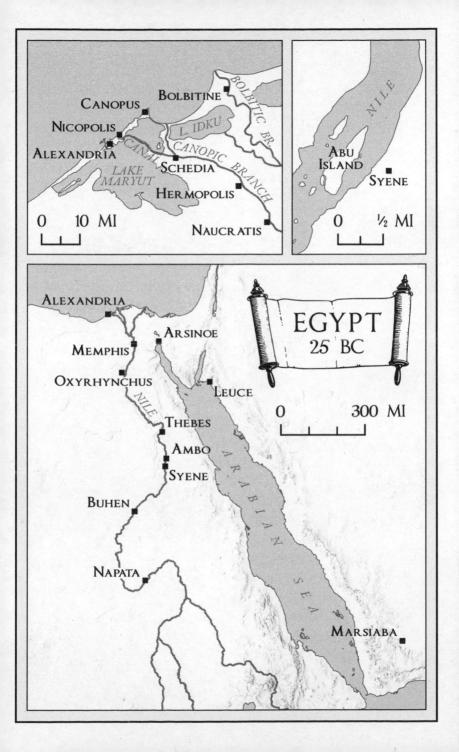

CANOPUS
BOLBITINE
NICOPOLIS
L. IDKU
BOLBITIC BR
ALEXANDRIA
CANAL
CANOPIC BRANCH
LAKE
MARYUT
SCHEDIA
HERMOPOLIS
NAUCRATIS
0   10 MI

NILE
ABU
ISLAND
SYENE
0   ½ MI

ALEXANDRIA
ARSINOE
MEMPHIS
OXYRHYNCHUS
NILE
LEUCE
THEBES
AMBO
ARABIAN SEA
SYENE
BUHEN
NAPATA
MARSIABA

EGYPT
25 BC
0   300 MI

PROLOGUE

One year previously: Arabia "Felix" – "the lucky"

Staring down at the stump that was all that remained of his left arm, legionary Titus Terrentius of the Twelfth Fulminata legion lurched and stumbled across the darkened sands as though the very gates of Hades were opening behind him, leaving an intermittent trail of crimson, glistening black in the moonlight. The burden, dragged in his good hand, occasionally burbled or moaned as it bounced off rocks or slid through the blood train.

Concentrating as he moved, Terrentius focused hard on anything innocuous that crossed his consciousness to help take his mind off the dreadful pain or his very real danger. Not for the first time in the past quarter-hour, or even in the preceding days, he couldn't help but wonder what god he'd crossed to end up in this situation.

The blame had seemed initially to lie squarely with Aelius Gallus, the commanding prefect, for his ill-considered action, or perhaps with the great Princeps Octavian of Rome for ordering the expedition in the first place. Now, however, he knew different. Even if the gods weren't against them, others were...

★ ★ ★

The orders from the man who effectively ruled Rome had come down to the Prefect of Aegyptus the preceding year: a campaign to be undertaken to annexe the Sabaean lands of Arabia Felix and their incense production centres, and to control by both land and sea the trade routes that supplied Rome with its expensive and rare spices.

The Twelfth, based at cosmopolitan Alexandria – along with their sister legion in the province, the Third Cyrenaica – had been pleased, eager even, at the news. Prefect Gallus had spent months carefully preparing his campaign. At Arsinoe, where the Arabian Sea came closest to the Nile's lush delta, he constructed a fleet of ships large enough to carry a vast force past the endless wastelands, rocks and mountains that the Aegyptians called Biau and the Hebrews called Sinai, across the narrow sea and on down the coast of Arabia. The legions had been drawn together in the north, leaving only two cohorts to control Aegyptus. There they had combined with an army of strange non-Roman auxiliaries, comprised largely of Aegyptian cavalry units, Jewish irregulars and Nabataean mercenaries from the deserts north of Arabia.

A goat had been opened and read and the omens pronounced good, and Gallus had smiled to the cheers of his men and given the command to depart. It had begun as a glorious and magnificent expedition, the valiant soldiers of Rome boarding bulky transports to the fanfares of the musicians and the cheers of the civilians. Terrentius himself had grinned like an idiot as he clambered down into the hold of the broad vessel and, along with his fellow legionaries, found a place to sit among the supplies, grateful that they had not been allocated space in those ships that carried the horses, oxen and camels as the unfortunate auxiliaries had been.

★ ★ ★

Terrentius' thoughts whirled for a moment as he stumbled in the dirt, the gravel in his boots rubbing his feet raw and adding to his torment. He'd been warned by his friends to wear socks to prevent chafing, but the Arabian heat was just too much to even think about such apparel.

Righting himself, he gritted his teeth against the agony of his severed arm, momentarily dropping the groaning figure, gripping his elbow and raising the forearm to prevent too much blood flowing free. His tourniquet must have loosened. A quick glance over his shoulder told him it was just about over. Now it was all down to him. Taking a deep breath, he gathered a handful of the man's tunic in his fist and staggered on, hoping he had remained unnoticed.

The catalogue of disasters that constituted Gallus' campaign had begun almost immediately. Rounding the tip of the Sinai, the fleet had encountered a freak storm at open sea and arrived battered and worn at the Arabian coast, only to discover that they would have to continue many leagues south along the rocky coast before finding a harbour where they could safely put in.

Of the one hundred and thirty ships that had slipped away from Arsinoe, fewer than a hundred arrived at the port of Leuce and, as the men clambered, wearily and distraught, onto dry land, many had found somewhere quiet to make offerings, libations or simple prayers to Neptune in fear or gratitude.

Among the legions, resentment began to rise towards the prefect's Nabataean guide, Syllaeus, who had insisted on this

SIMON TURNEY

disastrous route as the best entry point to the fabled lands of Arabia Felix. The Nabataean official had remained in the confidence of prefect Gallus, however, insisting that there had been no reasonable alternative.

What had been planned as a week-long sojourn at Leuce to allow time for any stray vessels to rejoin the fleet had then turned into months of waking nightmare as a sudden plague began to manifest itself among the men, an illness perhaps contracted at home and then spread in the cramped conditions of the ships, or possibly native to Leuce and virulent enough to move about the Roman camp like a sudden brush fire.

The pessimists among the common soldiery, initially a minority that had now grown into the majority, proclaimed the campaign a mistake, doomed and disfavoured by the gods. Truly, the size of Gallus' enormous force had almost halved by the time the disease had run its course and the segregation of the sick from the healthy had halted its spread.

The army that left Leuce the next spring, heading into the desert along ancient and mysterious nomadic trade routes, was a different force entirely to the one that had left Aegyptus. Brooding and dark, sick and tired, fewer than seven thousand men pressed on toward the fabled lands of Arabia Felix, the Nabataean Syllaeus once more leading the way, to the loathing of many.

Terrentius paused, his head spinning. The loss of blood was starting to affect him and he was beginning to feel distinctly faint, yet he had to press on, else all would be lost. Tearing off a strip of his russet-coloured tunic, he added an extra tourniquet, pulling it tight until the flow of blood slowed once more.

Gritting his teeth, he glared down at the barely conscious man in the long brown robe and growled. Changing his grip, he grasped the man's long hair and used that to drag him across the rough ground.

The next few months had been a blur of thirst, hunger, weakness, exhaustion and despair, punctuated by occasional violent bloodshed when the army of Gallus came across a small town or settlement that confirmed they were in the lands of Arabia Felix and under the watchful gaze of the Sabaeans.

The names of conquered towns went down in the prefect's wax tablets for later reports and to count toward the possibility of a triumph, though they meant little to the soldiers themselves: Neirani; Asca; Athrula. What constituted glorious expansion for Gallus meant the periodic loss of hundreds of comrades for his men.

And then finally, less than a week ago, they had reached the prefect's goal: the great mud-brick, powerfully walled city of Marsiaba, capital of the Sabaeans. Given the height and thickness of the defences and the almost unassailable rock upon which it sat, a direct assault would have been suicidal. Although a siege had seemed out of the question from the very beginning, the only water available being that which the army had brought with them on camels, there had really been no other option. The sparse dry wood in the area was largely unsuitable for the construction of siege engines and, as the army of Gallus created its perimeter and began to send out patrols, the water was placed under secure guard and the men put on half rations.

★ ★ ★

Terrentius glanced over his shoulder again. The camp of the Nabataean mercenaries and their Jewish companions lay brooding behind him, the torches and lamps twinkling innocently in the darkness. Had they been in collusion since the very beginning, or had their loyalty been only recently bought?

It had been less than half an hour ago that Titus Terrentius and his companions had set out from the camp of the Twelfth on their routine patrol. The century, already under half strength, had tramped off on their route around the perimeter, covering a quarter of the circuit where they would wait until the next patrol met them and exchange watchwords before turning and marching back.

"Pick your bloody feet up," the centurion had growled at him as they marched.

Terrentius, along with several of his companions, had grumbled quietly, glaring at their commander. It was hardly their fault that they were having trouble marching in the dark in this terrain. The other patrols had cut the route slightly short in order to stay on the low, flat ground below the walls of Marsiaba. His centurion, however, ever the strict disciplinarian, had led them along the precisely ordained route, crossing crests of rocky ground and scree slopes: a decision unpopular with the men.

A decision fortuitous beyond measure in retrospect.

It had been at one particular rocky ridge when the centurion leading them had suddenly waved them to a halt and dropped sharply behind a boulder. A man at the back had opened his mouth with a question but the optio, the centurion's second in command, had slapped him across the head and gestured him to silence. The thirty or so remaining men of the century had dropped into silent hiding among the rocks.

Terrentius had been close to the front, near the centurion, and rose to peer over the tip of the rock that obscured him. He had a moment to see a single lone figure on the sands perhaps three hundred paces from both the patrol and the nearby camp of the Nabataean mercenaries before the centurion's massive fist gripped his sleeve and yanked him back down out of sight.

"Get down, you prick. They'll see you."

But Terrentius was frowning. Something about the way that figure moved and the shape of his attire had been very familiar.

He shook his head.

"What is it?" the officer growled quietly.

"That's Syllaeus, the guide!"

The centurion's brow furrowed.

"You sure?"

"Positive, sir." Terrentius nodded vigorously. Beside him, the centurion released his grip and rose to glance over the rock.

"Bugger me, you're right. The question is: who in Hades are those others behind him?"

Terrentius and several of the other legionaries rose once more to peer over the boulders. The man was definitely Syllaeus. There was something snake-like and hypnotic about the way he moved, and he was attired in a brown robe typical of his people, yet elaborately decorated at shoulders and cuffs, and a strangely ill-fitting Phrygian cap. What Terrentius had failed to notice at first glance was the group of men converging on Syllaeus from the opposite side: more than a hundred men, armour and weapons glinting in the moonlight.

"Them's Arab types." The centurion frowned. "Got to be Sabaeans. No one else around here that looks like that. The Nabataean bastard's consorting with the enemy!" the centurion snarled. "Screw the patrol... I think we need to have a little word with our friend from Petra."

A few paces behind, the optio cleared his throat. "Should we not report this to the camp straight away, sir?"

The centurion shook his head. "Come on. I want him intact to answer a few questions. We need to get him before he's in with that lot."

The soldiers drew their swords as one, checking their helmet straps and hefting their shields, gripping them tight in their left hands.

"Run!" the officer hissed, rising from his hiding place.

As silently as possible, the only noise the crunch of the rock and sand beneath their hobnailed boots and the slight shush of mail or clunk of wooden shield, the surviving three dozen men of the century rose from the ridge and ran toward the unheeding nobleman as he watched the Sabaean warriors approach from the city.

The well-trained, disciplined and angry soldiers had covered fully half the distance from the rocky ridge to the lone figure before the alarm went up from the approaching knot of enemy warriors. A shout alerted the Nabataean and he turned, his expression unreadable in the night, to see the men of the Twelfth legion bearing down on him.

With a squawk of fear, the guide whirled this way and that for a moment in a panic, then, settling on his objective, tore off across the sands toward the group of warriors, dust billowing up around his heels.

"Faster! I want that bastard in custody!"

The men reacted to the centurion's shout, finding reserves of energy of which they had been unaware, picking up speed to try and overtake the running man before he could reach the safety of his co-conspirators. With shouts of rage, the Sabaean warriors poured across the sands toward the Romans. Armoured in cuirasses of small, interlinked bronze plates and with square, plain shields of hide and barbed spears or slightly curved blades: this was Terrentius' first sight of the enemy they had travelled so far to defeat.

A quick mental extrapolation made it clear that the traitor would reach the welcoming arms of his Sabaean conspirators before the century could catch him, and Terrentius turned to question the centurion on the wisdom of attacking a much larger force.

As he turned, however, he realised that the centurion had pulled his dagger from his belt, gripping his sword with trouble beneath his shield arm. With a mighty throw, the officer hurled the short blade. The Roman pugio *was a thrusting dagger, not weighted for throwing, but accuracy was not the centurion's objective. His aim was true and the heavy weapon struck the fleeing nobleman on the back of the head, bouncing off into the darkness. Syllaeus tumbled to the ground, the sense knocked from him, and a moment later the Romans ran across the prone figure and engaged the Sabaeans.*

Terrentius raised his shield desperately as the glinting tip of a thrown spear reflected the moonlight long enough for him to catch sight of it and defend himself. The triple-barbed point tore through the leather and wood, reaching three inches inside before it snagged, and carving a thin scratch across his wrist. The weight of the spear projecting from beyond the shield was enough to pull the heavy object down and away from him.

Gritting his teeth, the legionary let the useless shield fall away and instead drew his pugio from his belt, raising it just as the first warrior reached him.

The legions had been drilled mercilessly, even in the sun and terrible conditions on the desert march, and in full battle they would form into lines, defensive tortoises or squares without the need for more than a wave of the standard, precision and discipline their overriding advantage.

This was a different sort of fight, though, and Terrentius was grateful, not for the first time, that his centurion was a hard bastard and had also drilled into his men the need to be able to react individually without losing that strength they gained from unit cohesion.

"On me!" the officer cried, and the legionaries began to pull toward their centurion, each man fighting his own battle but equally aware of the general situation.

The nearest Sabaean warrior swung his sword around in a tight arc, using all the space he had available, the sharp outer edge of the wicked blade slicing toward Terrentius' ribs. Desperately, the legionary thrust down with his left arm, the dagger catching the swinging blade and sliding down the curved edge with a nerve-jarring screech, striking sparks that lit the night like small shooting stars.

The warrior's eyes were wild: not with fear, but rather with something akin to rage. The man was actually smiling, three missing teeth making his grin somewhat lopsided and strange. With a jolt, Terrentius' sliding dagger connected with the sword hilt and deflected the initial blow. As he lashed out with the gladius in his right hand, the man calmly knocked away the sword with his square wood-and-hide shield.

For a fraction of a second, the combatants stared at each

other, their arms both wide, but Terrentius' training overtook him. A gladius was a weapon and so was a dagger, and even a shield used correctly, but so were fists, feet, elbows, knees and…

The crunch as he head-butted the Sabaean with his reinforced bronze helmet told him without further need of investigation that the man was already out of the fight. A broken nose would give a small crack, but this was the sound of shattering jaw and cheekbones. If the warrior was lucky, he might die from a random sword blow now. If not, the next hour or more would be an agonising journey to Elysium for him, viewed through pulped eyes and a smashed face.

Already, Terrentius had turned away from the falling man, fixing his eyes on the next target as he stepped in beside the centurion. Other legionaries were now gathering in the centre, though the number of Romans was slowly being whittled down in the face of the greater odds. A distant roar drew his attention momentarily and he glanced off toward the Nabataean camp to see more armed men running toward the fray. These fresh warriors were, in theory, auxiliaries and allies of Rome, and yet the situation had changed. Syllaeus' true colours had been revealed and, with them, those of the entire Nabataean contingent.

"Shit, sir, there's a whole bloody army of them coming!"

The centurion grunted his agreement as both men stepped forward, parrying blows and avoiding the thrusts of a spear from somewhere behind their current targets. Terrentius lashed out and felt his blade tear deep into thick muscle, the enemy's shriek instantly lost in the barrage of wails and bellowed cries all around. In the impossibly low light, he couldn't even tell where he'd struck the man, but it must have been in the torso by the feel of it.

With lightning reflexes, he ducked left at the very last moment as the barbed spear of another warrior scraped and bounced along the cheek- and neck-guards of his helmet, drawing blood from the very tip of his ear.

"Crap!"

There were just too many of them. Where the one man had been in front of him just a moment ago, there were now three. Manically he stabbed again and again with his gladius, feeling the blows connect more often than not, his left hand waving defensively back and forth, the tip of the dagger occasionally touching something in the press.

He cried out as something struck his arm, and looking down he realised that his left hand had gone, the dagger lost somewhere in the dirt as blood pumped from his severed wrist. He gritted his teeth, trying not to scream, the shock and pain almost driving him to his knees and blessed unconsciousness.

Suddenly he was being hauled backwards. Panic surged through him as he saw the centurion stagger back, the barbed point of a spear, crimson and glistening, protruding from between his shoulder blades. As Terrentius stared in horror at the collapsing officer, the men around him pressing back desperately and fighting in an ever-tightening knot, the wounded legionary felt himself being hauled around again and found himself face to face with the optio.

The centurion's second in command was almost as long-serving a veteran as his commander and with as much experience of battle. The shorter, stockier man, a black beard highlighting his gleaming white teeth as he grimaced, pulled Terrentius to a standing position, holding him by the reinforced shoulder pads of his chain shirt. The legionary stared down at the constant stream of blood running from his stump.

The optio shook him ruthlessly.

"Listen to me, Terrentius!"

"Sir?" He was bewildered, in shock and so much pain it seemed almost distant: someone else's wound.

"For Jove's sake Terrentius, listen to me!"

Something about the familiarity of the situation, being bellowed at by the martinet of an optio, snapped him out of his daze. Dragging his gaze from the grisly remains of his arm, he focused on the officer before him.

"Yessir."

"That's better."

The man paused for a moment and ducked, pulling Terrentius down with him as a sharp spear passed through the space they had just occupied. The optio wrenched him to the left and pointed at the undulating desert off to the east. Terrentius stared at it in confusion. The deep grey-brown of the land met the deep purple of the sky in a haze and it was hard to distinguish the precise shape of the horizon.

He blinked and his eyes refocused, his brow furrowing. "What the...?"

"Sabaeans. Thousands of them!" the optio growled. "We've been betrayed and led into a trap."

"Oh shit. What do we do?"

The optio stared at him and shook his head sadly.

"What we do is fight these bastards here until the last Roman stands." He turned, dragging Terrentius round with him, hauled the unconscious form of Syllaeus from the dust and thrust it at him. "What you do is run back to the camp with this piece of shit and raise the alarm. The prefect has to retreat now, or both legions are lost."

"Legions... lost."

The optio gave him a slap on the side of the helmet that rang like a bell. "Go! If we fall, Aegyptus will be wide open; defenceless!"

Shaking his head, Terrentius turned and staggered away from the fight, dragging the treacherous Nabataean with his good hand.

After a few moments he paused to look back. The men of his century were gone. The optio appeared briefly, lunging into the air, and then disappeared among enemy warriors. Turning his back on the scene, grimly aware that he was the last survivor of a whole century of men, and also that he had to get his arm cauterised as soon as possible before he bled out, Terrentius stumbled on toward the camp to raise the alarm and deliver the traitor.

Arabia "Felix" indeed. Which humourless god thought of *that* bloody joke?

The one-armed legionary staggered on, the security of the eastern provinces riding on his shoulders.

Six months ago: Napata

Amanirenas, queen of Kush, daughter of kings, wife of kings, mother of kings, beloved of Atum of the curved horns, living embodiment of Iusaset, rightful pharaoh of all the lands of the Nile and general-in-chief of the Kushite armies, turned over in her bed, sweat soaking through into the sheets. She moaned in faint panic.

The two enormous mute eunuchs who stood guard inside the door of the sleeping chamber exchanged a glance, uncertain whether or not to wake their mistress. If they did so and she was in one of *those* moods, they could be decorating spear points by noon for daring to interrupt her sleep. But then if she was in one of those moods and she was having a nightmare and wished to be woken and they *didn't…*

They were saved the anguish a moment later as the queen sat bolt upright in her bed, her one good eye flickering wide open, the empty socket of the ruined one darker in the shadows. The two guards quailed automatically. It was hard not to in the presence of the living goddess who ruled the high Nile.

"Nedjeh!" she bellowed in furious tones. The two guards almost fell over each other to be the first out of the room and in search of the revered priest Nedjeh.

The Kandake – the warrior queen of Kush – bit her quivering lip and forced herself to calm, dragging down her breathing.

She reached up and ran a pointed fingernail down the long scar that bisected her eyebrow and had taken her left eye before leaving a cleft in her cheek and chin. It soothed her to do so, for it came as a physical reminder that it had been she who had walked away from that night, and not her opponent.

Amanirenas was no stranger to night terrors. Indeed, they were like old friends, flocking to her in the darkness and swaddling her through the night. But this was different. This was not a dream of death or blood or the killing of kings. This was not searching for her eye or tying off her leg to save it from bleeding out. This was new. This was... this was prophecy, she was sure.

Carefully, she lifted her sheet and wiped the sweat from her face. It would not do to be seen as weak by the priests. She rose, nubile, lithe, the colour of old carob seeds with hair of midnight black braided and tied tight around her brow. She was naked. She always slept naked. Her time of submitting to the lust of men was long gone with her husband and no Kandake could hope to rule the world if she could feel shame just for the air on her skin.

She was stretching and flipping her sword over and over by the time the priest arrived, watched rather nervously by the remaining guard at the door.

"My queen," Nedjeh said respectfully as he entered with an odd smile. He did not bow, as the feeble northerners did to their emperor. Priests in Kush bowed to no one. Sometimes in the past the rulers of Kush had even bowed to the priesthood, for those who spoke for the gods were the only ones in the world with the right to remove a person from the throne of Kush. She suspected that the current crop of priests – even wily Nedjeh – would never dare try such a thing with her, but it was always a threat, and a good one, for it kept Amanirenas on her toes.

"I dreamed. It was a truth dream, I think."

Nedjeh frowned and leaned against the wall. "The gods rarely send truth dreams to those who do not serve them."

Amanirenas gave him a withering look. "I serve the gods more than most. More than many of your brothers, Nedjeh. Do not lecture me on the nature of dreams and the priesthood. Just explain to me *this* one."

Nedjeh nodded and gestured for her to go on as he fiddled with the tassels on his leopard pelt garment.

"I saw a ram. It was a ram *and* a man, in the way of Atum. He was standing upon the back of an elephant, surveying his domain, when an eagle plummeted from the sky and tried to carry him off. The ram was too heavy and the eagle and the ram fought upon the elephant's back until both were wounded and exhausted. Then, finally, the eagle won out, raking the ram with its claws, and when it stretched out triumphant, its wings became arms and it was not only an eagle, but a handsome young man. What does this mean?"

Nedjeh cleared his throat. "Rome. The time has come to face the great empire of the north and take back what is ours, Kandake."

"Explain."

"The ram, my queen, is Atum, who the northern Nile-dwellers say is called Khnum. He is the ram god of creation, born as we know on the holy mountain outside this very palace. But he has another holy site for the Aegyptians, at a place they know as Yebu and the Romans call Elephantine, for it rises from the Nile in the shape of one of those noble beasts. The people of that land believe that Atum rose from that island, but now Elephantine is in the hands of Rome, plagued with statues of their emperor who looks down upon the gods. Atum will never be free from the eagle until that island is free of Rome."

Amanirenas frowned for a moment, then nodded. "Rome has withdrawn many of its soldiers from the land to go and fight in Arabia. Aegyptus is like an open basket of fruit, ripe and ready to be eaten. We will be all but unopposed. Go, Nedjeh. Tell Kalabsha to muster the armies. We travel north to Elephantine at dusk."

As the priest scurried off with an oddly self-satisfied smile, the one remaining eunuch guard who had stayed in his place in the room cleared his throat, emboldened by the energy and positivity of the queen.

"Kandake, will not Rome seek revenge if you enter their lands?"

His eyes widened as Amanirenas' sword punched through his front teeth, his tongue, tonsils and neck, cracking the spine as it passed, and pinning him to the wooden doorframe.

"Yes, Ama," she replied quietly. "I believe they will."

I

ALEXANDRIA

The trireme *Fidelis* lurched and bounced across the waves. Sailors kept their feet with the confidence of veterans as they went about their tasks, the banks of oars dipping in time to the piper and forcing the vessel to creep forward slowly once again from where it had languished this past hour.

Titus Cervianus, leaning against the rail in the prow, found himself jerked back, fighting to maintain his grip on the sturdy timber as the vessel got underway once more. Blinking away the spray thrown up by the oars, he glanced briefly back toward the rest of his century. The men were standing to attention in ordered rows at the centre of the deck, the optio and centurion beside the formation, glassy-eyed and aloof.

As usual, nobody seemed to greatly care where Cervianus was. It was at the same time both a curse and a boon, though he was grateful for his virtual ostracism right now as he leaned calmly on the rail, shifting his leather bag so that it stopped slapping against the timber. Better to be here and comfortably unpopular than standing in neat rows and trying not to fall over comically with every lurch of the ship.

The fleet of almost a hundred vessels had arrived in the waters surrounding Alexandria last night, guided true by the famous lighthouse that rose from its rock like a pillar holding up the sky. The decision had been made for the safety of all concerned not to begin the docking process until this morning and even then the whole procedure had been so slow that many of the triremes had been required to produce lunch for their passengers before a jetty became available.

It made Cervianus smile to see the vast number of merchant vessels flitting in and out of the city's great harbour past the waiting mass of military ships, priority having been given to the traders that were the city's lifeblood. Only when the mercantile traffic eased here and there did a jetty become free and one of the great triremes begin to manoeuvre into position.

Cervianus had enjoyed lounging around and taking in the atmosphere of the greatest city in the east during the interminable wait that had bored most of his companions, even though most of the place was not yet truly visible.

Though the *Fidelis* was currently at the front of the queue, much of the city was still hidden by the great island of the Pharos, the mole, or the headland upon which the royal palaces stood. Here and there, tantalising glimpses of the city on its hills appeared briefly as the ship rose and fell, giving momentary flashes of great colourful colonnades and colossal buildings. But the sea air and the warmth of the roasting sun, mixed with the smell of spices and wood that accompanied the view of the great lighthouse, had served as a wonderful welcome and introduction to this land that had ruled a vast empire when even Athens was a mere collection of huts on a mound.

He'd expected Aegyptus to be much hotter and drier than his homeland in Galatia, but at the moment everything was just comfortably warm. Things would be different, of course, away from the coast and its breeze. Writers spoke of the oppressive heat in the interior.

The ship lurched again and Cervianus gripped the rail until his knuckles whitened. Behind him he heard a metallic crash as several of the legionaries lost their footing and collapsed in a heap. The sound of Centurion Draco's voice snapping angrily at them served only to widen his smile, though he carefully kept his face hidden from view, gazing out over the water.

Even without looking, he knew that Draco was glaring at him.

Once more, as he settled back into his comfortable position, Cervianus was grateful he'd had time to brew up a jug of ginger and raspberry-leaf broth to allay the sickness that the bucking of ships always caused in him.

Had the other men of the Second century shown the slightest interest in speaking to him, he might have brewed up two jugs, but still, listening to the sounds of those men who routinely ignored him being violently ill during the night had been surprisingly soothing.

As the *Fidelis* picked up speed, the piped melody increasing in pace, he watched the city sliding past and the harbour entrance drawing toward him. Though he had never been here, he knew the layout of the great city so well that if he closed his eyes he could almost see what lay within. His mind furnished him with an image of the carefully drawn map of the city he had been viewing only last night.

His ability to read and to speak several languages, only one of the lesser of many reasons for his enforced solitude, had led to Cervianus cultivating a voracious appetite for books, as well as providing him with plenty of time to sate that appetite. On the journey he had devoted as much time as became available to studying the geography and history of this mysterious land and particularly of this great city that would be his home now for as long as Rome deemed it necessary.

Most of the section of the metropolis that *was* visible from here, marching out along the coast from the centre to the east and the Canopus Gate, constituted the Jewish Quarter: the largest concentration of that people outside their homeland. The eastern end of the city was therefore of little interest to the legion and to the Roman administration with the exception of the need to watch and control that ever-troublesome race.

His attention was drawn back to the direction of travel as the great temple of Artemis swept away to the left and the harbour entrance raced toward them, the *Fidelis*'s trierarch having lined up his vessel perfectly for the approach.

To the right, as the ship lunged forth, the magnificent Pharos rose up into the sky, a reminder that a man who was a god had laid the first stones of this city. To the left, the diabathra swept away to land, an artificial harbour wall that enclosed one of the largest port complexes the world had ever seen.

And then they were suddenly inside the reaching arms of Alexandria's great harbour. Regardless of the number of texts he had read in Greek or Latin, the images carefully transcribed and maps etched on bark-skin tablets, nothing had quite prepared him for this.

Ancyra, where what was now the Twenty Second had been based for decades, and the home of Cervianus and most of his compatriots, was officially a city; indeed a "Roman" city now, but the whole of Ancyra would fit into the enormous sprawling mass that was Alexandria many times over. Ancyra in its entirety could fit into Alexandria's *harbour*.

The port was simply breathtaking, enclosing a body of water over a mile across in every direction, spotted with myriad vessels of all shapes and sizes. The Pharos lighthouse at the entrance stood on the tip of its great island, largely bare and connected to the mainland by the heptastadion, a man-made causeway wide enough to drive multiple carts abreast. From there, the waterfront was a mass of buildings and people, jetties and ships, statues and temples, familiar in style and yet alien in architecture.

Directly ahead lay a huge, square building that was undergoing work, covered in scaffolding and men: the Timonium, a palace that Marcus Antonius had begun before his death. His rival and vanquisher, Octavian, was having the building reassigned and statues raised there in his own image to remove forever the taint and memory of that most unpopular Roman statesman.

The *Fidelis* swung to the left, adjusting its course for one of the many dock areas, close to the Timonium and the busiest area of the harbour. Once again, Cervianus had to tighten his grip as he watched the jetty striding out into the water toward them, welcoming him to his new home. He smiled.

"Cervianus, you waste of space! Get in formation!"

With a sigh, he gave a last look around at the city of Alexander. Still, no need to worry. The Twenty Second "Deiotariana" legion had been permanently reassigned to the province and Cervianus had eighteen years yet to serve under the eagle, so there would be plenty of time to explore the city and its wonders.

Turning, he caught the look in Draco's eyes, a mix of disdain, distrust and irritation, and hurried along the deck between the oarsmen. Falling in at the rear of the formation, near the optio with his vine staff, Cervianus tried to hunch down a little and fit in with the formation.

It wasn't easy.

At over six feet tall, Cervianus was half a head above the next tallest man in the century and a full head over most. Where the majority of the men of the Twenty Second were blond or light-haired and continued to grow moustaches or beards of various styles after the fashion of their Gallic ancestors, proud reminders that the legion had not always been Roman, Cervianus was clean shaven with raven black hair.

Adjusting the leather bag at his side, he became acutely aware that he was the only man not carrying a shield and pilum, his being stowed in the cart below with the rest of the century's equipment: standard practice in order to allow him quick access to the bag and room to work.

He tried various positions to hold his arm and settled with resting it casually on the top of the bag until the optio nudged his elbow with the vine staff, sliding his arm down straight.

"Try and at least look like a pissing legionary, Cervianus."

Sniggers hissed from some of the men nearby and the optio growled loudly.

"If any of you comedians think that's funny, I look forward to seeing you standing knee-deep in the latrines tonight. Get my drift?"

The sniggering stopped immediately and Cervianus sighed quietly, trying not to attract any more attention. He became aware that the man next to him was watching him, his eyes straining left while his head continued to face forward, expressionless. The man was frowning slightly. He was new – a replacement for the unfortunate Luguros, whose simple tombstone back in Galatia failed to adequately describe what they'd cremated after the bear had finished with him. Cervianus had seen the replacement a few times during the voyage but, both shunned and shunning company, he had remained separate as usual.

The man turned his gaze forward again, still frowning.

The centurion at the front started rattling out orders, but they were virtually inaudible this far back, particularly given the noises of the ship and the harbour around them, and Cervianus allowed his attention to wander again.

The trireme was almost at the jetty now, slowing its pace ready to dock.

What would this new assignment mean for them – for him in particular? They would presumably have a fortress of traditional Roman style now. There had been talk for the past few years about building one at Ancyra following its annexation, but the Twenty Second had been left in their former Galatian barracks for the time being, assuming they would soon be reassigned anyway. From what he'd read, Octavian's legions had a full range of facilities in their fortresses, including baths, hospital, shops, gymnasium and even training centres.

His attention was rudely drawn back to his current situation as the *Fidelis* thumped into the jetty, bouncing off and back again before slowing with the teeth-jarring noise of wood grinding on wood. The sailors threw ropes over the edge of the ship, where they were caught by tired-looking dock workers and fastened to posts.

"Right you lot. Look sharp. Follow me and keep in formation. No fraternising with the locals. Keep your eyes straight ahead and ignore everything but us."

Cervianus let out a gentle sigh again. There was little enough excitement and interest to be had in garrison life, and Draco was determined to knock even that out.

The soldiers waited patiently, sweating in their mail shirts and bronze helmets, while the unarmoured sailors ran a boarding ramp down to the timbers of the jetty and secured it.

"First cohort, Second century… Advance!"

Ahead, the standard waved slightly as the signifer started to move. The musician blew the signal for slow march on his cornu, and the century began to move at a stately pace along the deck, down the ramp and onto the jetty. Cervianus waited patiently for the men to move and realised with a start that the man next to him was giving him a sidelong searching look again.

"What *is* the problem?" he hissed.

"Shut up and pay attention!" snapped the optio behind, giving Cervianus a painful prod in the shoulder with his staff. "And I can hear all that sighing," he added ominously, just as Cervianus took a deep breath.

Evandros, the bully in their contubernium who had taken every opportunity for the last two years to make Cervianus' life miserable and difficult, and who stood in front of him in the formation, laughed as he began to step forward. Cervianus followed suit, grateful at least for the distraction. The half-speed march was not an easy step to master, used only for slow parades and ceremonies, and was particularly difficult on the ship and ramp with the slight rocking motion and the slippery coating of the timber.

Trying not to move out of step, he once more concentrated on the city, now so tantalisingly close. The stone quayside at the end of the jetty was thronged with people and activity, a strange-looking building behind rising over their heads. This much closer to land, it became disturbingly apparent that the tint of spice in the air that he'd smelled out to sea was actually the pungent aroma of horse and camel dung, sweetened with the scent of incense burning all over the city. It was a heady, slightly sickening mixture.

Negotiating the ramp with care, the century, a column of eighty men, four abreast, began to make their way at parade pace along the wet timber of the jetty, closing on the quay. A surreptitious glance around without moving his head confirmed that other triremes were at jetties in the same port. Off to the right, a military vessel was just departing, the century it had carried now mustering on the stone paving ahead. To the left, another had just arrived, the creaking and groaning as it scraped along the timber adding to the general din.

No one spoke as the century entered the city of Alexander the Great, home of wonders, capital of the infamous Cleopatra, port city of the most ancient empire the world had ever known. Cervianus was almost bursting with anticipation.

The cornu player blew the muster command and the men came to an ordered stop, standing to attention, while the centurion and the signifer conferred out front.

The crowd hung back, several paces from the century, tense, as though waiting to leap on them, but fearful and nervous. Cervianus wondered whether they had tried to accost the First century that landed this morning, trying to sell them dates and sweetmeats. If they had, their fearful gaze was entirely understandable. He could imagine the reaction of the commanders.

A figure appeared from the crowd, the citizens opening a path to make way for him as he moved out into the open with a strange swaying gait, like that of a great hunting cat. His head was covered with a white skullcap that fitted seamlessly to his dark brown, hairless head. His eyebrows had been removed and replaced with painted replicas, his eyes accentuated with galena and, though clean shaven, he sported a short, stubby false beard made from what looked like flax. His torso was bare, dark and thin with little to be seen in the way of muscle, while he wore a skirt of white linen with the pelt of a leopard tied around the waist as an over-covering.

In one hand he held a strange staff of whitened wood with a twisted top and in the other, a gold censer hanging by three chains, white smoke rising from it as it swung gently.

The man approached nonchalantly, swinging the censer and muttering in a low voice.

"What in Hades is this?" the optio grumbled.

As the man continued to advance, the optio stepped out from the rear of the column, his vine staff by his side, waving a hand and shaking his head.

"Piss off, fella. Don't need your help."

The man paid him no heed, seemingly intent on his swaying motion, the censer picking up a stronger swing. The optio stepped directly in his path.

"Look, fella, I'm a good religious man, but this isn't the time."

A voice from the front of the crowd cleared its throat and spoke nervously.

"He must cleanse and bless you. Sobek watches all armies in Aegyptus and his priests must tell him if you're a friend."

The optio frowned.

"Well I suppose we don't want to piss off this 'Sobek' then. Just don't try and involve my men. I'm watching you," he added, making a vaguely threatening motion with his fingers pointing at his eyes.

The priest turned with a complicated motion and began to sway along the line of men toward the front, continually muttering and wafting his incense, the optio keeping pace with him irritably.

Realising that he was temporarily free of trouble, Cervianus sighed again and rolled his shoulders.

"Why are you always on your own, then?"

Taken by surprise, Cervianus spun his head to see that the man next to him was still regarding him with interest. The legionary was considerably shorter than him, but powerfully built, broad across the shoulders and with a lantern jaw. His moustache was short and neat; a mousey brown.

"They don't much like me."

The man shrugged.

"Me either. What's *your* excuse?"

It was Cervianus' turn to frown.

"All sorts of things. People say I'm bad luck. Some of the others even wash their hands if they touch me. Evandros and his thugs make sure I remain as popular as a latrine sponge. And, of course, I'm not *quite* as thick as pig shit, so they don't really understand me."

The legionary laughed. "Yes. I can see how you might have difficulty making friends."

Cervianus narrowed his eyes. "You're new? A replacement for Luguros."

The man nodded. "Reassigned from the First century just before we set sail. Apparently I'm a bad influence and… how did the optio put it? Ah yes, 'a disruptive, evil-tempered and downright dangerous piece of shit'."

Cervianus shrugged.

"You should fit in well here then," he said, spitefully.

Again, the man laughed.

"Rumour has it that your centurion's a real piece of work, though I find it hard to believe he can be much more of a bastard than Nasica. I think they're expecting him to either knock me into shape or crucify me before the week is out."

Cervianus nodded despondently. "And he probably will. You might want to end our little chat there; else you'll find yourself in the same situation as me."

He gestured to the soldier on the other side of the new recruit. Petrocorios was giving the pair of them a stare of mixed contempt and haughtiness.

"Him?" the bulky new man laughed. "Hold this for me."

Cervianus' brow furrowed further as he took his companion's pilum.

In the flash of an eye, the man's arm shot out at groin height and he gripped the observer, squeezing hard. The contemptuous legionary's eyes bulged and a high-pitched squeak escaped his lips while his face went white.

"If I ever catch you looking at me again or even breathing heavily near me I'll cut these off and send them to your mother back at the menagerie. You understand?"

The legionary, his eyes dangerously bulbous, breath held, nodded vigorously.

Letting go of the groin, the shorter man retrieved his pilum.

"It's all about how you deal with people," he said with a smile. "I like to be fairly direct."

Cervianus blinked, his gaze lingering for a moment on Petrocorios, who had let his pilum fall away in order to grasp and soothe his painful crotch, causing grunts of irritation from those it bounced off before hitting the ground.

"Eunuchs aren't popular in the legions," Cervianus said quietly. Shaking his head as if to clear it, he stared at the newcomer. "I'm Titus Cervianus, capsarius for the Second century."

"Ulyxes. Legionary with 'mental problems' apparently."

Cervianus grinned. "I think that diagnosis is fairly sound."

"Ha."

The two stood in silence for a moment and then carefully returned their gaze to the front as the optio returned, smelling of incense. The officer fell into his accustomed position at the rear of the column where he lashed out with his vine staff and delivered a ringing blow to the helmet of the wounded legionary beside them.

"Stop playing with yourself, Petrocorios, and pick that weapon up."

Cervianus kept his face straight, his eyes watering with the effort of not laughing. Ulyxes made a "tsk" noise quietly.

Ahead, the cornu sounded again, marking the order to move on.

Titus Cervianus, capsarius of the First cohort, Second century of the Twenty Second Deiotariana legion, blinked the dust from his eyes, dust stirred up by the tramping feet of the rest of the legion.

The century had spent almost four hours standing in formation in the forum, gradually becoming more and more parched and bored and continually ogled by the locals, while waiting for the entire legion to disembark. By the time the last century had arrived and fallen in to their assigned position the sun was already well on its descent toward the western horizon.

Cervianus had watched the officers of the legion conferring at the front of the square before the mustered troops, and then engaging in conversation with an official in a toga, and had briefly wondered whether they intended to keep the legion on its feet in the square until even the carts and mules had been brought up and made to stand to attention.

Then, finally, another official had arrived, alongside a man wearing the decorative armour of a military tribune. A brief discussion had taken place and the legion had at last been moved off toward the eastern gate of the city.

The marvels of Alexandria had occupied Cervianus' attention and barraged his senses for only the first moments of the march before the shimmering glare of the setting sun reflecting on the cloud of dust that enveloped the column made it almost impossible to see anything around him. He would miss the canal and the hippodrome, the grove of Nemesis, a few temples and the squalor of the Jewish Quarter due to the eye-watering dust.

He chided himself for the irritation he felt, given that he was only in the First cohort's Second century with fewer than two hundred men in front kicking up the dirt. What it must be like for those at the back with almost five thousand ahead of them didn't even bear thinking about. For a moment it irritated him that the medical wagons carrying the dozen or so sick and wounded were back there in the worst of the dirt cloud and the baking sun.

Back in the old days of Galatian rule, when the army answered to King Amyntas and the influences on command were of Greek origin rather than Roman, great emphasis was placed on medical care and the carts of wounded men travelled separate from the army with their own guard, often slower and with extra supplies and attendants. Not so when one followed the eagle. The legions of Rome placed the emphasis on speed and military efficiency. A wounded soldier took second place to one who could dig or fight.

Again, he shook his head and squinted into the strange orange glow that was formed by the low, glaring sun reflecting off the haze of sandy dust.

It was no good brooding on things. His intense concentration and tendency toward introspection was yet another cause for his general unpopularity with the rest of the century. Indeed, the only time he could remember being remotely popular was during an outbreak of the flux last year when the legion was encamped near the north coast in Pontus. That it should take suffering bloody faeces to make most people converse with him was either hilarious or tragic, or possibly both. Of course, the most adverse influence had been missing at the time, with Evandros spending most of his time squatting over a trench and hoping his guts didn't leave him.

The simple fact was that Cervianus was too good a physician to serve as a capsarius, and he knew it. Trained by a Greek physician and with years of private service, even in matters of surgery and herbalism, before his enlistment with the army of Galatia, his medical knowledge outstripped even the commissioned medicus of the legion who ran the hospital unit and received a centurion's pay, let alone the rest of the field medics.

Moreover, with his gift for languages and learning, he had quickly fostered the resentment of his peers, many of whom had only been taught to read and write what was strictly necessary for military service.

All in all, he was as far removed from the common

legionaries as he was from the centurionate, many of whom had also undergone a less-than-thorough education.

But that wasn't the main reason for his virtual ostracism.

No, indeed.

As he'd intimated to Ulyxes, he was considered unlucky by the men of the Second century. Pure superstition, of course. Distrust fostered into dislike by the carefully placed words of Evandros. Just because he'd stated on more than one occasion that not *everything* was made so by the will of the gods and that some things could be explained with simple science and logic rather than because Jupiter or one of the other Roman deities had a boil on his backside.

As a physician, he could hardly believe otherwise.

Oh, he didn't *deny* the gods, of course. There was room in the world, even in Cervianus' world, for the gods. After all, where else could a man turn when he was crouched behind an earth bank while screaming Pontic archers tried to puncture him? It was just that more could be explained and achieved with human intellect than mumbling over a statue with an incense burner.

Such opinion was not, of course, popular with the common soldiery.

He'd learned this early on in his first year of service after a discussion over the cause of fog with Petrocorios had left him lying in his own sick bed, having been severely beaten with a small iron statue of Neptune.

A sudden inhalation of grit and dust led to an explosive coughing fit which elicited another poke from the optio's staff.

"If I were you," a voice muttered, "I'd wait 'til that prick was alone in the latrines and jam that thing up his arse."

Cervianus turned to Ulyxes and stared.

"Do you have a death wish? Keep your voice down."

The other legionary shrugged. "He can't hear us over the noise of the march. He wouldn't even know we were talking if you hadn't turned round."

"Shut up and march, the pair of you!"

Cervianus faced front again, but a sidelong glance afforded him a view of the grin plastered across Ulyxes' face.

The capsarius sighed deeply. This strange man was the first person to even offer an overture of friendship in the last year, since Luguros in fact, whose brief attempt to befriend him had been quickly forestalled by the others.

It would certainly be nice to have someone to speak to at times, and someone to "have your back" as they said was always useful, but something about Ulyxes worried him. The man did not seem to have any realisation of just how irresponsible and dangerous he was being. The optio would kick seven shades of shit out of a man just for looking at him in a funny way, and the optio was a cuddly kitten compared to Draco. Being seen to be too close to Ulyxes could very well be hazardous to one's health.

It was a puzzle he would have to think on: whether the pros of camaraderie outweighed the cons. Like so many things in Cervianus' life, even friendship came down to a mathematical equation.

A gust of wind sprang up seemingly from nowhere, the first he'd felt since arriving in Aegyptus, and wafted the dust cloud away from the column. For a long moment, Cervianus blinked, able finally to see ahead, past even the tribunes, standard bearers and musicians.

The sun was now almost at the horizon. He daren't turn to check how low, else he'd provoke another prod with the optio's vine staff, but the shadows the men cast on the beige landscape were long and thin. The heat was beginning to wane as the sun sank and the land began to feel more like home. Somehow, during that hazy, brown eternity that was the march from the city's forum, they had passed unheeding through the Canopus Gate, by the hippodrome, and past most signs of cultured civilisation.

Here, houses formed slums that huddled close to the glory of the great city, mud-brick structures with reed roofs that spoke eloquently of extreme poverty. The paved street continued out beyond the city, but this far beyond the walls the road was only discernible among the grey-brown grit because of the slight camber.

Blinking in the suddenly clear air, he reached up with his free hand and wiped the encrusted dirt from his face. Most of the century wore their helmets hanging on their backs, their green scarf providing the main head-covering, a simple concession to the heat allowed by the commanders, but Cervianus' helmet was stowed in the baggage along with his shield and pilum. He wiped the sweat from his neck and failed entirely to sympathise with the bully in front, who had salty water gathering in the bowl of the helmet hanging on his shoulders.

The land to the east of the city rose imperceptibly at such a low gradient that Cervianus hadn't even been aware they were climbing until the breeze afforded by the combination of height and proximity to the open sea had cleared the dust cloud. In fact, the breeze was stirring up more dirt, but this remained at knee level, allowing the entire column to heave a sigh of relief.

The houses, if one were generous enough to call them that, thinned out as the road climbed until finally, as the march levelled out once again, the view was clear to both sides.

Off to the left, perhaps three hundred paces away, the land fell into a sharp slope that ran down to meet the sea, glittering white and perfect blue in the last rays of the sun. Various monuments that Cervianus had been unaware of, even given his study of the area, dotted the coastline, each holding their own enigma that he couldn't wait to unravel as soon as duty allowed him time.

On the other side, though he had to peer past Ulyxes and two others to see it, the land sloped down very slowly for the best part of a mile, past the canal and to the Mareotis Lake. It would have been nice to set eyes on the Nile, that most ancient and majestic of rivers, but this far out of the delta only tiny streams would be found, the main channels lying away to the east where the ground would be green and lush instead of brown and dusty.

With mild surprise, as his gaze moved back to the left, Cervianus saw Aulus Vitalis, the senior tribune and effective commander of the legion, ride out of the line alongside the other officer who had joined them in the square. The pair sat together for a while on the rise as the legion filed slowly past, gesturing with sweeping arms and having what may have been a deep debate but looked to Cervianus a great deal more like a fiery argument.

The column crested a low hump in the road and, as the heads in front dropped out of the way, Cervianus, his height giving him an extra advantage, got his first look at their destination. Here, perhaps two miles from Alexandria itself, what appeared to be a partially constructed city lay in a dissembled state.

Off to the left, on the highest point and close to the sea, stood a low embankment with a solid, military wall complete with towers and parapet along only one side, the other defences standing to less than shoulder height at best and covered with wooden scaffolding. Cervianus gave a small smile. This was surely one of the new fortresses that had sprung up in the past few years, just like those he'd read about in the west – possibly even with a hospital.

This would be the home of the Twenty Second, then. He was a little surprised to find it under construction. He'd assumed it would be an extant building or that the legion would be building their home from scratch.

But the fortress was far from alone. A great monumental forum was taking shape perhaps half a mile further on, temples of the Roman triad almost complete with their columned porticoes and roofs, awaiting only the paint and decoration.

What appeared to be a bathhouse was also almost finished, along with a partially completed channel, diverting water from the Alexandrian canal to the new settlement.

The most complete monument by far was the triumphal gateway, a triple arch of marble, elegant and strong, covered with friezes and inscriptions and topped with a gilded statue of the Princeps Octavian in regal pose. It seemed that everywhere one went in the republic these days, the nephew of the great Caesar was busy looking down on you and reminding the people of his victory over Antonius.

"Looks like Alexandria's in for a challenge, eh?" Ulyxes grinned. "Probably too Greek for Octavian."

Cervianus contemplated commenting, but merely nodded. That was clearly the intention: a glorious, beautiful, strong city on a hill overlooking that metropolis that had supported the Princeps's enemy.

"There's the Twelfth, look."

The capsarius risked a glance around; Ulyxes was pushing his luck chatting in line. The optio, however, unnoticed by

Cervianus in his studies, had left his position, presumably on some task back to the next century.

Relieved at the sudden freedom from the ever-watchful officer, he frowned at his companion.

"The Twelfth?"

Ulyxes grinned. "Nobody tells you anything, do they?"

"Come on?"

The shorter, bulkier man shrugged. "The Twelfth Fulminata. They're the current legion assigned here."

Cervianus' brow furrowed further. "We're *sharing* the place?"

"For now. Rumour has it they're being reposted to the east soon. *Rumour has it* that we weren't supposed to be brought to Aegyptus yet; not until they'd completed this place and were ready to ship out."

The capsarius shook his head in exasperation. "And everyone knows all this?"

"Good grief. Did you not even wonder at the suddenness when we were moved out of Ancyra?"

Again, all Cervianus could do was shrug and shake his head. Concentrating his gaze in the rapidly diminishing light, he examined their surroundings with more care. Sure enough, the scaffolding and work sites were dotted around with workers wearing the russet-coloured linen tunics favoured by most of the legions.

As the Twenty Second approached the great monumental arch and the new, paved square before it, the groups of workmen stopped what they were doing to watch the new arrivals. Their gazes were, Cervianus noted, almost universally contemptuous. It was a look Cervianus was quite familiar with, but this attitude was clearly being displayed toward the whole of the Twenty Second and not just him.

"Friendly bunch, aren't they?" Ulyxes noted lightly. "I'm guessing they don't like us because we're Galatian."

"But most of them look like locals. Aegyptians. They're barely Roman *themselves*."

Ulyxes grinned.

"Ah, but they were recruited into a *Roman* legion, weren't they. We were an independent army first. Doesn't make us popular. We may have to break some heads in the coming weeks."

Cervianus glared at him. *Breaking heads*. Sheer idiocy. When differences could not be overcome with reasoned discussion, walking away was always the sensible course of action. Besides, who did Ulyxes think would have to fix those broken heads afterwards? "Just ignore them."

Ulyxes laughed. "Oh it gets better and better!"

"What are you talking about?" the capsarius snapped irritably.

"That one we just passed working on the cistern tank had a criminal brand." He shook his head and squinted as they passed another work party, who glared at them and spat in the dust.

"More of them: thieves and murderers. Even the odd *slave* mark. I'd love to know what's going on here. None of this lot are allowed to follow the eagle by Roman law."

Fuscus, one of the more reasonable men in the contubernium, craned his neck from the line in front and peered round at Ulyxes.

"I heard they got the shit kicked out of them in Arabia last year. Lost most of a legion. The dickhead who controlled Aegyptus drafted every man he could find that could walk into the Twelfth to make up the numbers."

"Great," Ulyxes replied. "And now we're going to be serving under a man who drafts horse-buggerers into the army."

The man shook his head. "No. New prefect in Aegyptus now. Only arrived a month or two back. Saw the shit situation he'd been left and sent for us. We're his new troops."

Cervianus sighed. "Wonderful. How long until we're sent into Arabia too, I wonder?"

"Shut up," Evandros snarled without turning. "Nobody's talking to you."

Ulyxes raised his eyebrows as Fuscus turned away. "Want me to sort that for you?"

"Hardly. It'd just provoke more trouble. Leave it be."

The heavy-set new recruit shrugged. "Your funeral."

Cervianus sighed and started as a voice behind him snapped, "Eyes front! Stop sodding around!"

He hadn't even noticed the return of the optio. Further discussion was impossible anyway, however, since at that moment the command musicians sent out a series of blasts on their cornua that were quickly picked up by those of each century, and the entire legion came to an abrupt halt and turned to face left with the thunder of thousands of stamping feet. The dust cloud billowed up to waist height once more before falling away and drifting off in the breeze.

The tribunes of the Twenty Second, wearing the green tunics and cloaks unique to the Deiotariana, along with their guiding tribune in his traditional red, gathered in a short line in front of the assembled mass. The senior tribune, Vitalis, sat on his horse in the centre, his ever-stony, miserable expression fixed on his legion.

"Men of the Twenty Second—" he bellowed, and immediately had to pause and cough noisily in the dusty atmosphere.

In the momentary silence the only sound to be heard was the background noise of construction as the Twelfth legion went on with their work, pausing only occasionally to make their contempt a little more obvious.

"Men of the Twenty Second, welcome to Nicopolis. While under the command of the noble prefect Gaius Petronius, governor of Aegyptus, this will be our home base and winter quarters."

In the brief pause the tribune left for effect, someone off to Cervianus' right muttered, "How will we *know* when it's winter?" There was low sniggering and the capsarius carefully kept his expression blank and his face forward. There was no doubt in his mind that the optio had already singled out the culprit to deal with later.

"As you can see," Vitalis went on, "the fortress of Nicopolis is not yet complete. It is being specially constructed to house two legions simultaneously and is a massive undertaking. As such, as soon as we are settled in, the Twenty Second will lend our arm to the construction work at any time we are not required for other duties."

Cervianus noted with interest how the tribune from the Twelfth suddenly snapped round to glare at Vitalis. Clearly something there had not been fully agreed. Vitalis ignored the man glaring at him and took another deep breath.

"While the work goes on, the Twelfth will remain quartered in the old Caesarean fort on the near edge of Alexandria and will be returning there when not involved in work. We, however, will be making our quarters in the buildings that have already been constructed in Nicopolis, along with some others that were commandeered when the settlement that previously stood here was cleared out. Any of you that are not assigned a structure will erect your tents in the standard manner as though you were on campaign until a building is completed and assigned."

Groans rose from the men, understandably. A leather tent would be too hot to touch by lunch time, cook the occupants as though in an oven, and offer insufficient protection from dust storms.

"Remain in formation until my adjutants have consulted with your officers and then you will be given further instructions and told to fall out."

He smiled, a rare occurrence and even now containing no humour.

"Make the most of tonight to rest and organise yourselves. You have a little over half an hour of light left yet and the entire legion will be mustering at dawn to greet the prefect when he comes to inspect us. If I see a single rust spot or crumpled tunic in the morning you'll wish you'd fallen overboard on the journey."

He paused to let his words sink in and then turned to a junior officer by his side.

"Good. Catilius? Confer with the tribune here and begin the assignments."

Cervianus allowed his eyes to wander as much as he could without moving his head. Twenty paces or so away, three legionaries working with adzes on a chunk of stone allowed the full weight of their scorn to pour down on him.

At least the Twelfth were going to be quartered separately for now. Trouble was definitely looming in Nicopolis.

The evening air wafted warmly past the piles of brick and stone, heaps of rubble and timber, coils of rope, bags of nails and tools abandoned to the elements. Cervianus stood beside the door of the partially dismantled mud-brick structure that had been assigned as the temporary quarters for his contubernium, shaking his head in disbelief at the mess.

It had been drilled into the Twenty Second, even in the old days, that tools needed to be cared for: oiled at the end of the day and repacked. They belonged to you and cost good money, so a man with any sense cared for his equipment. And in the two years the army had been a legion under Roman rule and Draco had been in command of the Second century? Well, drill and discipline had become the centre of everyone's life. This was just another sign of the rot that seemed to have crept into the Twelfth since the drafting of so many inappropriate or questionable soldiers.

Cervianus took a swig of water from his flask, acutely aware that there were limited supplies out here, this far from the city and with Nicopolis' infrastructure still incomplete.

A hand fell on his shoulder and he jumped, his heart pounding in his throat as he turned to see the nonchalant face of Ulyxes. The man was surprisingly quiet on his feet, given what Cervianus had seen of him so far.

"Never heard you come out," he breathed, deliberately calming his pulse.

"Clearly. Needed a break. So did my purse."

Cervianus raised an eyebrow and his companion shrugged.

"Used to be lucky at this game, but these lads are crushing me. I've lost a week's pay so far and promised half tomorrow's rations. I'm trying to decide whether to go back and hope for the best or quit while I'm behind."

The capsarius sighed. "They'll keep pulling you back in and working you. It's what they do with new people, you know that. That bunch in there have it all worked out; they don't play to win individually. They help each other and work the game so that it doesn't matter which of them wins so long as you lose. Then they'll divide the loot at the end of the night when you've gone."

Ulyxes nodded, sighing. "Guess I should have seen that coming. I may have to extract the money back from them later. It generally galls me to leave knuckle marks on a legionary, but I don't much take to being cheated."

Cervianus leaned back against the wall and folded his arms. "That would do nobody any good."

"It'd do my *purse* good!"

"Yes, but it would lead to reprisals and more beatings. Next thing you know I'm stitching wounds on five men and applying salve and then you'll be caught by a dozen of them in an alley when you least expect it and won't show up for roll call the next morning. I've seen it before."

Ulyxes shrugged again. "Better than just letting people walk all over you and take what they want. You've got to stand up for yourself, 'cause no one else will."

"Better to beat them at their own game," Cervianus said slyly.

The shorter man narrowed his eyes. "Go on…"

"It's easy to beat people at dice. Easier than beating them with a stick, for sure."

Ulyxes' brow furrowed further. "You're telling me you can beat them?"

"Easily."

"So how come you're not rich or in there?"

Cervianus gave him a level look. "Guess."

"Ah. Not welcome, eh?"

A nod.

"Is this another of those reasons you said about that people don't talk to you?"

The capsarius shrugged.

"It may be. In the first week after I joined up they tried several times to take me for everything I had. After five days I'd stripped more than two months' pay out of the bunch of them. Never been welcome since."

Ulyxes grinned. "How did you do it? You must be an impressive cheat."

"No cheating involved. It's a simple combination of being able to keep track of numbers and apply logic to the rolls, and being able to read people."

"Sounds harder than a dark alley and a plank of wood to me."

"Not really. It's incredibly simple. Count the occurrences of each combination of dice rolls. When it comes to your turn, go for the one that's happened least often and put a good stake down on it. If the rolls have been very evenly spread, don't bet high. You'll lose some here and there, but gradually, over the night, you'll find your pile building and building, and they won't be able to work out why. They simply don't think that deeply about the mathematics of the game."

Again Ulyxes nodded, thoughtfully. "You have to have a good memory then."

"It helps, yes."

"Mine's pretty good."

"Really?"

The shorter legionary closed his eyes. "When you fell into rank on the trireme, you couldn't work out where to put your arm. You rested it on your medical bag and the optio pushed it off. The bag needs repairing. It has a frayed strap that's tied tight. Your initials are burned into the bag's top, along with some phrase in Greek. I can't read Greek, but I could draw them for you."

Cervianus nodded. "Impressive, but that's observation, not memory. Let me try something."

"Alright."

"Remember this sequence." He took a deep breath and ran out a list of numbers at a rapid pace, breathing again when he'd finished.

Ulyxes shrugged. "Six, twenty-nine, three hundred and twelve, forty-eight, nine hundred and nine, four thousand three hundred and sixty-eight, nineteen, dog's testicles, seventy-seven, eleven, six hundred and seventy-two."

Cervianus stared at him.

"I think the 'dog's bollocks' in the middle just to throw me off was a bit mean," Ulyxes added.

"That's incredible."

"Maybe, but it's only so much use in the army."

Cervianus stood up straight and frowned. "And you've never used this at dice?"

"Never occurred to me you could."

"It's called an eidetic memory. They say Archimedes had it; could remember everything he'd ever read and quote it back."

"I wouldn't go that far."

Cervianus grinned. "You're going to take a month's money off them in one night."

"What about the 'reading people' bit?"

"You don't need it with a memory like that. Just play the odds and you'll walk away tonight with a sack full of denarii."

Ulyxes smiled. "And then I'll be almost as popular as you."

Cervianus shrugged. "Evandros and his pet thugs have the measure of me. You, I think they'll be wary of."

The capsarius continued to grin as his companion winked and then, turning, re-entered the building, heading back to the game. Cervianus, however, leaned back against the wall and sighed with relief after the day's activity. His helmet, shield and pilum and most of his kit had been stowed in the supply wagons and delivered to the camp a couple of hours after they arrived. While the other soldiers had washed their shields, carefully cleaned down their travelling kit, and spent an hour or more polishing the grit damage from their helmets, Cervianus had merely taken his from storage and laid them out ready. Now he stood, relaxing, while others rushed around preparing themselves.

"Hoy lads, it's one of the newbies."

Blinking, he peered across the street in the night air, the deep cerulean blue broken only by starlight and the guttering torches that marked the various occupied buildings. A group of legionaries in russet-coloured tunics appeared from an alleyway opposite.

Cervianus drew a deep breath, preparing to shout a warning but a voice from behind them in the darkness called, "Get moving. Back to barracks, you lot!"

The half-dozen dirty, messy legionaries slowed on the street as a man in an optio's uniform followed them out of the shadows.

"No loitering and causing trouble."

"Aww come on, sir. It's not like he's a Roman. It'll just be like kicking a Gaul. Caesar did plenty of that and they gave *him* a triumph!"

48

The man yelped as the optio's staff caught him a sharp rap around the ear.

"One more word and I'll have you working double shifts in the quarry. Fancy that, Mussius?"

The man fell silent and the group walked on along the street, casting hate-filled glances at the medic standing by the doorway. The optio stopped.

"Back to barracks and get yourselves washed, shaved and settled in. I'll be back shortly and I'm going to check in on each of you. If any of you is still up and moving I'll make sure you regret it."

Cervianus frowned, ignoring the soldiers as they shuffled sullenly off toward the city. The optio had stopped and was unfastening his helmet, brushing the crest that marked his rank and watching as the dirt and sand fell out of it. The man hoisted the helmet under his arm and strode toward Cervianus.

It was only as the capsarius peered at the helmet hooked under the man's armpit that he realised the optio was missing his left hand, just above the wrist. As the officer approached, he examined the missing appendage. The work was quite good. He'd have done a superior job, of course, but it was a better piece of work than most medics in the army would manage.

"Do you not salute an officer?"

The comment threw him and he realised he was staring at an optio's arm while slouching against a wall. Instantly straightening, he saluted and swallowed nervously. The optio grinned.

"Better. But you can relax now, soldier."

Cervianus continued to stand straight, lowering his arm.

"Apologies, sir. I was… thinking about your men." He winced

inside as he said it. Insulting an optio's men was tantamount to insulting *him* and his words, though carefully chosen, could be interpreted badly.

"I can imagine. The tribunes agreed to keep the legions apart for now, but there will always be times when contact can't be avoided. My work party was behind schedule, so I've extended their shift."

Cervianus nodded slightly. "They seem... they are recent conscripts?"

The optio nodded and leaned casually against the post on the far side of the door. "The Twelfth is full of them now: criminals, slaves, thugs and deserters. Even a bunch of the local auxiliaries were drafted in as legionaries. We were at less than quarter strength half a year ago. Now we're almost full again, but the quality of the legion has suffered. It'll take a couple of years to get this lot trained as though they were standard quality recruits."

"With respect, sir," Cervianus said quietly, "they don't like us. I'm not sure the tribunes' idea of a joint fortress is a good one."

The optio laughed. "Truly. But don't panic. After the campaign, the Twelfth will be moving on and the Third will come down from Thebes to join you."

"Campaign?" Suddenly Cervianus was alert and interested.

The optio shrugged. "Not been told, eh? Well it'll all be made clear in the morning no doubt. All I'll say is don't get too comfortable. You'll be moving on soon enough."

Cervianus fell silent, his mind racing.

"I was intrigued," the optio said. "They tell me that you men served for decades as a client army. You've only been a legion for a couple of years?"

"Yes, sir."

"Can't see much difference to the rest of us, apart from the green. Aren't your tunics expensive?"

"Not as expensive as the shields, sir. Green was King Deiotarus' royal colour, sir, and the shields have to be painted in the royal design."

The optio pursed his lips. "I shall look forward to seeing them, then."

"Excuse me, sir..."

"Yes?"

"Can I ask about the arm?"

The optio shrugged and shifted his helmet to his good hand. "If you like."

"Well, sir. It's been well attended to, clearly, but I believed that loss of a hand or foot was an automatic discharge?"

"Not when the legion's at quarter strength it isn't. Still got my sword arm and that was all prefect Gallus was interested in."

The optio realised the legionary was still examining his arm with a professional eye.

"You a medic by any chance?"

"Yes, sir." Cervianus frowned. "The wound was extremely neat. Very sharp blade?"

"You have *no* idea."

"Was it in Arabia, sir? I heard your legion suffered pretty badly out there."

The optio nodded. "Not just us, but the Third as well. We lost over eight thousand men all told, including a lot of the officers. Got my commission in the field at Marsiaba; got a phalera too for my troubles. Nice to have, but it's not as important as the pay increase, I can tell you."

Cervianus nodded sagely. Eight thousand men! That meant that the two legions had lost most of their troops. Arabia had clearly been brutal. And now the optio had intimated that another campaign was in the offing. He peered again at the man's stump and an involuntary shiver ran up his spine.

"Anyway," the officer said, taking a deep breath and straightening, "I must get back and make sure the lads have behaved themselves on the way home."

Cervianus saluted and the optio returned the gesture.

"Bear in mind with the Twelfth, and the Third when you meet them, that the veterans have all been through Hades and back this past year, and a lot of the rest of our men are crude and still barely house-broken. They all need someone to take their anger and frustration out on, and your legion's new, so it's going to be you. Just weather the storm for a while and things will settle eventually. You're only temporary outcasts. Have a good night's sleep, soldier. You'll need it."

As the optio turned and strode off back toward Alexandria, Cervianus sighed and leaned back again. If only it were that simple. Even when the others became accustomed to the Twenty Second, little would change for Titus Cervianus. Rolling his shoulders, he turned and entered the building. Unless the optio was winding him up, which seemed unlikely, it would be best to be well rested.

Strolling into the front room, he could see the light and hear the sound of the dice game going on in the back chamber. Shaking his head, he walked on past and to the bare, mud-brick room where rough sleeping pallets had been installed for four men, the rest of the contubernium being in the room next door. His blankets looked surprisingly inviting, spread out welcomingly on the pallet.

After a few moments spent stacking his gear by the wall nearby, Cervianus unlaced his boots, removed his belt and slipped under the blanket. He would wear his spare tunic in the morning and stay warm through the night in his well-travelled clothes.

Lying back in the near darkness, his mind whirled with the images of his first day in Aegyptus: the Pharos and the great port, the temples and forum, the strange priest with his stick and incense casting spells over the legion as if it would make any difference. Then Ulyxes: a man who actually seemed to be genuinely offering friendship. Of course, that would change. Over the next week, Evandros would gradually drive a wedge between the pair of them and draw the stocky psychopath over to their group. In a week's time, Ulyxes would be just another man to avoid in the latrines; another henchman of Evandros.

And the slip of information from the one-armed optio? A campaign? Surely not back to Arabia after what had happened to the Twelfth? Would the new governor really be eager to repeat the career-destroying mistakes of his predecessor? No; not Arabia. Besides, the optio had not seemed bitter or worried, so it was something else, for certain. But what?

The morning would tell: a parade with the new prefect of Aegyptus and probably an announcement.

In a way it was saddening to think they might be moving out straight away. He'd hoped to have plenty of time to explore the great city of Alexander, but that now seemed unlikely. Of course, there were still so many other things he would love to see in this land that the chance to move could be a blessing in disguise.

If...

He turned as he heard footsteps.

Frowning into the gloom, he made out the shape of a person in the doorway to the small room. He tensed. What now?

"Cervianus?"

He released a relieved breath as he recognised Ulyxes' voice. "Over here. I'm going to get some sleep. How's the game going?"

The legionary padded across the room in bare feet and crouched next to the pallet. Cervianus waited until his eyes could focus in the gloom and realised the man was smiling.

"Good, then?"

"Oh Titus, you have no idea. I'm going to need to commandeer a cart to take the winnings away. I suspect I may have to break a nose or two tonight when we finish and I try and leave the game and take my money, but I'll be careful not to do anything that'll cause you extra work."

"Thanks," Cervianus replied drily.

"Anyway," Ulyxes grinned, "I owe you. Here."

He flicked something with his thumb and Cervianus blinked as the spinning metallic object caught the faint light of the oil lamp out in the front room and flickered. The disc landed on his chest.

"My lucky coin." Ulyxes grinned. "Had it since I joined. I suspect you need it more than me. Besides, I have a lucky 'medic' now instead."

Cervianus blinked, trying to focus on the coin. In the gloom he could just make it out. It was one of the Galatian commemorative medals that had been struck around forty years ago to celebrate the part the army had played in the victory of Pompey over Mithridates. Probably worth a small fortune to a very nationalist Galatian these days.

"Thank you."

Ulyxes patted him on the shoulder and rose to return to his game, leaving Cervianus in the Stygian room, contemplating the coin and the man who had given him it. He was aware that in other peoples' eyes, he was probably something of an enigma, but so was Ulyxes. Life was certainly going to be interesting with him around.

Two rooms away there was the sound of shouting and a punch and Cervianus grinned as he rolled onto his side and waited for sleep to descend.

He was still clutching the polished silver disc when the oil lamp guttered out an hour later and the room fell into full darkness.

II

NICOPOLIS

The Twenty Second legion stood stiff and silent in the great paved square of the new city, the triumphal arch of Octavian casting the only real shadow in the locale, a shadow that fell tantalisingly short by a distance of mere feet from where the legion stood.

Cervianus tried to shrug his shoulders to shift the sweat that had pooled at the base of his neck where it met the tunic and mail but without moving noticeably, the optio standing behind watching his men intently for any movement or infraction.

The legion had begun to muster in the warm dark morning before the eye of Ra had risen over the delta to cast its burning gaze on the Roman forces. By torchlight, Cervianus and the others of his contubernium had scrambled into tunics, run out to the temporary latrine and wash building that had been set up, and then gathered their full parade kit, the men affixing crests to their helmets and brushing down their linen tunics, giving their shields a last moment polish and then checking one another for any mistakes.

The capsarius had struggled to examine himself in the bronze plate he carried as a mirror until Ulyxes had finished a mutual check with one of the others and then obligingly came over to look the medic up and down before pronouncing him ready.

By the time the golden disc rose in the east, the legion was already assembled.

Cervianus glanced at the rising sun, keeping his eyes narrowed and not lingering for fear of damaging his sight. The eye of Ra: that's what the ancient people of this land called the sun. Back home it was Helios, and in Rome: Sol. A man of science could see, just as Anaxagoras had, that the sun was no more the whim of a god than was the olive tree or the forging of steel. Superstition was the bane of all reasoned thinkers. Yet it was hard, particularly here in this land that was so closely tied with the sun, not to be swept away in the mysticism of it all.

It was said that the Aegyptians had worshipped that disc for more than five millennia, and in the great swathe of history, would this land even notice the presence of Rome or the Twenty Second legion?

The great golden sphere burned the white stones of the square and the legionaries that stood upon them.

The wait, over an hour thus far, had been excruciating. The strain on the legs and back was enough on its own, but combined with the heat, which increased with each passing moment, and the fact that no one could move or remove their helmet, things were beginning to look worrying. Even back in Ancyra the heat was intense during the summer and the officers had been sensible enough not to keep the men standing in formation for too long without water or rest.

Yet the legion had been mustered at dawn for a prefect who had not yet put in an appearance and tribune Vitalis stubbornly refused to allow his men to fall out while they waited. With a practised eye, Cervianus scanned the ranks in front and around him and counted roughly one man in four already showing the early signs of heat exhaustion: swaying slightly, slumped shoulders, glazed eyes, the occasional leg twitch as cramps set in. Somewhere off to the right he heard someone retching.

Something would have to be done soon or half the legion would be lying on the paving in their own vomit when the prefect arrived.

"Optio?"

"Eyes front and shut up, Cervianus."

"But sir… the men are starting to become faint."

"You deaf, soldier?"

The capsarius ground his teeth. Pushing the officer further would likely win him a sound blow with the staff. His mind raced, trying to find a way he could persuade the officers to reason. Of course, when men started falling over, *then* they would notice, but then he would likely be blamed for not warning them in time.

Every cohort of the legion had its own capsarius, universally unimaginative men capable of stitching a wound or applying a dressing but little else. Certainly none of them would stand up for medical reason in spite of the officers. They were primarily soldiers, with a little medical training at most. Even the medicus and his staff, safely back in their shelter with the few wounded or sick, and mercifully saved this torment, would think twice before arguing with the centurionate.

For the thousandth time Cervianus cursed his decision to sign on with the army: no spur of the moment decision, but rather an act to which he had been driven in desperation. If it hadn't been for that *damn woman* and her rigid superstitions, he would likely still be in a very lucrative private surgery in Ancyra. Instead, here he was, watching men slowly roasting.

If only…

His attention was distracted by the distant sound of horses. A number of heads turned to identify the source of the noise.

"Eyes front, you lot. Don't make me start handing out charges."

The men, steaming and exhausted, faced forward once more, the silence in the square pregnant with disaffection.

Moments later, the riders came into view: half a dozen senior officials and officers, escorted by the prefect's own cavalry guard. Three men wore white togas adorned with a purple stripe, while the other two, looking considerably more tired and hot than their companions, wore the decorative cuirasses and armour of tribunes. The prefect himself bore a cuirass of burnished bronze, decorated with impressive figures that Cervianus could not quite make out at this distance, a crimson ribbon tied in a Hercules knot around the waist indicating his rank as the commanding officer.

The prefect dismounted, removing his helmet with the ivory-coloured plume, and pushed the brilliant white cloak back over his shoulders as he handed the helm to one of the tribunes.

Gaius Petronius, Prefect of Aegyptus and commander of three legions, a tenth of Rome's entire standing army, was a man of below average height, with almost fully receded wispy grey hair, a prominent nose and wide ears. In some circumstances, such a figure bedecked in the garb of a senior officer could cut a somewhat comical figure, but there was about Petronius a presence that belied his physical appearance.

Cervianus realised he was already in awe of this man, and for no identifiable reason.

The prefect strode forward and stepped onto a large, uncut marble block, tribune Vitalis of the Twenty Second standing respectfully back from the commander's shoulder.

The prefect scanned the silent ranks of soldiers.

"Men of the Twenty Second Deiotariana... stand at ease, remove your helmets and for the sake of Minerva, drink some water before you fall over."

Cervianus noted the look that crossed Vitalis' face and made a mental note not to be around the tribune for the rest of the day. To have his parade formation shattered by the command of his superior without a single inspection would irritate him and drive him to take out his discontent on his own men later on. Vitalis was not an inherently tolerant man.

The prefect waited a moment or two for the legionaries to gratefully remove their helmets and swig from their canteens. In a gesture that took Cervianus by surprise, the prefect swigged from his own canteen and then crouched and passed it to one of the men at the front of the cohort. The capsarius's initial impressions seemed to be being borne out: this man carried with him an aura of authority and power, and with it he seemed to think of the men first. Cervianus smiled.

Petronius stood once more and smiled a relaxed smile that lit his countenance and seemed somehow to lessen the comic effect of his nose and ears.

"Men of the Twenty Second, welcome to Aegyptus and to Nicopolis, the city of victory. I am only sorry that you have been drawn here ahead of schedule and that the fortress was not ready for you to settle into. You will, I'm afraid, have to make the best of an uncomfortable situation, but then, given your history, it is clear that your legion is accustomed to handling change and discomfort with a stoic nobility."

The exact words would have been wasted on the majority of legionaries, who had likely never studied philosophy or heard of Zeno and his stoicism, but the feeling behind the words sank into the crowd and warmed them to him.

"I'm sure you've been told," the prefect continued, "a certain amount of what you are about to hear already, and I expect the rumour mill has been working and you will have gleaned a lot from gossip. Some of it may even be true."

The prefect smiled as a few laughs rose from the crowd, then clasped his hands behind his back and rocked on his heels.

"I am only recently arrived in the province myself and it will take some time for me to find my feet as governor. However, I find that, due to a number of... *unfortunate* decisions made by my predecessor, I have a great deal to do to put this land in order, in both the civil and military sectors.

"I recognise your Galatian origin and that you are only recently citizens of Rome, and therefore you may not be aware of the importance that the senate places on this province. Aegyptus is the source of much of Rome's wealth and food and, as such, she needs to be protected and nurtured like a new-born, despite her advanced age."

He smiled.

"In the area of civil works, which are not immediately your concern but will become so in time, when the Twenty Second may be required to join in the construction work, I have already drawn up plans for new canals and irrigation works. The tribune of the Twelfth continues to concentrate on the fortress here and the defensive works."

He straightened again, his face becoming suddenly serious and even sombre.

"However, for over a year, while the armies of the province were tied up in Arabia, Aegyptus was left open with woefully small defensive garrisons. While the legions fought in the east, the south of this province came under attack and the paltry defensive force was overwhelmed almost instantly.

"While the two legions based here are slowly making their way back to full strength, it will be some time before they are capable of undertaking any sort of campaign and so I have brought forward the transfer of your legion. With your help, we will consolidate our hold on the province and punish the invaders for their actions; we shall make them think twice before ever crossing the border under arms again."

A rumble of agreement rolled across the men.

"To the south of Aegyptus lies a kingdom called Kush, a land that has vied with this one for millennia and looked north at the fertile Nile valley with jealousy and hunger. The Kushites, under their queen, Amanirenas, took advantage of the lack of legions last year to push north and into the province. They sacked the city of Syene, the southernmost metropolis of Aegyptus, took thousands of slaves, and pillaged anything of value, including the new bronze statues of the great Princeps himself. Our latest reports suggest that the bulk of the queen's army has returned to Kush, but that an occupying force remains in Syene, as well as a number of smaller garrisons in installations around the border zone."

He clapped his hands together, startling those whose attention had begun to wander.

"In four days the Twenty Second will march south, under your tribune Vitalis, to restore to Rome control of the southern regions and to drive the Kushites from the land. Since you are new to the province and do not know the land or its people any more than I do, I have released two cohorts of the Twelfth to accompany you. This is all that legion can currently spare but, as you travel south, you will pick up two more cohorts of the Third legion at Thebes, as well as a number of local auxiliary units. It will not be the largest force ever mustered in the province, but should be more than adequate for the task at hand. I would have liked to have led the force myself, but there is more that needs attending to here than the greedy queen of Kush, and so I find myself forced to leave the campaign in the hands of my trusted tribunes."

He straightened.

"For the glory of the Republic and its Princeps, you will succeed where our predecessors failed and the legions will once more be so feared by our enemies that they would charge the gates of Hades before crossing voluntarily into Roman territory. The Twenty Second will make its mark here in Aegyptus!"

A roar of approval flowed across the crowd. Cervianus raised an eyebrow. These men considered themselves Galatians first and Romans second, if at all, and yet, without any noticeable effort, the prefect seemed to have reached something inside them and tied them to him. The Princeps had been careful this time in selecting the right man for the task.

"For the senate and the people of Rome!" Petronius bellowed.

Another roar, this time far louder and longer.

Petronius stood for a long moment, smiling at the legion, and then lowered his hands as the noise slowly faded.

"I am confident in the glorious Twenty Second, children of Galatia. Now, spend the next three days preparing yourselves.

Your officers will attend to the general organisation of the legion and, in conjunction with my staff, will arrange the necessary support units and wagons, maps and equipment. Acclimatise yourselves. Get used to Aegyptus and get some rest after your long journey from Ancyra. Do what you need to do to be prepared and at your very best when the army leaves. The blessings and favour of myself and of Rome will go with you."

He turned to Vitalis, who nodded, his face stony and betraying none of the irritation that Cervianus knew he must be feeling.

"Fall out, men."

Cervianus stood for a moment, emotions tumbling around inside him, mostly conflicting. A born and bred Galatian, he had an inherent distrust of the bureaucracy of Rome and yet as Petronius had spoken, he had had to fight the urge to cheer wildly with the rest. The news of a campaign to come was nerve-wracking and meant great peril and a lot of work for medical staff, but at the same time, would he ever again be given the opportunity to travel up the Nile and see the heart of this ancient world, right the way to the southern lands?

"You coming?"

He blinked and shook his head, realising that most of the men were dispersing from the square. Ulyxes was watching him expectantly. Fuscus, standing close by, tapped the stocky soldier on the shoulder.

"Come on. Let's go get a drink."

"I'll be along in a bit."

The legionary glared for a moment at Cervianus and then shrugged at Ulyxes. "It's your funeral. Jupiter'll probably send you knob-rot just for being near *him*."

Ulyxes grinned. "Well at least *he* can probably cure that."

Cervianus smiled and turned to leave along with his companion. Ulyxes was tapping his finger on his lower lip as they made for their rooms, the men of the Twelfth legion now on-site and beginning to work on the buildings of the "City of Victory".

"Vitalis is leading the legion on campaign," the heavy-set soldier mused. "What happened to our legate? I mean, he's the *commander* of the legion, so shouldn't he be here and doing it? I haven't seen him since before we embarked in Anatolia."

Cervianus narrowed his eyes. "He'll have been reassigned. No legates in Aegyptus."

"Not even of the Twelfth or Third?"

"No legates at all," the capsarius replied. "No full governors either. Tribunes in charge of the army and a prefect in charge of the country, by dictate of the senate."

Ulyxes frowned. "Why's that?"

"Nobody of senatorial rank is allowed a level of control in the province. I suspect our great Princeps is trying to avoid what happened here with Marcus Antonius and Cleopatra. No one with enough authority to cause trouble will get the opportunity again. Got to hand it to that Octavian: half a dozen years since Actium and he all but rules the republic now. He's every bit his great-uncle's successor."

The stocky legionary shrugged. "That's not necessarily a good thing to be. Look at how Caesar ended up."

The two men fell silent as they walked. The republic was currently in a state of flux and, while the senate still nominally held control of the government, alongside the appointed consuls, the slide toward monarchy that had begun with Sulla and continued with Caesar seemed to be set in stone now, with

Octavian following the trend. A crown would not be a surprise in the near future.

A sudden blood-curdling scream made the pair jump and stumble to a halt.

"What in Hades was that?"

Snapping their heads this way and that, the two stragglers quickly spotted the source of the yell: three soldiers from the Twelfth were stacking heavy blocks of stone using an A-frame and pulley, but something had clearly slipped and one of the men was thrashing helplessly at the base of the stone.

"Shit. His hand's trapped."

Cervianus did not reply as the two ran toward the accident. Instead, all military and political matters fell away from his mind, his professionalism taking hold. By the time they had reached the scene, he had already identified the trouble and decided on the course of action.

"Help us!" one of the men shouted, trying in vain to heave the massive granite block away from the wounded man. The other joined him and Ulyxes ran over to lend his hefty arms to the task.

Cervianus shook his head sadly. "You'll not move it and even if you do it won't help him."

"We've got to free him."

The capsarius shook his head again. "No use. The fingers are crushed beyond any healing. All we can do is save most of the hand."

The man's eyes widened. "My hand?" he said shakily, his face ashen.

"Sadly, we can do nothing about your fingers, but your thumb is free and we can perhaps save down to the middle knuckle on the rest."

The man's mouth fell open in a mix of horror and despair.

"You'll be able to grip things, given time and the right care in recuperation."

Ulyxes pointed at the medical bag. "Give him something for the pain, then!"

"I've nothing that will work that quick. We need to deal with this now. Every moment risks further damage and we stand to lose more of the hand while he bleeds out."

Ulyxes nodded unhappily. "Soldier?"

The wounded man twisted to face the speaker, his eyes hollow and panicked and, as his head turned, Ulyxes hit him with a punch that would have laid out a donkey. Cervianus stared.

"Get on with it," the stocky man grunted, rubbing his knuckles. "He's out of pain for now."

"Hold him."

Ulyxes gestured to the other two workers and the three men crouched around the capsarius and supported the wounded man while Cervianus delved into his bag and withdrew a wooden block marked with long gashes and a roll of leather. Unrolled, it revealed a selection of knives of varying weights and thicknesses. Carefully, he selected a heavy, cleaver-like blade and passed the wooden block to Ulyxes.

"Place it under the hand and hold it very steady. Don't move it."

The shorter man nodded, his eyes wide as he followed his instructions. Cervianus waited until everything was in position and, his tongue poking from the side of his mouth in concentration, brought the blade down in a heavy, perfectly accurate, blow. The fingers came away at the second knuckle with the razor-sharp edge, wobbling where they protruded from the block, as blood ran from the open wounds and fell to the sand.

"How are we going to burn them? Anyone got a flint and steel?"

"We're not," Cervianus replied. "Cauterising is quick, but it kills off the ability to feel. I'm sure he'd rather retain sensation once he's healed."

Ulyxes dropped the wooden block and continued to support the unconscious patient, watching with fascination as Cervianus worked. The capsarius made several small cuts, creating flaps on what was left of the fingers, which he then stretched and pulled together, effectively sealing the wound.

Holding the wound shut, he reached into the bag again, withdrawing a small leather wallet. Holding it in his teeth, he removed a small metal pin with his free hand, expertly sliding it through one flap of skin, bending it, and then pushing it through the other before twisting it so that it lay flush with the severed finger. A small bottle from the bag was then opened and drops sprinkled onto the freshly pinned finger.

"What's that?"

"Vinegar. Good for slowing the blood."

Ulyxes whistled through his teeth as he watched the procedure repeated on the other three fingers.

"That's impressive."

"Fairly simple, really. Now we just bind them and in a week or so his own medicus can remove the pins and the fingers should stay closed and safe. So long as there's no infection he should be able to start working on gripping and manoeuvring his hand in a month or so; maybe even sooner. At least with no burning he'll be able to feel everything."

Quickly, he wrapped the four stumps in lint and sponge, also soaked in vinegar, and then bound them with linen.

Leaving the hand, he opened his bag again and rifled through a set of small leather pockets, pulling out small, wrapped bundles until he found what he wanted. Taking out a tiny jar, he passed it over to the remaining man from the Twelfth, his companion having left to vomit copiously when the fingers came away.

"This is barbarum, pre-mixed to a specific strength. Unwrap his dressing every two days and apply this to prevent infection. Here is centaury and henbane, again pre-mixed. Just add a pinch of it to a cup of spiced wine and give him it whenever the pain gets too much, but... and remember this... never more than three times in a day, and never more than a pinch."

"Shouldn't the medicus be doing all this?" the soldier asked uncertainly.

"Personally, I wouldn't bring a dog with a blocked rectum to most of the medici in the legions. Follow those instructions and then in a week's time take him to your medicus to remove the pins. He can't do too much damage by that time."

Ulyxes gently passed the unconscious man to his friend and then stood.

"Thanks," the crouched soldier said, simply. Cervianus nodded, packed his equipment back into the appropriate places and then joined Ulyxes as the pair strolled off toward their lodgings.

"That," the stocky legionary said as they walked, "was amazing. I've seen similar wounds in the past and the capsarius would just hold him down while a soldier cuts the hand off and burns the stump."

Cervianus gave a humourless laugh.

"That is because while Rome likes to think of herself as the centre of all things civilised, when it comes to medicine, they are still *barbaroi*. It takes a Greek to teach true healing."

The two men walked on in silence for a moment.

"Stop staring at me."

"Sorry."

Cervianus frowned down at the sleeping pallet. The contents of his medical bag were distributed across the blanket in neat, ordered rows: herbs at the top, divided into those for poultices, for open wounds, for varying forms of disease or for burns. Miscellaneous wadding, lint and so on in the centre. Below those were the leather ties for tourniquets, the linen bandaging, various wound-closing equipment, and then the surgical gear at the bottom, including the cylindrical case of tools, the roll of knives and a bag of collyrium sticks.

All in all, the kit was beginning to look a little light on content. He'd intended to resupply back in Ancyra before all of this started, but the legate there had put a hold on all equipment and supplies, since the army was about to pass into the financial control of another governor. Resupply would be the problem of the Prefect of Aegyptus.

Well, the prefect wanted everything ready before the army moved out, so he would have to produce a list of what was needed to bring the kit up to scratch, and then go and visit the quartermaster to sort it all out.

Perhaps this afternoon, since they were apparently being given miraculous free time to put everything in order.

He frowned.

"Where are my pins? Don't say I left them at... no. There

they are. Getting very low on henbane too. Have to mix up some new batches of everything before we travel."

Adjusting the neat rows of equipment, Cervianus straightened everything and swapped them over until the order was perfect.

"There..."

He stood and folded his arms, satisfied with the result of his labours. Now he would need a wax tablet to make out his list. Strolling across to the window ledge, he became vaguely aware of raised voices and laughter outside. Grasping the tablet and stylus, he leaned into the window alcove and peered through the iron grille.

In the street outside, three men in the russet tunics of the Twelfth, busily working on the construction of a drain across the thoroughfare, were laughing and pointing. Cervianus moved to peer at an angle and could just see a figure standing in the main doorway of the building they were currently using as a barrack block. It took only a moment before he noted the build and shape of the figure and realised it was Ulyxes.

Shrugging, he opened the wax tablet and, leaning on the window ledge, began to make marks on the surface.

"Centaury?" he mused. "Wonder if they have reasonable stocks of it here? In fact, I wonder if they even use it here? Have to go sparingly if not until I can get supplies brought in."

He frowned as he tapped the tablet, peering across the room at his carefully organised medical kit.

"I'll need some mandragora too, but they must have that."

He blinked irritably. The voices outside had become louder and more taunting, intruding themselves on his thoughts. He leaned into the alcove again and listened.

"Gauls? Nah… they're all Greek over that way," one of the soldiers spat.

Again, the capsarius lowered the tablet and frowned out of the window. As one man dug, the other two were grinning and pointing at Ulyxes.

"That explains it. The Greeks have always been a weird lot. Obsessed with young boys, I heard."

"Yeah. That one looks like he's seen a *lot* of young boys, too."

Cervianus shook his head. "Don't push him," he said under his breath, willing the three soldiers to get back to work.

"Hey? You? You all lonely here? Maybe we can send someone into the city and find you a eunuch?"

There was an ominous silence as Cervianus made a mark in the wax with his stylus, his breath held. Then there was a slow scraping noise near the door.

"Oh, shit."

Snapping the tablet shut, the capsarius flung it down onto the pallet and rushed out of the chamber into the main room. The stocky, quick-tempered legionary was no longer in the doorway. Dashing across, Cervianus grabbed the doorframe and peered through, nervously expecting to see Ulyxes already standing in a pool of blood and a pile of body parts.

What he actually *did* see made him stop and stare before breaking into a wide helpless grin.

Ulyxes had stepped down from the doorway, lifted his tunic, and proceeded to urinate with a powerful flow into the half-constructed drain. The liquid rushed and burbled down the dry, dusty stone channel toward the three workers, who had stopped, their faces enraged.

"You barbarian shit!"

Ulyxes sighed deeply as he lowered his tunic. "Ahh... that's better."

"You..."

Cervianus watched with a sinking feeling as events began to unfold with distressing predictability. The nearest of the three men, a reedy, thin man with greasy hair and a burn mark suspiciously located where a slave tattoo would be, looked back and forth between his companions and this newcomer. Clearly the man was unsure of what to do. Given time, Cervianus could have put that to use, but time was unfortunately up.

Behind the thin ex-slave, the other two men were clearly veterans of the Twelfth with the muscle tone of practised soldiers and the haggard faces of men who had stared into the jaws of death and lived.

The larger of the two, a veritable ox, slapped the head of the mallet he held into the palm of his other hand meaningfully, and stepped out of the gutter just as the trickle of urine washed past. Next to him a tall, wiry and muscular soldier with a stubbly chin cracked his knuckles and followed his friend, grabbing the ex-slave as he stepped up and turning him toward Ulyxes.

"Three of you eh? Sure you don't want to go back for some friends first?"

Cervianus swallowed nervously.

"Err... Ulyxes?"

The stocky legionary from the Twenty Second turned to glance over his shoulder and grinned.

"Two of *us* now,' Ulyxes corrected himself. 'The odds are definitely against you."

"Ulyxes, I'm not sure—"

He never managed to finish the sentence as his friend let out a loud roar and ran at the three dirty workmen.

Cervianus stared in mild panic. It wasn't that he was a coward; he'd seen action more than once since he joined the army of Galatia, though he was not strongly built and not naturally inclined to violence. The problem was more one of logic, a force that ruled the capsarius with more zeal and focus than either his heart or his head.

They were to campaign in the south against an unknown enemy in a few days' time and here was the mad bastard Ulyxes trying to get them beaten to death by their own side while they were still in camp.

Momentarily he dithered, wondering whether it would be better if he just ducked back inside the building and ignored the problem. Ulyxes would soon start ignoring him along with the rest anyway. It was surely a waste of effort to try and look after a man who would simply ditch him soon.

It was with some surprise that he realised he was running out into the street before he had arrived at a solid decision, as though some hidden part of him had commanded his body to become involved while his brain was busy.

Ahead, there was a bellowing noise and an almighty thump as Ulyxes and the ox-like soldier met at a run. The enemy was a good two feet taller than Cervianus' friend, and yet the two were a match across the shoulders.

At the last moment, before they met, the man had raised his mallet ready to bring it down in a powerful blow, a choice that surprised Cervianus. A brawl with bruises and even broken bones was not unknown in the army and would likely result in fairly harsh punishments, but to attack with a hammer was to risk killing a fellow legionary, and the sentence for *that* didn't bear thinking about.

The blow never came, though. As they had closed and the man raised the mallet, Ulyxes instead dropped and turned, presenting his powerful shoulder at navel height.

The meeting knocked every last gasp of air from the big man and he was thrown aside easily despite his size. Behind him, the wiry soldier braced himself to withstand similar punishment, but Ulyxes came to a halt.

At that moment, Cervianus lost track of what was happening ahead. His running feet had brought him to the enormous legionary who was bent double, wheezing, his mallet hanging by his side. Cervianus' eyes widened as the man took a deep breath and began to straighten. He clearly hadn't noticed the arrival of the capsarius and was quickly recovering.

Panicked, Cervianus dithered again. Should he really be getting involved? If he did and he didn't lay the man out, that mallet would likely end up wedged in his head.

"I'm sorry about this," he said to the big man in a sympathetic voice.

The legionary looked up in surprise and then frowned as he began to straighten, changing his grip on the mallet.

His expression remained furrowed as Cervianus delivered him a powerful kick between the legs, putting every ounce of strength he had into the blow. The man was tall and the attack had been awkward, and the capsarius found himself twisting and toppling, ridiculously overbalanced.

As he hit the ground, the dust rising around him, he rolled onto his back, watching for the hammer blow that would be coming, prepared to roll out of the way, but the huge legionary was still standing in exactly the same position, his expression changing, the frown melting away to be replaced by a look of intense shock, his face slowly turning purple.

Cervianus lay there for a moment until the big man staggered backward, dropping his mallet to clutch his privates. With a sigh of relief, the medic clambered to his feet and turned to see Ulyxes up to his neck in trouble. Two more workers from the Twelfth seemed to have appeared from somewhere among the rubble and his friend was in danger, beleaguered by enemies and defending himself against the blows of three men.

Three men? Then where...?

He was turning to try and locate the reedy ex-slave when the man popped up behind him with a length of wood and delivered a sturdy whack on the back of the capsarius's head.

Staggering forwards, Cervianus concentrated as hard as he could through the flashing lights in his brain and the roaring noise in his ears, trying not to fall over and leave himself prone and at the mercy of this sneaky slave.

His head screamed at him and somewhere inside, his logical, reasoning mind detached itself from the situation.

Look what you've got yourself into, Titus Cervianus. You're risking disciplinary proceedings at best, and death at worst, and for what? To try and protect a man who clearly has no interest in personal safety or his future prospects. And now you're out of it all and probably concussed. The little one can finish you off at leisure and, even if he doesn't, the big one will recover soon and will want to deal with you personally. With a hammer!

"Shit."

He reeled, his head lolling forward, and noticed the long line of blood-coloured drool dangling from his mouth. *Classy. You're a classy man, Cervianus.*

With extreme difficulty, he raised his thumping head slowly, with what he hoped was a defiant expression, only to see that the smaller man had turned and run, already twenty paces down the street and accelerating.

Confused and panicky, he turned to try and take in the situation. The huge ox-like man was leaning heavily against a wall, his hand under his tunic. Momentarily, the medic in him wondered whether he had done some serious damage to the man's reproductive system. It was quite possible, given the strength of the blow. Still, at least the man wasn't here and about to drive him two feet into the ground with that big mallet, which was a plus.

Ulyxes, on the other hand, was in distinct trouble. One of the three men lay on his back, unmoving, but the other two were beating the stocky legionary mercilessly with fists and feet. Occasionally their barrage lifted for a moment and Ulyxes landed a couple of return blows, his face a mask of rage, spattered with blood and caked with dust.

He was putting up a good fight, but wouldn't last much longer.

Cervianus took several deep breaths and shook his head gently, trying to clear his throbbing, jumbled thoughts. Once again, before he had a chance to reason through the situation, he found himself stumbling, half blind and fully confused, in the direction of his beleaguered companion.

In the strange half-conscious stagger, he realised with irritation that he had just trodden in the drain and Ulyxes' urine had splattered up onto his boot, mixing with the sand that was ever-present at Nicopolis to cake the leather.

"Oh damn."

One of the two remaining men had turned to face him, leaving Ulyxes fighting a much more reasonable single opponent. As Cervianus, his mind still spinning, watched in consternation, wondering how he would manage this, he noted the man stoop and pick up a hammer.

"Oh no…"

He raised his fists in what he hoped was an impressive, defensive manner but was, in truth, a comical gesture with flopping arms, as his mind spun.

And pain suddenly lanced through his hands as something struck him across the wrist.

Panicked, Cervianus turned to identify this new threat.

Quintus Scribonius Nasica, the primus pilus, or senior centurion, of the entire Twenty Second legion, stood glaring at him, vine staff raised for a second blow.

"Disengage this fight at *once*!" he bellowed, his face inches from Cervianus' own.

The capsarius, his mind still fuzzy and confused, noted with interest the pungent stink of cheap wine on the centurion's breath. Clearly the hushed rumours were true and Nasica *did* turn to the drink while on duty. It was a rumour that stayed low and never reached a tribune's ear, though. For all the primus pilus might be a slave to the vine, it had never yet been noted to adversely affect his military performance and no man in the legion would dare stand against him. Nasica had earned his commission and a corona decoration under Caesar, withstanding the famous elephant charge at Thapsus. A man who could look a charging pachyderm in the eye and not flinch was not a man to question.

Desperately, Cervianus tried to swing round and come to attention with a salute. Unfortunately, concussed and confused, the attempted manoeuvre finished instead with him floundering on the ground in the dust.

Nasica paid him no further heed, reaching out with a powerful ham-fist and grasping the attacking man from the Twelfth by the neck. The tendons in his wrist stood out and the leather of his wrist band creaked as he lifted the man from the ground with no apparent effort, bringing his grizzled, scarred face to within an inch of the panicked soldier.

"You're not one of mine and, unless you drop that hammer, that makes you an enemy. Care to try your luck, soldier?"

The legionary, his eyes bulging in terror, made a squeaking noise, all his constricted throat would allow, and dropped the hammer, waving his open hands around to emphasise how unarmed he was.

Cervianus stared up from the dust. He'd never been this close to the primus pilus. The men of Nasica's century, the first one in the First cohort, called him *Invictus*, the unconquered. Cervianus could imagine how a century might feel with this man leading them. Pride and panic vied for control of his whirling brain.

Over at the end of the unfinished gutter, Ulyxes and his opponent had separated and come to attention, both covered with blood, dust and urine.

"You two are a disgrace to the Twenty Second. Brawling in the gutters? Where do you think you are? Some shithole tavern in the Subura?"

He turned to look at the man in his grasp and lowered him to the ground. As his grip released, the man collapsed onto his backside, desperately gulping in air.

"The rest of you should know better too. You've got until I count to five to be out of my sight or I'll deliver you to your own primus pilus... *in a bucket!*"

Cervianus scrambled around, trying to get to his feet,

realising with distaste that he had landed once again in the gutter. By the time he was standing, there was no sign of any member of the Twelfth legion around them – just him and Ulyxes and a man with the authority to have them crucified if he so wished it.

"Srr…?" his mouth didn't appear to be responding correctly to his thoughts.

Nasica turned his baleful glare on the capsarius. "You don't know when to stay quiet, do you, soldier?"

He turned and yelled over his shoulder.

"*Curtius*?"

A man wearing the crest and harness of an optio appeared as if from nowhere, three legionaries with him in immaculate condition. "Yes, sir."

"Curtius, take these two hooligans and throw them in the stockade while I go and see the tribune. If either of them opens their mouth on the way, have them flogged. No food or water until I return, either."

He paused.

"Ulyxes! I might have known. Draco's not kicked the stupidity out of you yet, then?"

Turning back to the optio, he pointed at the blood-spattered stocky legionary.

"If Ulyxes even looks at you wrong, nail him up for the crows."

Cervianus stared in dismay and had to force himself to stay quiet.

The primus pilus regarded him once more with a steely look. "Get going; and if I find out it was you who started this, and not them, I'll tie you to a boulder and drop you in the harbour."

Nasica turned, not sparing them a further glance, and strode off, hands behind his back, gripping his staff, toward the unfinished fortress where tribune Vitalis had his headquarters.

The capsarius stared at his hand. His fingers had gone numb following the blow from the centurion's staff. Not a good sign. There were things he could probably do, but his mind didn't seem to be working properly.

Ulyxes fell in next to him. The optio was barking orders, but it sounded vaguely muffled. In fascination, Cervianus gingerly touched the back of his head and, when he brought his hand back round to look at it, there was matted hair and blood on it.

"*Ahh*—" He opened his mouth and bit his tongue to stop the involuntary speech that rose from his throat.

Clamping his mouth shut, he concentrated on staying upright as the optio strode out forward, one of his legionaries at his shoulder while the other two followed along behind.

Ulyxes grinned, blood coating his chin, and spoke quietly out of the corner of his mouth.

"We showed the bastards, eh? Thanks for wading in, mate."

"*Snrfl.*" His mouth clearly still wasn't in working order.

With a sigh, he raised his eyes to the partially constructed cistern, the lower half hollowed out of the hillside, which currently functioned as a stockade.

He had known consorting with Ulyxes would be trouble, and yet he kept on doing it.

In this man's company, the question was whether he would live long enough to actually go to war.

Cervianus probed the back of his head gingerly. Minor damage really; very lucky. The concussion he'd been suffering was still fuddling his thoughts but was relatively light and he should be recovering fully by evening.

Ulyxes was more of an issue. While Cervianus had taken a single, heavy blow to the back of the head, his companion was covered in cuts and contusions and held his arm as though it was causing him trouble. Quietly and under his breath, in case it provoked the ire of the guards, he cursed the fact that his medical kit was still in their quarters, spread out across the pallet. He hoped that the other occupants of the house were not taking the opportunity of his absence to mess with his supplies – it was just the sort of petty mischief Evandros would get up to.

Behind him, the ladder that had been dropped into the huge, rectangular cistern to allow them access was being drawn back up by the guards. Cervianus looked around himself grimly. The unfinished water tank was perhaps eighty feet long and twenty wide, the walls reaching up at least twice a man's height, hacked smoothly from the solid rock. At this point there was no roof, and piles and drifts of dust and sand spoke eloquently of the unpleasant conditions occupants would be under whenever a strong wind blew.

Half a dozen legionaries in reddish-brown tunics, stained and faded, sat in a small group at the far end of the structure, eyeing them cautiously.

"Great," Ulyxes said, his voice slightly indistinct as he spoke through a split lip. "We get jumped by bastards from the Twelfth and to punish us they put us in a sealed room with more of them."

Cervianus gestured silently for his friend to lower his voice.

"Well…" Ulyxes grumbled back at him, "I can probably take two more, but six is pushing it. You up to another scuffle?"

"My head feels like someone moored a trireme in it and I think I can taste my own brains. Don't start anything or we'll both get killed."

Ulyxes shrugged and gave a sharp intake of breath at a lancing pain in his side.

"What's up?" Cervianus asked, his eyes narrowing.

"Just a pain in my side. It'll be fine."

"Lift your tunic up and let me look."

Ulyxes stared at him. "Cervianus, we're in the stockade with half a dozen psychopaths and you want me to show them I'm a shirt-lifter?"

"Just do it."

Muttering, the short, stocky soldier painfully and slowly raised his tunic up to his armpits and the capsarius leaned down, his eyes rolling with the sudden confusing change of perspective, and looked at his companion's side. A large patch around his lower ribs was already turning purple and blotchy.

"I think you've got a cracked or broken rib. Possibly two."

"Had 'em before. They heal."

The medic straightened.

"I don't think you're in any mortal danger, but you look a mess. I could really do with getting my kit and treating you."

Ulyxes graced him with a grin that the capsarius thought contained more than a hint of lunacy.

"You wasted no time, then!" a grizzly voice called across the cistern.

They looked up to see that one of the other occupants had risen to his feet and was sauntering slowly across toward them. Cervianus took a deep breath, preparing himself for the worst.

"Looks like you had a fight with an ox cart and lost," the man chuckled.

Ulyxes shrugged and winced again. "A few of your friends decided to try their luck."

The man laughed. "Ah, legionary pride. A punch up with a new arrival's nothing new."

As the man closed on them, Cervianus realised that this was no ex-slave or conscript criminal, but a longstanding veteran perhaps approaching fifty years of age. The man had stubbly grey hair and a chin to match. Judging by the growth on his face and the state of his clothing he could have been here for a week or more.

"We're not popular, apparently," Ulyxes said, flatly.

The man grinned as he approached and came to a halt in front of them.

"Newbies never are. Plus wearing that green sort of makes you stand out. Makes you a bit of a target."

Ulyxes glanced down at his tunic and then back up at the man, his eyes narrowed. "What's a man of retirement age doing in the stockade, then?"

The soldier laughed. "Improprieties. Dishonouring the legion and committing sacrilege."

"Sacrilege?"

The man's grin widened.

"I took a leak in the chapel of the standards. What can I say? Mars came to me in my time of need and told me it was alright."

Cervianus rolled his eyes.

"Gods do not appear to legionaries and tell them to piss in a shrine."

"Mars did. The chapel's only just been built and it's not consecrated yet. Besides, we owe the bastards nothing."

Ulyxes nodded sympathetically. "Sounds familiar. What about your friends?"

"All sorts. Nothing serious. We're not popular men, you see."

Cervianus' ear pricked up. "Oh? Why's that?"

"We're due our muster out, but neither the last prefect nor the new one will allow it. Say the legion's too far below strength to let veterans go. We fought at Pharsalus and helped save the republic from that knob-nosed turd Pompey, and this is how they repay us. Anyhow, it's worth pulling the odd prank to stay in here and not have to heave blocks of stone around."

Ulyxes nodded. "It's a bastard business for sure. But you're doing yourselves no favours kicking your heels in here, really."

The soldier shrugged.

"We'll be back out in the next few days. Word has it our cohort's going to be marching south and centurion Sempronius won't leave his veterans here when he needs them."

The group fell silent for a moment as each man's thoughts turned to the planned campaign.

"You lot been in Aegyptus for a while then?"

The man nodded. "Since the dawn of time, I think." He grinned. "A decade or so under Marcus Antonius, here and off on campaign, and then ever since under different prefects."

"Ever been up the Nile?"

"Only as far as Thebes. It all gets a bit weird when you leave Alexandria. The locals inland are about as Roman as the Parthians are. You might as well be outside the borders of the republic altogether. Wrapping the dead in bandages and ripping out their stomachs. Burying them with boats for their afterlife. It's all pretty odd stuff."

Cervianus cleared his throat. For some reason the comment offended him, and it had nothing to do with his own non-Roman origins.

"Don't forget these people ruled an empire the size of the republic when even Romulus was a twinkle in his father's eye."

"True, but it's still a weird place. They have a healthy respect for gods, but for some reason they stick animal heads on them all. I'm happy to bow before any god if it means getting through the next scrape unmarked, but I'm buggered if I'm going to kneel and give offerings to a bloody dog!"

Ulyxes grinned. "Keep talking. You'll get on famously with Cervianus here. He apparently thinks gods are a waste of time."

"I never said that," the capsarius snapped defensively. "It's just that not *everything* can be attributed to them."

The soldier made a strange gesture with his hand, wobbling it and then pointing at his eye.

"Careful what you say then in this place. The locals here don't do anything without the gods' say so. They used to think their kings and queens were gods too. Even bulls, birds, cats and crocodiles. Everything here is *something* to do with the gods."

Ulyxes laughed. "You're going to be a popular man, Cervianus."

"Oh, sod off."

The capsarius folded his arms grumpily and leaned back against the wall while the other two talked. After a moment, Ulyxes cast him an apologetic look and then strode over to join the other occupants. Cervianus, however, stayed where he was, his mind, still slightly befuddled, roving back through the details of the gods of Aegyptus he'd read about.

This land was still much more arcane and mystical than Rome or most of the more northern lands. Spells were said over both the living and the dead; the practice of mummification was a fascinating meeting of the science of medicine and the strange mysticism of the local religion. The great tombs of the pharaohs were monuments to the difference between this culture and any that Cervianus was familiar with.

It was going to be a strange journey upriver, obviously.

Time wound on with no method to mark its passage but the gradual descent of the sun. Ulyxes spent the afternoon in deep conversation with the veterans from the Twelfth, playing dice with them and laughing. Cervianus felt that he should be irritated or disappointed at being left to himself and not invited into the group, but the time on his own had been useful to sift through his gleaned knowledge of the country and he was more than familiar with simple solitude.

As the afternoon wore into evening and the golden glow disappeared with a surprising turn of speed, the brilliant twinkling stars came out. Everything here was in the same place as the night sky at home, but somehow it looked different; stranger. Cervianus couldn't have said when it was that he drifted off to sleep, but it was certainly after the night sky was displaying its full glory.

He awoke with a start as the ladder was dropped down the cistern wall, landing with a thump close by. His head spun for a moment in confusion and then realised what was happening.

"Legionaries Cervianus and Ulyxes?"

The capsarius looked up.

"Yes?"

"Yes *sir*, you piece of shit. Get up here… and your friend."

With a little care and difficulty, Cervianus climbed the ladder and stepped out onto the rocky surface where he waited for his companion to join him. Ulyxes seemed unreasonably happy; the man was incorrigible.

"Straighten up, you two, and follow me."

The two men fell into position, standing to attention, surrounded by neat legionaries in green tunics and the optio that had led them to the stockade hours earlier.

"Where are we going, sir?" Ulyxes enquired.

"Shut up and walk."

The two prisoners shared a questioning look and walked in silence down the slope and across the main thoroughfare that led into the construction site that would become Nicopolis. On the rise at the far side stood the fortress that would one day be the home of the Twenty Second, a dark purple shape against the indigo night, dotted with twinkling yellow stars.

Cervianus paid careful attention as they approached. The fortress had been well sited on a slope with the sea protecting one side. A series of posts hammered into the ground marked out the location of what would be three defensive ditches surrounding the walls. For a moment he found himself sympathising with the poor devils that would have to hack those ditches out of the rock but then realised that, timing and the situation being what they were, he himself could end up being one of those very men.

A dozen or so men worked at the gate even into the night and, as they approached and passed across the threshold, Cervianus was impressed at the precision and care the soldiers were taking with their work, the light from guttering torches revealing the smooth lines of the stone. There was something about the mind of a professional architect that echoed the neat order of a physician's thought processes and Cervianus always held in a certain awe a man who could take a chunk of stone, look carefully at it, and then craft it to fit perfectly with its companions with no need for a second attempt.

Passing the great stone blocks being levelled and chipped at, the piles of timber and ropes and A-frames, the two men, with their escort, entered the fort proper.

Surprisingly, the legionary fortress was a great deal more complete inside than first impressions had suggested. While the main defences were still being constructed, the granaries, headquarters building, stores and workshops were all nearing completion. The barracks would come in last.

The legionaries marched the pair along the Via Principalis and to the corner of the enormous headquarters building. Cervianus had seen the equivalent structure in smaller Roman forts across Anatolia, but this was something else: a sight to behold. It was, for a start, perhaps ten times the size of the buildings he had previously seen, the façade with its new, crisp colonnade stretching over two hundred feet away, punctuated halfway along with a decorative gateway. Sections of the roof were still being tiled, work having stopped overnight, but the roof remained covered with scaffolding, baskets of tiles attached to ropes and blocks and tackle hanging loose.

Already the building was almost complete, white and red paint applied to the outer wall. Cervianus noted with interest that the antefix tiles at the roof's edge were stamped with the thunderbolt emblem of the Twelfth legion. They might be moving to another province in the very near future, but clearly the Twelfth were leaving no doubt among the Twenty Second as to who it was that had built their fortress.

"Stop sightseeing and pay attention," the optio barked from behind and Cervianus turned his head forward once more.

They approached the monumental entranceway, the columns of Marmaris white and expensive Numidian yellow marble indicating the importance of the building, and turned to enter.

The courtyard inside was every bit as impressive as the exterior. Already completed down to the paintwork and the wooden balustrades, the huge colonnaded square was large enough for a cohort to stand to attention, a podium for the officers rising in one corner, close by a bronze statue of the Princeps Octavian. The doorways of countless offices led off the main forum beneath the portico, perhaps one in five glowing with the light of torches or lamps. The starlight was enough in the beautifully clear sky to make out most detail regardless.

Ahead, another ornate doorway led into the main basilica where the principal offices of the legion's commanders would be, along with the shrine of the standards and the various pay offices and senior clerks' rooms. The legionaries escorting them, however, veered off to the right and marched them to a doorway indistinguishable from the others.

As they reached the colonnade, the escort came to a halt and the optio strode past them to the entrance, leaning around the door jamb.

"Prisoners from the Twenty Second as ordered, sir."

A voice from within asked that they be sent in and the optio looked at them and jerked his thumb at the door.

"Be quiet, obedient and respectful or I'll return you to the tank without using the ladder this time."

Cervianus and Ulyxes looked at one another nervously, and then strode in through the door, leaving the purple night and entering the golden light within. The office was surprisingly large and well appointed. As their eyes adjusted to the change in light, Cervianus took in the salient points: the desk, chair and cabinet that had clearly only just been installed, the smell of fresh paint, the hanging portraits of a middle-aged woman and a young boy, painted with great skill on wooden plaques, that hung on the walls.

And the occupants.

The prefect Gaius Petronius, governor of Aegypt and overall commander of the army, sat in the only chair, his fingers steepled on his chest as he regarded them. To either side of him stood a man in a tribune's uniform. Vitalis of the Twenty Second bore a look of barely concealed loathing, but his gaze still seemed friendly beside the glare they were receiving from the tribune in the red tunic and cloak, presumably the man in charge of the Twelfth.

"You would be Cervianus and Ulyxes of the Twenty Second, then?"

"Sir."

The prefect continued to look them up and down, his eyes sparkling.

"We have been discussing the situation. There appears to be some doubt over with which party the guilt for this incident lies. I have, however, commanded legions many times and am quite well aware that it is a rare fracas in which *some* guilt does not exist on both sides."

He leaned forward.

"Do you have anything to say on the matter?"

Cervianus opened his mouth, but Ulyxes, standing directly next to him, shifted his boot slightly and trod hard on his companion's foot. Cervianus took the hint, his eyes watering with the sudden pain, and his mouth closed again.

"Good." The prefect smiled. "At least you know when to sit quiet and take what's coming. I only hope you remain as stoic in the coming days."

The prefect glanced quickly at the men to either side.

"I am informed that the pair of you are the only men from your legion involved and that there were several more from the Twelfth that have melted away into the sand unnoticed. I expect they will surface at some point when their officers notice black eyes and split lips and they will be dealt with in their own time."

His face became serious.

"I am inclined to harsh punishment, I have to say. I have three legions in Aegyptus: two currently under strength and with poor recruits, and one new arrival that is, as yet, an unknown quantity. I have a province that is the most important in the republic outside Italia, an enemy force occupying the southern regions, threatening overtures from the peoples of Arabia in retaliation for Gallus' abortive campaign, and a mountain of civil administration problems to attend to, including the danger of low production yield due to poor irrigation systems. Given all of that, just how much do you two think you are improving the situation?"

Again the pair stood silent.

"I need the legions to become a more cohesive army, working together to rebuild what Gallus allowed to fall apart. What I do *not* need is argumentative soldiers trying to drive a wedge between their legions. Do you understand me?"

The two men nodded. For a moment, Cervianus felt panic rising. This was a clever man and he was absolutely correct in every way. He could quite reasonably and legally invoke flogging or extended imprisonment.

"However," the prefect said with a sigh that filled the two prisoners with relief and hope, "I am somewhat tied by the delicate balance I am forced to maintain between the legions. I cannot punish you two heavily without inflicting a similar punishment on those other guilty parties that are currently unknown. If I punish you, likely there would be reprisal attacks by your fellow legionaries in the Twenty Second. Circumstances drive me to unaccustomed leniency."

He stood.

"Legionary Cervianus. You are, I am given to understand, a duplicarius, receiving double pay for your medical duties? I am dropping you to standard pay grade for two months. I cannot imagine where you would spend your wages while you're on campaign in the south anyway, but along with this goes the loss of your excused-duty status. You will be expected to dig, build, toil and portage like the rest of the men. Be grateful that's as far as I go. If I hear your name again, I will have the whip at the ready."

Cervianus nodded hurriedly. It was considerably better than he'd expected.

"Legionary Ulyxes? I am given to believe that you have only recently been moved into this unit in an attempt to try and break your rebellious tendencies. As such I am at a loss as to how to effectively deal with you, short of simple dismissal or execution, neither of which helps me with my manpower issues. I would personally have had your pay stopped from now until the end of days, but Vitalis here tells me that your new centurion is a martinet and a very inventive man and so I have decided to leave your fate to him. You will report to centurion Draco each day two hours before the morning call is sounded and you will follow his instructions to the letter.

This will go on until your centurion decides that you have been punished sufficiently, should that ever happen."

Ulyxes stayed still and calm, but from his close proximity, Cervianus could hear his teeth grinding angrily.

"Very well. The records will be amended to show your punishments and status. Now get out of my sight."

Cervianus and his companion gave a sharp salute and then turned and marched out of the office into the great forum square.

"Just fabulous," Ulyxes grunted as soon as they were out of earshot of the room. "Draco's going to lead me around by the balls and make me dance on nails for months. *You*, you lucky bastard! Standard pay for two months! The hardship, eh?"

Cervianus shrugged. "Just be grateful. We could have been given a flogging. Imagine how much effort some of our century would put into swinging the lash. We got off lightly. And remember that those lot from the Twelfth will probably get worse when they're found."

Ulyxes shook his head angrily. "Don't be an idiot, Titus. They'll not reappear. Hades, they won't even look for them. Did you see their tribune's face? He'll probably find them and buy them a drink."

The capsarius sighed. "You've got to learn to control your temper. We're going on campaign in a few days and I'd rather we didn't do it covered in bruises and on quarter rations."

Ulyxes sighed. "Let's get back to the barracks. I have a jar of wine that I can hear calling me."

III

CORRUPTION

Nicopolis was in a state of organised chaos. The next morning would see the entire Twenty Second legion, along with sections of the Twelfth and a number of auxiliary units that were expected at the fortress by lunchtime, marching south against an enemy of unknown number and capability; an enemy who had displayed temerity and sheer nerve sufficient to invade the territory of Rome.

The noise was dreadful and reminded Cervianus of the great market of Ancyra on the Dies Mercurii which brought traders in every variety of goods, both living and inanimate, from the mountains around. The streets of the unfinished metropolis were packed with wagons transporting goods from the surrounding land and from Alexandria, piles of grain sacks, stacks of weapons under guard, penned oxen and horses and camels, legionaries trying desperately to get everything in order, engineers and artillery officers collecting ropes for the torsion weapons or packing dissembled siege engines into wagons, and every other manner of activity known to the military mind.

Among this seemingly chaotic world, which Cervianus knew from personal experience to be in truth carefully organised down to the last sack of grain, other people milled.

Traders from the nearby city attempted to ply their wares, some useful, some irrational and pointless, taking every advantage of the soldiers' burning desire to spend their money while they still could. The legionaries with more foresight were buying spare water flasks, blankets and extra grain. Those with less sense bought wine, rude or amusing knick-knacks or other frivolities.

Whores also plied their trade, taking advantage of the lack of walls and pickets around the huge, unfinished camp and city. Many soldiers would be spending much of their remaining wage on a little companionship prior to the campaign and Cervianus could find no reason to blame them for that; certainly less than for those who were busy getting drunk and would seriously regret their actions in the morning.

In the midst of this, those men of the Twelfth who were remaining behind in Nicopolis to continue the building work watched with barely concealed hatred.

Cervianus peered out of the window and almost banged his head on the lintel as the weather-beaten, wrinkled face of a speculative local merchant appeared from nowhere, gazing back in at him.

"Crap. Where did all these merchants *come* from? It's as though every dodgy trader east of Carthage has descended on Nicopolis."

Ulyxes, folding his newly purchased blankets, shrugged. "It's just like it always is, but here there's no walls around the camp to keep them out. Normally we'd have to go outside to find them."

The capsarius nodded as he closed the shutters on the inquisitive merchant.

"I've got my list ready, so I'm off. Anything you want me to requisition for you?"

The stocky legionary shook his head. "Got everything I need. Have fun with the bureaucracy."

"Ha."

Collecting his medical bag from the bare pallet and slinging it over his shoulder, Cervianus snatched his tablet from the ledge and snapped it shut, pocketing the stylus. "See you in an hour or two."

Ulyxes nodded, standing straight then suddenly jerking with a sharp indrawn breath.

"Your back again?"

"It's just a bit tender."

Pausing, Cervianus frowned. "When I get back I'm going to go over this with you. What Draco's doing to you is nearly killing you."

Ulyxes shrugged. "It's just a bit of extra hard work. The bastard could easily do worse. What I need is to buy one of those cute but dirty little girls out there and get her to walk up and down my back first."

Cervianus shook his head. "That's just plain dangerous. Try and keep your recuperation and your libido separate. They're not a good combination."

The stocky legionary grinned at him and Cervianus turned once more and strode from the room, out into the main chamber of the building. Two other legionaries from his contubernium glanced up as he entered and, realising who it was, ignored him and went back to their preparations. Passing them, he walked out through the door and into the bright, already searing Aegyptian morning.

The noise, heat and smell combined to hit him like a punch

in the face. Over everything, even the incense sellers' stalls, the overpowering aroma of camel dung pervaded the air.

Closing his mouth, he pulled his green linen scarf up over his nose and set off toward the fortress.

The work was already heavily underway around the site, legionaries sweating and swearing as they adzed stone, hauled ropes, planed timber and lifted blocks. Here and there an optio or a duplicarius engineer shouted orders or barked angrily, whacking men with their sticks or pushing the ever-present nefarious traders away from the work.

"Soldierrrrr."

Cervianus turned at the light, purring voice, sultry and sweet as honey.

A young woman of Arabian extraction threw her arms around his shoulders and fastened herself tight.

"Sorry. In a rush. Much to do," he said, his voice cracking slightly.

The young lady smiled and moved slightly, her gauzy shift leaving little to the imagination. "We can be fast if you prefer?"

Cervianus swallowed nervously. "I *really* don't have the time right now." Something in the back of his mind kicked him and called him a coward.

"Perhaps later?" she purred.

Before he realised he was doing it, Cervianus found himself fumbling in his purse. Biting his tongue, he withdrew several copper coins. Smiling, he dropped one into her hand and held up the others.

"Call it a deposit. Find me at nightfall by the triumphal arch and I'll make it a lucrative night for you."

The girl smiled and her hand dipped beneath his tunic and

brushed his inner thigh with a light touch. He made a strange, squeaking noise.

"I shall be there, my master," she sighed happily and blew him a kiss as she moved on in search of more ready business.

Cervianus shuddered and squeezed his eyes shut. It would be nice, after all...

Shaking his head, he drew a deep breath, trying not to think of her shapely breasts.

Angrily, he snapped open the wax tablet and ran down his list as he stalked purposefully toward the fortress. Concentrating on the goods he needed, he mentally compiled a catalogue of quantities and a list of the compounds and lotions he would have to brew up this afternoon and tonight in preparation for the off.

So wrapped up was he in his thoughts that he almost walked into the tall man before he realised he was there. Startled, he dropped his tablet and stooped to collect it. Straightening again, he realised that the man was regarding him with a strangely penetrating gaze. Clearly a merchant of some variety, he was taller than Cervianus, which alone was a surprise. His beard was long and dark and his hair was wrapped up in some bound covering of beige linen. His robe, an ankle-length blue affair, decorated with gold-coloured embroidery, was dusty and worn.

He smiled, revealing a number of missing teeth.

"You need charm."

It was said with such matter-of-fact certainty that Cervianus was at once both taken aback and offended before he realised the man was offering religious odds and ends rather than merely personal abuse. He shook his head irritably, brushing the dust from his wax tablet.

"I don't want a charm, thank you."

The man's piercing gaze narrowed and he collected an item from his cart without even looking at it, his eyes remaining locked on Cervianus'. "I not ask you *want* charm. I say you *need* charm. *This* charm."

The capsarius focused on the object dangling on a leather thong from the man's hand. "What is that?"

"Crocodile tooth, from sacred crocodiles in temple at Ambo. Worth many more coin than you have."

Cervianus shook his head again. "I don't need a crocodile's tooth. Excuse me, but I have *real* things to attend to without this mumbo-jumbo."

He stepped around the man, but the merchant grasped his shoulder.

"I would advise you to let go. I am not a man who is patient with charlatans."

The merchant smiled again and released his grip. "Any coin. Give any coin; I give you charm."

Cervianus frowned and stepped back. "*Any* coin?" He was well aware that, while such trinkets were entirely frivolous and held about as much divine power as a shitty sponge, the minimum going price for them was quite high and was kept so by the superstitious legionaries.

"Any coin. Here."

The man dropped the charm on its thong into Cervianus' palm. The capsarius shrugged. At the very least he could resell it and make a considerable profit. Or perhaps give it to Ulyxes, who was more superstitious and really could very much do with a little extra watching over. Fumbling in his purse once more, he drew out two copper coins and dropped them into the man's hand.

Turning, he pocketed the charm and wandered on toward the fortress, trying not to acknowledge that the man was still staring at him, that strangely piercing gaze boring into the back of his head as he walked away.

The fortress was as busy as the rest of Nicopolis, if not more so, and Cervianus found he had to fight his way through the crowds in the main gateway. The Via Principalis thronged with men working on the construction or gathering goods for the campaign, guarding stock piles or loading carts.

Ducking and weaving his way among them, he made once again for the great headquarters building, if anything even more impressive now with the bright sun lighting the dazzling white and brilliant red walls and the terracotta tiles.

Following the same route the legionaries had taken after the earlier fracas and their sojourn in the cistern, and the directions received this morning from his optio, Cervianus entered the inner courtyard with only a passing nod of approval from the men of the Twelfth standing guard outside. Counting in his head, he identified the seventh door from the end on the left side of the colonnade and made for it.

The courtyard was packed with people and animals, the noise and the smell as unbearable as anywhere else in Nicopolis today, and the particular office he was making for seemed to be one of the busiest.

Gaius Calidius, the quartermaster of the Twenty Second Deiotariana, had been given an office and various stores in the fortress immediately following their arrival and, looking at the queues, that office was immediately next door to his counterpart from the Twelfth Fulminata. The lines of legionaries waiting impatiently outside were perfectly colour coded for the visitor, a fact that appealed to the logical mind of the capsarius and made him chuckle as he crossed the square and fell in at the rear of the queue of green-clad soldiers, who were sharing glares of mutual distrust with the russet-clad legionaries of the Twelfth in the next line.

The following hour was among the most tedious that the medic had ever encountered. The sun beat mercilessly down on the queue of men, only the front three of whom stood in the shade of the portico. It seemed to take an age for the queue to shift forward a single step, all the time standing under the baleful gaze of the men from the Twelfth. Once more, Cervianus found himself resorting to mental games to keep his mind sharp, re-working his list mentally, first alphabetically and then in reverse, and then ordering the list by number of syllables and so on.

The sun was already high in the sky, marching toward midday, when finally he moved into the blessed shelter of the colonnade and made the last few shuffling steps forward until he stood outside the closed door of the quartermaster's office.

At last, the door opened and a legionary exited, clutching a chitty for the supply depot tightly in his hand. He strode past Cervianus and off into the square as a voice called from within.

"Next."

Taking a grateful breath, the capsarius strode into the room blinking as his eyes, accustomed to the brightness of the courtyard, slowly adjusted to the gloom of the office. Two open windows to the rear provided a through-draught that kept the temperature in the room bearable.

Calidius sat in a comfortable chair at the opposite side of the office, behind a long counter that bisected the room, stacked with tablets, chitties and piles of small bags. Behind that counter and the quartermaster himself, shelves filled the rear wall, containing the more immediately accessible goods that might be required. A door at the very rear led off into the back of the building where a corridor ran along the outside wall of the range, connecting all the offices.

Calidius was a man in his mid-forties, portly for a soldier and with a florid complexion, constantly mopping his face in the heat. Having abandoned his armour and the marks of his rank, he wore only his tunic and a leather smock.

Cervianus had only met the man twice, and neither time had he been particularly forthcoming. When the army of Galatia had been reorganised and reformed as the Twenty Second Roman legion, a number of the more senior Galatian officers had found themselves demoted or simply surplus to requirements, while their duties were taken over by veterans from Rome, supposedly tying the new legion to its government. Calidius was a newer addition still, having joined the Twenty Second only as they waited to take ship at Tarsus. He was from northern Italia, high in the mountains, and his metabolism was suited to high altitudes and frequently chilly climates. He had not flourished in the temperatures of the eastern reaches of Rome's republic, and was positively wilting in Aegyptus.

"Name?"

"Titus Cervianus, capsarius of the First cohort, Second century."

"Cervianus," the man repeated quietly, flicking through his lists. "Cervianus? Oh yes. Here you are. What are you here for?"

"I've a list of components from my medical kit that are exhausted or in need of resupply. There shouldn't be anything extraordinary there, I think."

Calidius frowned.

"You don't have privileges beyond that of an ordinary soldier. I can replace blankets, pots, tools and so on, but only with evidence of damage to the original article. Need a blanket?"

Cervianus blinked. "I'm a capsarius. I need medical supplies."

"Says here you're an ordinary soldier. I see you've lost duplicarius status recently and had your special privileges revoked."

The medic stared at the officer behind the desk in disbelief. "Alright, I've had a two-month status and pay reduction, but I'm *still* a capsarius. I *still* need to treat the wounded. I'm fairly sure when the prefect changed my status he didn't intend to prevent me from doing my job!"

Calidius frowned again. "I really should have a written authorisation from your centurion or optio if you don't have the authority yourself. Perhaps you can arrange…"

Cervianus strode forward and placed his hands on the table, palms down.

"Look, sir, I really don't want to cause trouble. I just want standard medical supplies. If I have to go find my centurion and get written confirmation, then stand in this queue again all day there won't be time left to actually get the supplies. Can we find a way around this? Perhaps I can get my centurion to confirm with you later?"

Calidius frowned for a while, staring down at his ledgers.

"Well it's most unusual. I can't say I'm very happy about it, but we'll have to go with that, since I'm not going to be the man who gets in the way of supplying the campaign. You really should have come along a lot earlier if you were going to be a difficult case."

Cervianus blinked in disbelief again, but remained quiet as the man thrust out a hand.

"Give me your list."

Silently, the capsarius handed his wax tablet over and the quartermaster snapped the wooden casing open and ran his gaze down the scrawl within.

"What is it with you medici? Your writing always looks like someone got drunk and threw a bag of nails at the wax."

Cervianus sighed. "Perhaps I can help?"

"What's this say?"

"That one is 'mosulum'."

"It says 'musglub'."

Cervianus sighed again. "Definitely mosulum."

The man's finger ran down the tablet again. "And this?"

"Amaracinum. It's used in post-surgical poultices to help prevent flesh rot," he added helpfully.

"Charming. I have actually heard of these things though. I've been supplying them to supercilious know-it-all medici for over a decade. I know what the damn things are, I just can't read your writing. What's this?"

"Metopium ointment. I could make it from the raw ingredients, but it saves so much time to get it ready-mixed."

The quartermaster leaned forward and reached the bottom of the tablet with his probing finger. Finally, he slapped the wooden case down on the desk, took out a stylus and put a mark in the wax against some of the more common and simple ingredients.

"I'll save you some time, soldier. I can give you about a third of the items on this list. The ones I've marked you can collect from stores in about an hour."

Cervianus stared at him again.

"But these are required for the health and efficiency of the army. You should be able to supply *all* of these!"

Calidius shrugged.

"Some of those are just too expensive and would overrun my budget, which has been set by the new prefect and authorised by the tribune. Some are simply too hard to get hold of. Where, for instance, am I supposed to find metopium ointment here?"

Cervianus' eyes narrowed, aware now with absolute certainty that he was being cheated. "Where can you find it? Reach out of a bloody window! The Aegyptians invented the stuff. It's made in every village and available on most markets."

"Perhaps," Calidius snapped, glaring at this insolent newcomer. "But not on markets authorised for supply of the army."

"So what am I supposed to do for supplies? The army needs medical support on campaign."

The quartermaster leaned forward and Cervianus noted the greedy twinkle in the man's eye. "Perhaps you could supplement my budget? Supply the excess funds to purchase the non-standard supplies?" His palm twitched meaningfully.

"A bribe, you mean," Cervianus said flatly. "You can get everything on that list. I've seen medici and capsarii from the Twelfth with them," he lied smoothly. "If *they* can have them it's simple obstruction that I cannot."

Calidius ignored him and marked out a chitty, stamping it with his seal. "Here's the list of what you can have. Go to the stores and draw them."

"I—"

"That's the end of the matter," the quartermaster stated. "If you persist in arguing with a superior officer, I may be tempted to call in the guards and report you to the tribune.

Given your recent demotion, I wonder how he would look on you then?"

Cervianus glared at him, his teeth grinding in irritation. There was quite simply no way to win. If he continued to badger the man, he would end up on report and the tribune would have no option but to order a flogging.

"Thank you, sir. I will try not to let too many men die through the shortfall."

He saluted and turned to walk out. As he reached the door, unlatching and swinging it inwards, he started to step through the threshold, but stopped partway, as the door in the back of the office opened simultaneously.

A man in a centurion's uniform, wearing the red of the Twelfth legion, leaned into the room close to the quartermaster and the two exchanged quick, quiet words and a small pouch that jingled expensively. Realising he was in increasing danger, Cervianus filed the dubious exchange away in the back of his mind and strode out into the sunshine.

Something was going on here, and it was causing him trouble.

Titus Cervianus, demoted capsarius and irritated legionary of the Twenty Second Deiotariana, kicked at the gritty ground angrily as he strode back along the street toward the building that served as their temporary quarters for one more night, cursing as he stubbed his toe on a particularly stubborn stone.

The sun was already approaching the horizon, its glow having descended from brilliant white through bright yellow to warm gold and now deep orange. Before it touched the land it would become blood red, an ill omen for any campaign if one was to listen to any of the superstitious rubbish the bulk of the army babbled about.

It had been after lunch when Cervianus had stormed angrily out of the headquarters building and made his slow, irritable way to the huge temporary store house that would eventually be a warehouse when Nicopolis' port was more than just a dream of architects.

The queue at the stores had proved to be every bit as long and slow-moving as that at the quartermaster's. Two hours spent standing in the queue to receive little more than a quarter of the goods he needed had pushed the medic's mood ever deeper into impotent anger. The discovery, once he had left the building and strode away across the sandy ground, that even the goods he *had* received were of the lowest possible quality, old and dry and badly stored, had done nothing to improve matters.

An enterprising local had set up a large tent and stall, selling alcohol and some dubious herbal concoctions that Cervianus would heartily recommend against, and with his mood still stomping around in the gutter, he took advantage of the stall and purchased some thick, cloying, and surprisingly strong, date wine. He had tarried in the tent for four cups of the potent beverage, allowing his ire to gradually fade a little, though it remained simmering in the background.

And finally, as the sun began to sink, he had made his way back toward the barrack house. As he approached the low, mud-brick building, he noted the shape of Ulyxes sitting beside the door on a rock, running a whetstone up and down the blade of his gladius with rhythmic strokes.

"You would not believe the bloody day I have had."

The legionary stopped his sharpening and looked up in surprise. "Where in Hades have you been?"

"Visiting the most corrupt bastard quartermaster this side of the senate house in Rome. Apparently, if I want to be able to actually save lives and heal wounds, I'm going to have to treat the man to a healthy injection of sesterces!"

Ulyxes carefully placed his sword to one side. "Forget about quartermaster troubles. Draco's been on the warpath looking for you."

"Oh shit. What's up now?"

"No idea. He just left a message that if you ever show up, you're to go to his quarters immediately with your kit."

Cervianus' heart jumped. Just what he needed right now: an angry centurion. "I'd best get going, then."

As Ulyxes nodded, the capsarius turned and jogged back along the path toward the house at the end of the street that currently sheltered the centurion and optio of his century. He had barely reached the doorway when Draco's voice bellowed out from somewhere in the depths of the building.

"If that's Cervianus, tell him to get his arse in here, sharp!"

The capsarius ducked nervously inside, just as the optio was striding across the room to the doorway.

"I trust you heard that?"

Cervianus saluted and ran through into the back room to find Draco in just his tunic, tucking into a plate of meats and cheeses. The man stopped, a chunk of bread halfway to his grizzled face.

"About bloody time you showed up. Where have you been?"

The capsarius swallowed nervously, standing to attention and saluting. "I've been struggling with the quartermaster and the stores, sir. I need to discuss the issue with you if you have time, sir?"

Draco raised an eyebrow. "From the smell, I'd say you've been *struggling* with a few cups of the local brew. No time to take issue now, though. Get your skinny arse up to the fortress and report to the guard on the gate. They'll take you to the tribune."

Once again, Cervianus' heart skipped a beat. The tribune? Had quartermaster Calidius actually reported him to the staff? What was going on?

"Sir?"

Draco slowly lowered the bread to the plate and glared at him.

"I notice you're still here. Any reason for that, before I have you beaten?"

Hurriedly, Cervianus threw a last salute and, turning, ran from the room. He managed a second salute, while running, to the optio in the outer room and was then gone outside into the street beneath the fading, rust-coloured sky.

As he ran toward the fortress, which stood a quarter of a mile distant on the raised patch of land, his mind raced. If Calidius *had* tried to drop him in it, he had to have all his arguments marshalled ready to defend himself, but he could see no real reason why the man would do so. What advantage would he gain? No. More likely it was some new angle on the brawl he had been involved in. Perhaps new evidence had come to light? The perpetrators from the Twelfth had reappeared? Who knew? But even if that were the case, would it be a good or a bad sign?

It was with a passing, brief regret that he ran past the edge of the town and spotted the great triumphal arch of Octavian out of the corner of his eye, realising that a charming and very experienced young lady would be leaning against its marble pylon at that very moment, waiting to do extraordinary things to him.

Cursing, he ran on.

The two legionaries in their green tunics who stood by the gate of the fortress angled their pila so that the heavy iron points barred his way.

"What's your business here?"

The capsarius shrugged. "I'm not really sure. I'm Titus Cervianus. I was told to report here?"

"Ah, you're the medicus?"

"Capsarius, yes," he replied.

"Come with me."

As the other guard returned to his attentive position, the speaker propped his pilum against the wall and strode in through the gate. Cervianus followed at his heel, nervously.

"Can I ask why I was sent for?" he enquired of the legionary, quietly. At least this man was from another cohort and didn't know him enough to dislike him on principle.

"Don't know, mate. There's a bit of a do going on in the tribune's house, though. There's a lot of big nobs there, including the prefect, so be on your best behaviour."

Cervianus' eyes widened in the failing light as he was marched swiftly to the only complete tribune's house in the fortress. In future years, of course, tribune Vitalis would make his home in the praetorium, a grand villa purpose-built for the legion's commander, while his juniors would take these buildings, each a large, well-appointed townhouse in its own right.

Two more men stood on guard at the house's main door onto the Via Principalis.

"Capsarius to see the tribune," his escort announced.

One of the men nodded and opened the door. "Follow me."

Leaving the others outside, Cervianus nervously stepped inside with this new escort. The floor of the house had been completed very recently in black and white marble, a pattern intricate and beautiful. The walls had been freshly painted, though most were still plain white, awaiting final decoration. Ahead, a small atrium contained a square pool with a fountain. There was no water at this time and, imagining the quantity of rainfall the area must get, it seemed unlikely there would ever be more than that supplied by pipe.

Voices echoed through the fresh hallway from ahead and left. The legionary led him across the atrium, where the last rays of the sun cast a feeble beam in through the open roof above the pool, lighting only the capitals of a few columns on the eastern side of the room with a crimson glow.

The conversation was coming from a beautifully appointed triclinium, where men in togas and women in beautiful, brightly coloured stola and expensive jewellery, their hair in intricate waves and delicate curls, lounged languidly on couches, servants and slaves attending to their needs.

At the rear, two slaves in white tunics played tibia and lyre, issuing delicate and sweet melodies that contrasted jarringly with the chatter of the women, some of whom had high, irritatingly scratchy voices.

As Cervianus and his escort arrived at the entrance to the charming room, the legionary cleared his throat.

"The capsarius Cervianus of the Twenty Second, sir."

Tribune Vitalis looked up from one of the couches and beckoned. "Ah, good."

As he walked nervously over toward the commander of the legion, Cervianus took in everything he could about the occupants of the room. Vitalis he knew, and the woman lounging on the next couch with the green stola and the long hair dropping in curls by her ears, picking at something roasted on a wooden stick, was likely his wife.

Though currently out of uniform, he recognised the face of the senior tribune in command of the Twelfth legion, lounging with his wife on couches at the far side of the room, and the Prefect of Aegyptus was immediately recognisable at the end, his own spouse close by. Other occupants, male and female, he did not know, but were clearly either important civil dignitaries or other tribunes.

He was interested to note the simmering anger that was evident on the face of the Twelfth's tribune as the man watched his counterpart across the room. Clearly the animosity between the two legions had reached even the highest ranks. More interesting yet was the new but slowly blooming black eye the man was sporting, though he had positioned himself so that that side was in the shade and partially hidden.

The prefect's penetrating and intuitive gaze roved back and forth between the two senior officers, radiating disapproval.

The women seemed oblivious to the undercurrent of seething resentment that lingered in the room, laughing and chatting, squawking even, though the other men seemed to be well aware and were staying prudently quiet.

"Oh my dear, this place is simply ghastly. I have not been able to do a thing with my hair since our arrival. How ever do you cope?" The tribune's wife snapped her fingers and a slave brought across a plate of grapes and citrus fruit.

The prefect's lady gave a carefree laugh. "I've had similar

problems, Cornelia, though fortunately I had the foresight to bring some wonderful wigs with me."

"Wigs are definitely the answer."

"The climate is very good for the skin, though," another woman chimed in. "I follow the regime of three baths a day and I try to take a dip in milk every three or four days. They say Cleopatra did it, you see."

"But remember what happened to her. She slipped and fell on her asp!"

There was a chorus of laughter from the women, sounding like nothing more than a flock of crows. Cervianus tried not to instantly dismiss the women as a vapid waste of space as he reached the tribune on his couch. He failed.

"Sir. Can I be of assistance?"

Vitalis gave him a grizzly look and nodded, proffering a hand. Cervianus peered at the appendage and noted with interest the two fingers, index and middle, that had already swelled and were beginning to turn purple and discoloured.

"I fell and stopped myself with my hand," the tribune said flatly, his eyes searching out any question or mirth in the medic. They found only professional interest, and the officer relaxed a little.

Cervianus gently turned the hand, causing a sharp intake of breath. "It hurts when I do this?"

A slight twist and another hiss.

"And this?"

The tribune grunted.

"I'm afraid that as well as two broken fingers, you have sprained your wrist, sir," he said quietly, trying not to think too hard about that blossoming black eye across the room.

"I thought that might be the case. I am relying entirely on your discretion here, legionary Cervianus. I have had cause to discipline you recently and yet, despite that, I am informed that you are the best practitioner of medicine in my legion. My medicus is an effete snob with a single-minded approach to healing and a love of folkish medicine. He would likely hang a dead mouse from my nose and bleed me, and I would rather avoid all of that. I want you to tend to the hand and wrist and make no mention of these circumstances hereafter. Do you understand me?"

Cervianus nodded professionally. "Yes, sir."

"Good. If I hear talk, I will know it was you and your two-month punishment may well become a permanent career change. Bear that in mind."

"Of course, sir."

While the tribune lay there, his arm draped over the end of the couch, Cervianus began to dig in his leather bag, drawing out several compounds and his binding kit.

"Without wishing to anger you, sir, just the tiniest bit of bleeding might not be a bad idea too; the medicus would have been correct there. I would say that of the four humours, your yellow bile is out of balance. A small emetic to aid with purging could even be an idea, too?"

From between gritted teeth, the tribune spoke with a low voice. "If I have to listen to much more of tribune Ventidius' bullshit, I'll need no help to vomit." He sighed. "Fine. Bleed me a little if you must, but get this done quick and with the minimum of stinking salves."

Cervianus tried not to smile as he carefully worked on the hand, applying the small amount of amaracinum paste that remained in the pot and then carefully binding first the fingers and then the hand, being certain to keep the wrist at the correct angle.

Finishing the bandaging, he sealed it with bee's glue and carefully ran his hands around it, smoothing the dressing flat.

Fishing around once again in his bag, he found a parcel wrapped in silk and tipped a small quantity of the powder contained within into a piece of linen, folding that into a package and then replacing the silk container. He reached across with the folded linen.

"This is a powdered mix of henbane, mandragora and cinnamon, sir. It's a fairly mild mix, heavy on the cinnamon. If you find the ache becomes too much, add just the tiniest pinch to your drink and swill it to mix. Do not use too much, though, as even the mild mix can be quite potent."

The tribune narrowed his eyes at the packet as he took it. "I've had this before from the medicus, but he gave me it as a solution in a small bottle rather than a powder. Is it not easier to keep track of appropriate dosage in that way?"

Cervianus nodded. "Yes, sir. It's more common to dose in oil, but that requires several extra ingredients and, unfortunately, I don't have them to hand at the moment."

The tribune turned and frowned at him. "But you're on campaign in the morning! I hope you are not intending to travel lacking essential supplies?"

Cervianus swallowed, aware of the danger of his situation. To deliberately accuse the quartermaster, a man of centurion rank, in front of the tribune would likely cause a tremendous backlash. However any trouble between the two officers might turn out, the chances were that Cervianus would suffer either way.

"I will endeavour to have my supplies full by the morning, sir," he said, finally, keeping his face deliberately straight. Tribune Vitalis narrowed his eyes, as though reading the thoughts straight from his mind.

"See that you do."

Cervianus nodded as he tied the leather cord around the tribune's upper arm and unfastened his surgical cylinder, selecting the bleeding knife.

"Are you ready, sir?"

The tribune placed his cup down on the table before him, nodded, and clenched his teeth as Cervianus gave him a short, neat nick and placed his collecting tin beneath as the crimson flow trickled down the arm and fell into the dish with a metallic ring.

"I think," the tribune said loudly to the assembled officers, "that we should make sure the stores are all correct before we leave in the morning. I shall be gone for some time with the Twenty Second and I would like to be sure we have not left too few supplies in stock for our sister legion."

He locked gazes with the tribune of the Twelfth.

"Perhaps we should order a pre-march check on them before dawn tomorrow?"

Tribune Ventidius sneered.

"If you feel it necessary, Vitalis. I find I can trust my men to keep things in order."

Cervianus moved the tin around under the trickle of blood as Vitalis' arm twitched in irritation at his opposite number.

The prefect leaned forward. "I find this intolerant attitude between the pair of you both tiresome and puerile. If you have any fears for the state of the stores, arrange your inspection, but then forget the subject for now. We have beautiful music, beautiful ladies, good company and excellent wine. It would be a shame for you to mar this last chance for a social engagement in months with childish argument."

Vitalis nodded slowly, though his face showed that he was less than ready to let the feud fade. Turning to Cervianus, he fixed him with a gaze that carried some unspoken suggestion.

"I think that's enough blood, don't you? Bind the arm and get going. You need to have your kit full somehow and be ready for the morning."

Cervianus nodded hurriedly, reaching for his bag. Quickly, he found his oil of ephedron and scattered a few drops on the cut, watching for a moment until the coagulant took effect, and then wadding it with lint and vinegar and quickly sealing and binding the arm.

"Good," the tribune said. "Now go and put things in order. I shall expect to see you on the parade ground with the rest at dawn, fully prepared. We have a long journey in the morning."

Cervianus stepped back, dropping his equipment into his bag, and saluted.

"Yes, sir."

"Run along, then."

Cervianus turned and hurried from the room, trotting back through the atrium and to the front door of the house. The two legionaries on guard there grinned.

"Been sworn to silence?"

"Sort of."

"You should have seen it. Like a proper soldier's punch up, it was. We had to drag 'em apart on the prefect's orders. Vitalis would have *had* him, though. He was proper leathering him. Would have punched his face inside out if we hadn't been quick. Makes you proud to be in the Twenty Second, I'd say."

"If you say so," Cervianus sighed.

The two men stared at him and shook their heads as Cervianus strode off toward the fortress gate. While he hardly approved of two grown men beating each other to near death whether they be Ulyxes and the giant or the two tribunes, he had to admit one thing: the nature of the wounds suggested that Vitalis had inflicted the harm rather than receiving it. He frowned. Also, the tribune seemed to have understood what he *hadn't* said about the supplies. His manner; the strange, shared look; the announcement of a supply inspection. It was all part of Vitalis telling him something.

He was close to the fortress gate, the two guards stepping aside from him, when he decided on his course of action; a course that made him smile broadly. For a moment, as he passed the guards, he dithered. The plan was not without its dangers and rewards, but there was still the chance of meeting the girl by the arch. Perhaps she had waited? He had promised her much, after all.

He sighed and shook his head. Ah well. It was dark now and the girl would likely be gone, seeking more reliable clientele. He had other matters to attend to now. Turning to the guards, he grinned.

"Nice night for a jaunt."

The two men looked at each other and shrugged as Cervianus walked off with an unusual spring in his step.

Ulyxes grabbed Cervianus' tunic and the two came to a halt.

"Are you really sure you want to do this? Bear in mind how much trouble we're already in."

The capsarius nodded. "I need those supplies."

"But there's better ways. If the tribune knows you've been stitched up by the quartermaster, go through channels and drop him in the shit. Better that way than we get caught and beaten to death for theft."

"No. There's not enough time. I need the supplies and the quartermaster wouldn't give me them. Anyway, he'll be safely tucked up in his bunk with some woman from the streets now and the storehouse has been closed for hours." He grinned. "But I *am* going to leave him in the shit anyway. I'm sure the tribune was hinting at something like this."

Cervianus shook his head, adamantly.

"*How* sure?"

"Shut up and come on."

The pair ducked low and ran on, past the low shell of a granary that had grown little higher than the raised floor and a foot of wall, nipping between a water tank and lid that were awaiting placement and a rectangular structure of unknown designation. Ahead, their target stood bulky and looming against the indigo sky.

The pair dropped down behind a pile of uncut stones and peered nervously over the top, the bright moonlight giving them such a clear view it might as well be midday. Two men stood guard by the huge warehouse doors, which remained shut and locked. The colour of their tunics was not clear from here, but they would be green; the Twelfth had left all guard duty to the new legion.

"You'll be dropping the guards in the crap too, and they're our own."

Cervianus shook his head. "All the blame will fall on Calidius, and possibly, hopefully, his counterpart in the Twelfth too. I'm pretty sure he's just as corrupt and dirty as our own."

The warehouse was a new and solid construction, but was far from secure, given that it would eventually be only part of a large complex of similar buildings all within their own walled enclosure. Shuttered windows around six feet up dotted the walls, offering a difficult, though possible, point of access.

"Come on."

Ducking down, Cervianus sidled along the wall of the unfinished building until he reached the end and judged that he would be out of sight of the two men guarding the main door. It was not, after all, the front entrance that they were after.

Peering out from his hiding place, as Ulyxes arrived behind him, he carefully scanned the surrounding area for any movement or sign of life. It was almost like a different place to that which he had traversed earlier in the day, fighting off merchants and prostitutes and having to push his way through crowds of people. The streets would still be thronged with drunken soldiers and those opportunistic locals back near the barrack areas, but out here toward the shore, where only half-constructed warehouses and piles of stone punctured the barren ground there was nothing to attract either soldier or civilian.

No sign of movement.

Taking a deep breath, Cervianus rose and loped across the dusty ground silently, coming to a halt next to the wall of the huge warehouse, beneath one of the windows.

Ulyxes jogged across the ground behind him and fell into position by the wall, pointing to their left.

"If it's medical supplies you're after, you want to be another two or three windows down for ease. I had a good look around the place earlier while I was bored and waiting for my new dolabra."

The capsarius smiled in the darkness. His friend's phenomenal memory would come in very useful, he decided. Shuffling along three windows, he stopped again and raised his eyebrows. Ulyxes nodded.

With the advantage of height, Cervianus raised himself on his toes and peered between the shutters. The interior was pitch black, which meant that some illumination was necessary after all, but would also mean they were unlikely to be interrupted. Clearly the stores, once locked up, remained closed away until the morning.

Turning, he nodded at Ulyxes and, drawing his dagger, readied himself. The stocky legionary appeared in front of him and crouched, cradling his hands. Gritting his teeth, Cervianus stepped on them and his companion pushed him up to the height of the window, grunting quietly with the effort.

Around the corner, perhaps twenty paces away, the two legionaries muttered in low conversation, keeping their spirits up through the stupefyingly dull night-time vigil. They would do a quick circuit of the building every few hundred heartbeats, but there should be plenty of time to effect entry between sweeps. On this, the eve of the campaign, soldiers were inevitably getting drunk, whoring or praying and managing a few extra precious hours of shut-eye. No trouble like this would be expected.

As his bulky, strong friend held him aloft, Cervianus inserted the point of his dagger into the gap between the shutters and raised it slowly until it hit the catch. With infinite care, he pushed it gently further, raising the iron hook until there was a gentle "clunk" and the barrier gave way. Slowly and as quietly as humanly possible, the capsarius eased the shutters outwards, grateful that the building was a brand new construction in a dry land and there had been no chance for noisy rust to set in.

The iron grille that formed the main window inside the shutter was also affixed with a single latch in much the same fashion but now that the shutters were open and visibility was aided by moonlight, it was much easier to prise the grille catch open.

As the iron point of the pugio unhooked the latch and he drew back the blade, it caught the grille and made a short, sharp scraping sound. Both men held their breath, aware that, should they have been heard, there was not enough time to get away before the guards rounded the corner and saw them.

Fortunately, whatever discussion the two soldiers were involved in was animated enough to keep their attention focused there and they failed to appear, running and angry, around the warehouse's corner.

Cervianus heaved a sigh of relief and fumbled in his pocket, producing a small square of felt and busying himself, brushing the iron scrapings from the sill into the material and folding it.

Grunting under his weight, Ulyxes whispered urgently. "What are you *doing*?"

"Collecting the iron. It's good for wounds. Saves me scraping a spear tip later."

"Will you hurry up and open the bloody window?"

Filing away the packet of iron flakes, Cervianus examined his pugio. There was an unsightly nick halfway down the blade. If the centurion found that, he would likely make Cervianus pay for a new one. The nick would be a big job to polish out, too.

Grumbling, he swung the iron grille inwards and within moments he was scrambling through the portal and clambering as quietly as he could down onto the wooden racking within.

As soon as he found a secure foothold, he reached down and grasped Ulyxes' hand, hauling him up and through the window. Pausing only to shut the wooden boards and remove all outward evidence of their entry, the pair dropped down into the interior.

"Remind me again why I actually agreed to this?" Ulyxes whispered.

"Because you know we might need these things on campaign, because you and trouble are the closest of friends, and because I couldn't manage it on my own."

He could sense the brow furrowed in irritation, even in the darkness.

"There are labels on all the shelves and, knowing Roman quartermasters, everything will be organised with thorough and perfect logic. I've got a list."

In the oppressive gloom there was a lot of sudden shuffling and activity and finally, with a few flicks and clicks, Cervianus managed to light a small oil lamp with his flint and steel. Handing the terracotta lamp to Ulyxes, he drew his wax tablet from his tunic and examined it.

Since the episode with the quartermaster earlier, he had rewritten the list, omitting the few items that he had received that were actually of usable quality.

"This way."

With Ulyxes following close behind and holding the oil lamp up to cast a glow on the racks ahead, the pair crossed the warehouse, passing shelf after shelf of scarves, cloaks and tunics, mostly russet and red, with small piles of green here and there. Leather shield covers for three shapes and sizes of shield stretched away on a whole rack into the darkness.

"A man could get rich with a night's pickings from in here."

Cervianus pursed his lips and frowned at his companion. "We're not here for petty theft. I'm after medical equipment only, not something to sell for a private income."

Ulyxes shrugged. "Just a thought."

Cervianus locked his eyes on the shelves ahead, trying to tell himself that he hadn't just seen Ulyxes grab two tunics and stuff them down the neck of his own.

"Here we go. This is the medical supplies. The quartermaster clearly has no idea about how to keep these things. Some that should be kept well apart are stored close together, and some of them should be stored in a moist environment. Half this crap will be of little use anyway."

Ulyxes growled and raised the lamp.

"Can we stop complaining and just get the damn stuff?"

Cervianus nodded and began running his finger down the list, which he placed open on a shelf, his arm repeatedly darting out and swiping an item from the store, or picking through a stack of jars looking for a specific oil.

Behind him, as he collected his small pile of loot, Ulyxes glared at him, his arm beginning to quiver with the effort of holding the lamp above head height.

"Hurry up."

"I have to be careful to get the right things. It'd be a shame to get the wrong jar and rub oil of nardus into your wound, rather than metopium, eh?"

"I haven't a bloody clue, since I've never heard of either of them. My arm aches."

As he continued to select items, the tall medic grinned. "Metopium you would *want* on your wound. Nardus in a drink would help stop you farting, though."

Ulyxes sniggered. "Should get some of that. We could feed it to Vibius. I wish he would move to a different room. He keeps me awake sometimes. Makes a noise like a cow snoring and makes the room smell like the inside of an old boot."

Cervianus couldn't help but grin as he worked. The flatulent nature of Vibius was a common theme in jokes in their century. About the only time Evandros ever let up from his bullying in close quarters was when the subject of Vibius' posterior arose in conversation.

"Nearly there. Must be jars of honey here somewhere."

"We're not here for a snack."

Cervianus smiled as he found the jars. "Honey has many uses my friend, other than to smear on bread."

Ulyxes changed hands with the lamp, wishing he could rub his aching elbow.

"That's it," the capsarius announced. "Full kit." Reaching to his side, he opened his leather medical bag and carefully filed away the supplies, closing the top and buckling the one good strap, tying the other tight. "Alright," he said quietly, "when the tribune pulls the inspection in the morning, the medical supplies will come up short and Calidius will be hauled over the coals."

Ulyxes frowned at him, grateful to be able finally to lower the lamp. "But Calidius will know it was you because of the medical supplies. He'll just blame you and then come down on you like a ton of bricks."

Cervianus shrugged. "I'll just have to trust that the tribune was expecting this. He'll certainly understand."

Ulyxes was grinning.

"What?" the medic asked suspiciously.

"The med supplies would pale into insignificance beside some of the stuff in here."

"I told you I'm not here for petty theft."

"Then we'd best make sure it's not 'petty'."

Cervianus frowned. "I saw you take those tunics."

"Tunics are only the beginning…"

There was a pause in the dark and the stocky legionary took a deep breath.

"In the rear right corner, ordered by type. Over there…"

"Helpful, since I can only barely see *you*, let alone where you're pointing," Cervianus whispered gratingly.

"The weapon stores."

"Are you mad?" Cervianus stared at his companion, whose eyes were full of conviction and mischief. "Is this the sort of thing that got you disciplined and moved down a cohort?"

"This and more."

"I'm surprised you've never been flogged."

Ulyxes merely fell silent.

"You *have* been flogged?"

"Twice. Both times I stayed silent until the optio ran out of breath swinging the damn thing. It'll never happen again, though. I'm sharper now and I have this clever mate, you see…"

Cervianus sighed and shook his head, but the idea was starting to insinuate itself into his thoughts. He would have to replace his pugio soon anyway after that incident with the window. And he could only imagine the quartermaster's face as he tried to explain away the absence of costly armaments in the warehouse. Better still…

"Alright, but if we're going to commit major, punishment-inducing theft, we have to leave no other trace we were here. That means replacing the medical supplies too."

Ulyxes frowned. "That defeats the whole object of coming here."

Cervianus grinned as he opened his bag again. "Not if I put my empty jars and packets in place of the ones I've just taken. Unless they actually open them, which they won't, a standard inspection will come up showing full medical supplies. Only a medicus would be able to tell."

The stocky man grinned. "You're a devious bastard, I'll grant you that. Alright, get going." Changing arms again, holding the guttering lamp high, he watched as Cervianus carefully restocked the supplies with empty packets and jars.

"That one went further to the left."

"Thanks."

A moment longer, with the added guidance of Ulyxes' phenomenal memory, and the medical section looked as though it had never been tampered with.

"Right. Let's go look at the weapons."

The two men crept across the huge warehouse, staying close in the dim circle of light. The way the lamp was guttering they wouldn't have long before it ran out.

"I take it we want the smallest and most valuable?"

"Yes. The pugios, I'd say." Ulyxes replied. "Maybe a gladius or two if we can carry them."

The racks and shelves toward the rear of the warehouse, where the important supplies were kept, were largely empty, given the sudden flurry of supply activity in the past two days preparing for the campaign. Many shelves were bare and the weapon racks barer than most. He could just make out the pila standing in their racks, iron points gesturing defiantly at the roof. Beyond them, small piles of weapons were ordered by type, though again, there were few examples remaining.

Ulyxes stopped and pulled a sack from his belt, shaking it

out so that it billowed, and then folding the edges and clutching them tight.

"You brought a *sack*?" Cervianus enquired, incredulous.

"Just on the off-chance, yes."

"You may very well be completely insane, did you know that?"

"Come on," Ulyxes hissed.

Cervianus moved over to the shelves.

"The ones for officers are on the next shelf along," his companion noted. "They'll be the ones you want."

Shifting along one shelf, the capsarius searched around with his hands in the shady recesses and, squinting with the bad light, his fingers brushed the tips of sheaths.

"Pugios," he whispered.

"Put them in, but slowly and quietly."

Feeling around, he realised that the ones to his right were in plain leather scabbards and smooth hilted, much like the one at his waist. The one under his left hand, however, clearly felt embossed; the tips of his fingers traced designs across the scabbard. This was a decorative dagger, like the ones the centurions and optios wore. Just one of these would be worth more than everything he had noted on his requisition list.

As quietly as he could, he gathered the five decorative weapons on the shelf, hesitating every time there was the faintest metallic noise from his handful. Turning, he took two steps and lowered the pile into the sack, placing them in the bottom as quietly as he could.

"What else?" Ulyxes asked quietly.

"I think that'll do. They're expensive ones; worth a ton of coins. Let's get out of here."

As Ulyxes gripped the top of the sack, the pair slipped

silently back across the room. Once again, Cervianus tried not to pay attention to his companion's acquisitive arm that continually lanced out to the shelves, grasping a pile of scarves, a small bag of salt, or other handy articles here and there, and dropping them into the sack as they moved. It took a while in the guttering light of the dying lamp to identify their entry point, with the grille standing open, and it was with a tremendous sense of relief that Cervianus swung his medical bag round onto his back and set his foot on the lowest shelf, reaching to pull himself up.

With a little quiet scrambling, the pair hauled themselves to the top of the wooden racking, lifting the sack of goods with difficulty. Cervianus couldn't imagine what his companion had secreted away in the container that could possibly weigh so much. Bricks, perhaps?

As he crouched on the shelf, Ulyxes moved past him, extinguishing the lamp and leaning close to the window shutters. The shorter legionary held up his hand and put his finger to his lips, visible in the scant light cast by the cracks between the wooden covers, and put his eye to the slit. Cervianus held his breath; he could just hear the murmured conversation as the two guards made their circuit of the stores.

The thieves crouched silently for a while, Ulyxes' hand raised in warning, and then it dropped.

"Ready?" he whispered.

Cervianus nodded in the faint light from the crack.

"Come on."

The short, stocky man pushed open the shutters, leaving the sack on the shelf beside him, and dropped lithely to the dusty ground with a quiet thump. Cervianus leaned forward and looked down to see him already holding out his arms. Gently, he lowered their prize into his friend's hands and then edged to the sill and dropped to the ground.

As Ulyxes sprinted quietly off toward the nearby structures, Cervianus turned and conscientiously closed the grille, manoeuvring the two sides slightly so that the catch dropped back into place. He then closed the shutters and made them fast before throwing a vigilant glance toward the guard post at the front of the building. The distant murmur of conversation confirmed that the two legionaries were back in their accustomed place by the door. Dropping to a crouch, the capsarius loped across the open ground and joined his friend among the shells of future buildings.

"What now?" Ulyxes asked quietly.

Cervianus reached across to the bag in his friend's grip, opened it and drew a decorative dagger out. In the brighter moonlight, it was clearly a fine piece of work, with a carved ivory handle and bronze sheath hammered out and worked into a scene of a stag hunt. The sheath alone was worth a fortune.

"Back to quarters and we pack all this stuff deep down in our travelling kit. None of this can see the light of day until we're at least a week from Nicopolis." He grinned. "At least we'll be long gone before Calidius can order a search of the barracks. The fat old bastard's in trouble tomorrow. He may have to take his own advice and supplement his budget from his savings to account for the shortfall."

Ulyxes took a deep breath. "That, Titus, was what I call *fun*!"

"You have a strange sense of entertainment. Come on."

The two of them dodged between the buildings and piles of stone and work goods, occasionally spotting a hopelessly drunk legionary lying in a pool of his own vomit in the lee of a wall, or the rhythmic movements of a soldier with his rented companion in a more private location than the busy barrack area.

"Some of these men are going to be in deep shit tomorrow," the capsarius noted. "Some might not even get to dawn muster."

"You'd be surprised," Ulyxes replied with a grin, and Cervianus had to agree. Faced with the possibility of a thrashing from their centurion, no amount of drink would prevent most men from rising with the first call and falling into place blearily in the square with the rest.

"This is it. Tomorrow morning, we march," Ulyxes said, scratching his chin as they neared the house.

"I'm actually looking forward to it," Cervianus replied, his mind filling with remembered images of great pyramids and colossal statues in the mystical land of the upper Nile. The ancient kingdom of pharaohs was about to unfold before him.

IV

DELTA

Cervianus choked in the cloud of dust and, quickly checking around to make sure the optio wasn't watching him, shuffled his furca, the pole over his shoulder from which all his kit hung, into the hand that also held his shield – a delicate balancing act. Taking advantage of the free hand in the few moments before he began to fumble the heavy burden, he pulled up his scarf and wiped his eyes before settling it over his nose and mouth again and passing the pole back to his right hand.

He hadn't realised how much sheer hard work his excused-duty status had saved him until he had lost it and was now required to carry his full kit on the march, along with the added weight of the medical bag.

The Twenty Second had mustered at the dawn call in that great square before the arch. Prefect Petronius had attended and given an appropriately rousing speech on the subjects of Roman honour, the glory of the legions and the duplicity of barbarians, at which the majority of the legion present had roared approval. Here and there a man who had spent the night drinking too heavily and lying in a ditch or testing his flexibility with an Alexandrian whore winced at the noise.

Calidius, the Twenty Second's quartermaster, stood close to

the senior centurions and tribunes and alongside the legion's eagle, standards and musicians. He wore an expression like thunder and regularly snapped his head round, his eyes red-rimmed through lack of sleep, casting his gaze suspiciously across the crowd. Cervianus could have sworn the man had actually still been shaking with rage.

What exactly had transpired between the tribune and the quartermaster was not public knowledge, but those men who had stupidly and unfortunately left it until the last moment to collect urgent provisions had found the storehouse still locked up after the wakeup call, while the world was still indigo-painted. Surrounded by the tribune's guard, there had been both light and shouting blaring angrily from within.

Two cohorts of the Twelfth legion had mustered alongside them in rusty-hued tunics on the square and the Twenty Second, resplendent in their green tunics and crests, their glorious shields as yet still enclosed in the leather covers that would protect them from the weather, stood impatiently while their sister legion were set on the march first. The thousand or so men of the Twelfth would lead the way, their familiarity with the land giving them a supposed advantage, the distance between the two legions reducing the likelihood of trouble.

The Twenty Second waited some time after the last of the Twelfth had left the square before their buccina sounded and the signifers and centurions gave the orders to march. The wagons and artillery of both legions would follow on behind.

And so the army had begun the epic journey into the heartland of Aegyptus, the Twenty Second marching wearily in a huge choking cloud of dust kicked up not only by their own legion, but by the two cohorts of the Twelfth less than a quarter of a mile ahead.

The sun had still been bright and comfortable during the first hour of the march but, gradually, as the great fiery orb rose ever higher, the heat increased until it felt as though the gods had shut the world in an oven. The mail shirt that each man wore quickly became too hot to touch and every few heartbeats seemed to add a pound of weight to the men's kit.

Nasica, the primus pilus of the legion, had informed his men of the journey's planned first leg as they watched the Twelfth depart the square. Five days would take the army across the great delta of the Nile and to the city of Memphis, where they would take one whole day to rest and resupply. Those five days would be spent marching from dawn until late morning, with a four-hour stop during the worst of the heat, and then back on their feet until a little before sundown when they would set up their marching camp. This allowed for a little over twenty miles a day, spread over five hours in the morning and four in the afternoon, a necessarily slow pace, given the speed of the ox carts accompanying them.

As the legion crested a low rise and took in, at last, the glory of the Nile's great delta, separated from Alexandria by a few low hills and the Mareotis Lake, there had been a collective sigh of relief and a feeling that the oppressive heat was about to be alleviated. The army would reach the first major tributary of the Nile, the Canopic, at the end of the first day, and would follow it all the way to Memphis.

After the dusty, dry, brown land of Nicopolis and Alexandria, the sight of the lush green of the delta was truly welcome as the entire legion descended in its personal dust cloud to the intensively farmed land of the Nile.

The anticipation of losing the choking sand was soon shattered, however. For all the general lush green formed by the strips of farmland and their irrigation channels, the paths and roads between, along which the army would travel, were still hard-packed dirt tracks, covered in dust, sand and grit and every bit as choking and harsh as the hill they had just left. At least the view, such as it was, would be different.

The capsarius, struggling under his unaccustomed weight, cast his gaze around the new surroundings, fertile and busy, wishing the Nile were closer.

The great river flooded each year, torrents of life-giving water flowing from mountainous lands far to the south, and for four months, over what was winter time elsewhere, the farmland of Aegyptus lay beneath the water before the inundation receded and farmers could sow their crops in the fresh silt deposits. The deeply superstitious Aegyptians still called it the "Tears of Isis" and thanked their gods for the inundation, while Cervianus found it easier to place his faith in rain causing floods than the grief of goddesses.

Carefully organised channels criss-crossing the system of fields extended the effects of the inundation beyond the season and into the planting time.

By now, however, in "Shemu", the season of harvest, the land was already drying out, the last traces of even the stored water long gone, sheaves of barley and grain stacked in the fields awaiting collection and storage.

Cervianus knew from his reading what that meant for the low folk of Aegyptus: the months that followed the collection, leading into the great inundation itself, saw the common people working on great projects, once for their kings and gods and now for their Roman overlords, constructing the great tombs, monuments and temples of the land.

The farmers stood in their fields wearing only short skirts of linen, sickles lowered, sweat peppering their brows, and stared with fascination as the glittering might of Rome marched past. Some farmers grinned; others glowered. Rome's fresh grip on Aegyptus had been met with varying reactions, though, in truth, the change in rulers made very little difference to the common man. Such was usually the case with a conquered or annexed nation; such was certainly true back home in Galatia.

Soon, though, the fascination with the change of scenery wore off. Mile after mile of seemingly identical fields, punctuated by narrow channels full of reeds, weeds, and still water, and occasional hamlets of mud-brick houses, rarely more than a single-room affair with a pen for animals built alongside. It was repetitive and even for Cervianus, with his voracious appetite for culture and knowledge, it began to pall after a while.

A further irritation began to surface among the fields, adding discomfort to the journey: the insects. Occasionally, they passed a small marsh of reeking slime or stagnant water that swarmed with flies. Down here in the delta, where the fields were separated by the streams of the Nile and the irrigation channels full of still, tepid water, flies abounded; great bulbous ugly insects buzzed around the marching men, moving freely and irritatingly in and out of the dust cloud alongside myriad smaller flies that landed on any exposed patch of skin, biting and causing red swellings and violent itches.

Cervianus grumbled to himself, wishing he was still one of the "immunes" and had a free hand with which to swat away the endless flow of harrying insects.

"S'a lot of grain, eh?"

Startled from his quiet irritation, Cervianus turned his head, sweat running from his helmet, down his forehead and cheeks and pooling inside the green linen scarf, soaking it yet further. Ulyxes was peering to the side of the road, along which the army marched eight abreast, at the interested farmers and their stacks of produce.

"They say Aegyptus can produce more grain than even the old lands of Carthage – enough to keep Rome fed for a thousand years," Cervianus replied as though reciting it by rote from a text, then gave a thoughtful frown. "I'm not convinced on that last. The hunger of Rome seems unending to me."

Ulyxes gave an exasperated laugh. "You think too much, you know that?"

Cervianus grimaced at him. "And there are times when you don't think *enough*."

The smaller legionary grinned and glanced about them again at the rich greenness of the landscape, heavily muted by the thick billowing grey cloud that surrounded the army.

"It's so flat. Back in Nicopolis I assumed the whole of Aegyptus was going to be hilly, kind of like home. I reckon if I stood on your shoulders I could see a hundred miles from here."

Cervianus nodded. "It'll be like this right over to the far side of the delta at Clysma, and that's over a hundred miles east of here. There's mountains beyond that, separating us from the lands of the Jews, but it's flat most of the way across the delta."

"Shut up, you know-it-all prick," cut in Evandros' thick voice from two men across in the line. His favourite thug, the enormous Batronus, chuckled humorously and made motions at Cervianus suggestive of a beating. The capsarius tried to ignore the pair and the threat of constant low-grade violence they represented and smiled weakly at his friend.

"Anyway, the delta is very flat, yes."

"Will it be like this down south?" Ulyxes asked, showing an unusual interest in the land. So far, in Cervianus' eyes, his friend had rarely cast a thought more than a few moments ahead and the change was refreshing.

"I don't believe so," he said, warming to his subject. "The descriptions I've read tell of great rocks, ridges and even mountains as you head south. The delta pretty much finishes at Memphis; after that, the green strip along the Nile's only about five or six miles across in most places. Make the most of the flat and the green. It won't last long."

Ulyxes grunted noncommittally. "I can't believe it's so bloody sweltering here. Now that we're away from the coast, it feels twice as hot."

"Again," Cervianus said quietly, "make the most of that. We're still getting a little breeze because the land's flat, and the water channels and greenery are helping cool us down. That's going to be gone in a few days, and *then* it'll begin to get warm."

Again, a grunt issued from his companion. "I hope Draco's going to lay off me in the mornings, then. I'll probably drop dead of exhaustion if he has me repeatedly loading and unloading trenching tools for an hour on my own *then*. I need to get on his good side so he'll stop being a vindictive bastard at me."

"You and me both," Cervianus replied with deep feeling, changing the angle of the furca carrying his kit away from the rapidly forming bruise on his shoulder.

The hours dragged on, the seething heat and choking dust a constant in their lives, partially obscuring the endless identical fields with their inquisitive workers. Though it was only mid-to-late morning when the buccina for each century called the rest break, it felt to the men as though they had marched for a week.

The Second century formed up and stood in parade rows as Draco and the signifer stepped to the side of the road.

"The tribune has called the midday halt. I have been informed we will not be preparing defences, despite the four hours we will abide here, but I will be setting pickets. There will be eight men on guard duty at a time, and shifts will change each hour. The tesserarius will pass among you selecting the men for guard, issuing the day's passwords and detailing the latrine duty. The rest of you will move over to the left, off the road, into that field, where you will remain in your contubernia and prepare meals. Make the most of this. After the heat dies down, we march on to the river near Hermopolis."

The men made appreciative noises. The chance to remove boots and helmets and sit with a sip of water away from the constant, cloying dust was an attractive opportunity.

"Alright. Fall out."

Ulyxes and Cervianus dawdled at the rear of the contubernium as their compatriots wandered off the track and into the green field. The farmers here had finished with their gathering and the green shoots in the almost dry dirt beneath them were soft and welcoming. Whatever it was that was grown in this place was not wheat, at least. Small thickets of trees, bushes and dense undergrowth surrounded the field's edge, likely the location of a now-overgrown irrigation channel that had not been dredged following the last flood.

"Not sure I can wait till they've dug the piss-pit," Ulyxes announced. "I've been bursting for at least the last hour."

Cervianus shook his head and rolled his eyes. "Can you not hold it another quarter-hour for the latrines to be dug?"

"Not a hope. Here."

With a groan, Ulyxes handed his furca to Cervianus, who took it, staggering under the extra weight of his friend's entire marching kit. Unable to continue with their contubernium with the unaccustomed load of the two kits, the medic staggered uncertainly in the wake of his companion, who stepped away from the rest and into the undergrowth at the edge of the field.

Muttering and grumbling about the weight and his friend's assumption that he was happy to stand holding half a ton of gear, Cervianus stood impatiently six feet or so from the undergrowth into which Ulyxes had gone.

Birds squawked and flies buzzed and, despite the close presence of thousands of men, everything was surprisingly quiet. The capsarius felt curiously alone, all of a sudden. Something about this place was beginning to make him twitchy. He couldn't say what it was but something kept sending small chills up his spine. He shook his head irritably. It was just a field, for Ceres' sake. It wasn't as if—

"Shit!"

The sudden cry from the trees made Cervianus jump and, forgetting about the need to keep their kit inspection-clean, he dropped the two furca onto the muddy ground and rushed across to the undergrowth.

"What is it?"

The shout had not been the mere consternation of a legionary who had accidentally urinated on his own foot, but a genuinely startled or panicked call.

He rounded the bulk of a bulbous bush to find Ulyxes, his

tunic still in place, leaning against the bole of a tree, heaving in deep breaths.

"What happened?"

"Got... a shock." Ulyxes pointed off into the undergrowth and Cervianus turned to follow his gaze. What he saw made him grin and then laugh out loud.

"It's not funny. I almost shat myself!"

Chuckling, Cervianus stepped forward and parted the undergrowth to get a better look at the thing that had so spooked his friend.

The statue was perhaps eight feet tall, though mostly obscured by the greenery. In a pose that suggested it walked with a long stride, the huge basalt image of a man's body was surmounted with a bird's head, its long, curved beak pointing accusingly at the pair of them, deep, piercing eyes above it boring into their own.

"It's Thoth. The Aegyptians see him as a sort of balance between good and bad, I think. A god of learning and understanding; my kind of god. See the way his arm's held out? I've seen pictures of him where he holds an ankh in that hand. Obviously someone's stolen that. He didn't see *that* 'bad' coming, did he?"

Ulyxes stood back from the tree and took a deep breath. "Whatever it is, it scares the shit out of you when you find it in the trees! What's a statue of a god doing hidden in the undergrowth out here?"

Cervianus shrugged. "I honestly have no idea. I guess there's a temple somewhere round here, though. Perhaps he's some sort of guardian statue at the edge of the precinct or something like that. I don't think he'll eat you, though, so go ahead and piss."

Ulyxes gave him a strange look. "I don't think I need to any more, if you get my drift. Besides, even if he does look like a stretched goose, he's a god, and it never does a man good to piss on a god!"

Cervianus shook his head. "It's just a statue, and apparently not even an important one if it's abandoned out here. Don't let over-piety cause you to go in your own tunic."

Yet, despite his own words, Cervianus found his gaze drawn back to those eyes and, as his friend turned and made his way back out to where their gear lay, he found himself reaching deep into his tunic and clutching the crocodile-tooth amulet the merchant back in Nicopolis had all but forced on him. Turning with a strange frown, he shuddered despite the extreme heat and slipped the leather thong around his neck, tucking the pendant into his tunic.

Back in the green field, Ulyxes had picked up the two furca and held one out to him, with a curious, questioning glance.

"What was that?" he asked quietly.

"Just a pendant. Some merchant back in Nicopolis wouldn't leave me alone until I bought it."

The explanation was straightforward enough as to his ownership of the smooth triangular charm but hardly rationalised his willingness or desire to actually wear it. He grumbled and collected his furca, aware from the look on Ulyxes' face that his companion clearly didn't consider his question answered.

With a shrug, the shorter man turned and strode off toward the patch of ground where the other six men in their contubernium lounged, their kit propped together as they unpacked the food and cooking pots.

Ulyxes wandered across and sat with them, though Cervianus hovered, uncertain for a while, and then sank to the welcome, soft greenery a few feet removed from the group. Ulyxes gave him an irritated glance and jerked his head toward the rest, but Cervianus shook his head. He knew how things were with his compatriots. They would make enough food to supply him with a portion on the unspoken understanding that he remained apart from them for the duration. In the sharing of the tent they had no choice concerning proximity, but in the open, this was the way it had to be. Besides, staying safely out of reach of Batronus might be a good idea if the big moron was spoiling for a fight.

"What is it with you lot?" Ulyxes asked the others as they began to knead the bread and build the small fire in a carefully excavated pit.

"Eh?" Vibius questioned, and Cervianus closed his eyes, biting his lip. No good ever came of bringing up the issue and he silently wished Ulyxes' mouth shut.

"Why the cold shoulder for Cervianus?" the legionary pressed, despite the capsarius's fervent wish for silence. "I mean, I know he can be a bit arrogant and he's got all the social charm of a pond newt, but beyond that I can't see how he deserves this much enmity."

Behind him, Cervianus shrank into himself, trying to become invisible. This was the turning point. He'd seen it several times in potentially friendly compatriots. Now the others would begin the task of turning Ulyxes against him. Indeed, one of the six men opposite had once been just such a potential ally, half a year ago.

"He's a prick," Evandros said flatly.

Petrocorios shot him a warning glance.

"It's not that. He's dangerous; and unlucky. Bad things happen around him."

Ulyxes laughed derisively. "Bad things happen around me too. Bad things just happen; it's that simple."

"No," the other man countered. "It isn't. That one denies the power and will of gods. Gods don't like that." He lowered his voice conspiratorially and leaned closer. "Last year we were all standing on a parade ground, the whole cohort. There's this almighty rumbling noise, see, and the ground opens up under us."

Ulyxes nodded, transfixed.

"Vulcan's hammer blow, of course. But understand me, here: this was *aimed* at Cervianus. The bloody great crack starts at the river's edge, causes the granary building to collapse and sag in the middle and tears a great big line across the parade ground. Where does it first strike, you reckon?"

Ulyxes said nothing, but his eyes shot to the capsarius.

The legionary nodded.

"Opens right under his feet and goes on in a straight line, along the row of men. That's us, by the way: his contubernium. The bloody great hole tries to swallow all eight of us and the crack stops at precisely the other end of the parade ground."

He nodded knowingly.

"Oh, the rumbling goes on for a while, but that's 'cause Vulcan hasn't quite got his target, see? Cervianus is at the front of the line and he sees the hole coming quick enough to jump out of the way."

He leaned back.

"The crack was about twenty feet deep and three feet wide. Swallowed two men. One of 'em is now pensioned out, 'cause of the leg break he got that day. Other poor bastard landed on his head at the bottom. You've never seen a mess like it."

He sat back as though he had wrapped up a mystery.

"All 'cause we're stood in a line behind him."

Ulyxes frowned. "And you don't consider the possibility that it was a coincidence?"

"Not a chance. He'd spent the previous week arguing that the lodestone is somehow a natural thing and nothing to do with Vulcan at all? A rock that attracts iron? And it has nothing to do with Vulcan? No wonder the god got pissed off at him!"

Petrocorios made a superstitious gesture in honour of the blacksmith god and Cervianus rolled his eyes and leaned back.

As the argument deepened, he closed his ears to the ensuing torrent of abuse that washed over them, past Ulyxes who stood as an inquisitive rock amid it. Sooner or later, the sheer pressure of needing to appease his peers would drive a wedge between him and the medic. Either that or Batronus and Evandros would beat him to a pulp one night.

With a sigh, Cervianus lay back on the green carpet and let the warmth of the Aegyptian sun soothe him, washing away all his insecurities and issues. Life would go on; it invariably did. And yet he suddenly realised he was clutching the crocodile-tooth amulet again and pulled his hand away in exasperation.

Titus Cervianus, tired and sore legionary of the Twenty Second Deiotariana, stumbled out of the tent, allowing the heavy leather flap to fall back into place, muting the thundering snores, coughs and intermittent breath-stealing farts from within. Countless stars twinkled above, holes in the canopy of night, giving the landscape an eerie tone, particularly in the almost silent night.

The breeze rustled among the scattered trees and bushes, a sound akin to a legion of secretive whisperers. The strange silvery light turned the grass grey and the mud black, the sky a dark blue. He shivered in the breeze.

The legions had finally reached the Canopic branch of the Nile as the great disc of the sun picked up speed in its descent toward the horizon. Rather than the majestic waterway he had been hoping for, it seemed that here, and at this time of the year, the Nile consisted more of a channel of slow-flowing water barely twenty feet across and even that was largely hidden by the myriad reeds on both banks.

The welcome relief at the cool of the water as they arrived had soon turned to dismay at the vast clouds of biting insects that swarmed above the river at dusk, while the legions busied themselves in the raising of a temporary rampart and palisade formed of the sudis stakes that each man carried – a defence that surrounded three sides of the camp, the river providing the defence of the last, for speed of construction.

The town of Hermopolis stood tantalisingly close, perhaps half a mile away, the roofs of its buildings and the great temple edifices rising above the greenery of the delta, partially obscured by the levee that protected the settlement from the annual floodwaters. Due to an agreement between the Roman governors and the town's council, the legions were forbidden from camping within a certain distance of the built-up area and so the army's camp had to be located on the flood plain beside the river and not safely dry behind the great dyke.

Still, despite everything, the appearance of the river and the next sizeable town on their journey had refreshed the hope and interest of the men. What felt like endless days of the dry, brown world of Nicopolis had given way to the green flat landscape of the delta, and now to the Nile itself and signs that things were changing again.

Cervianus sighed and stretched in the open air. A gentle sound like the rumbling of siege engines across gravel was borne of seven thousand or so men snoring or murmuring. Row upon orderly row of plain leather tents stretched off toward the centre of the camp where the senior officers made their home for the night. The cohorts of the Twelfth shared the defences of the camp that they helped to construct, but their units lay on one edge, almost segregated, a wide road keeping them apart from the Twenty Second. The few auxiliary units they had picked up were lodged in the far corner, near the supply wagons and far from the superior legions.

Enjoying the play of air on his face, the capsarius rubbed his hair vigorously, wincing as the dust, dirt and dead insects fell out of it. It would likely be at least another four days before he could hope for a good bath. He could dip in the river, but the mix of latrine waste, insects and possibly dangerous animals made dirty hair a preference.

No. He would settle for relieving himself and then heading back to bed.

The nearest of the eight latrines that had been dug to support the camp stood on the flattest part of the riverbank at the downstream end, at the terminus of the thoroughfare that separated the two legions. It would be unpleasant now, after serving perhaps a couple of thousand men for the past six hours, but it would also be unoccupied at this time of night, well past midnight and marching on toward the dawn.

Huge spare leather tent sections had been tied to posts jammed in the ground, forming temporary walls that provided a modicum of privacy and prevented the worst of the smell from filtering into the nearby areas of the camp.

With trepidation as to what horrors lay in wait, Cervianus

turned into the wide street and strode down the last few paces toward the leather latrine building. As he closed on it, the powerful aroma of dung and ammonia began to curl his nose hairs and he had to bite down hard to prevent the bile rising as he reached the entrance and a malicious gust of wind sprang up, carrying the worst of the pungent stink straight into his face.

Swallowing and wondering whether it would be possible to hold his breath for the entire duration of his visit, Cervianus pushed his way into the miasma, his eyes stinging in the acrid air. While the leather shields prevented the smell from penetrating much of the camp, they also prevented the breeze from stirring the air within.

Stumbling forward in the gloom, he turned the corner, setting his eyes on the temporary wooden seat formed from planking and erected over the stinking trench. Once more, he wondered whether he might be able to wait, and cursed himself for not having been able to go earlier when the pit was still relatively fresh.

Wandering over to the seat, he looked down and was dismayed at the smears on it. For a moment he gagged and desperately had to hold down his evening meal. Turning, he surveyed the area to see if there was any better seating.

The body took him entirely by surprise and he was so taken aback that he gasped and found he'd taken a deep breath of the stinking air. His astonishment at the crumpled shape lying on the foul ground with an arm in the trench was momentarily interrupted as he busily emptied his stomach onto the floor.

As he stared down he noted with a professional eye, despite everything, the trail of rusty colour among the rest of the detritus on the floor. His head swinging back and forth, he realised that the stains on the wooden seat were not what he'd initially thought but were, in fact, blood – the same blood that trailed and smeared across the mucky grass and ended with the prone form in the russet tunic.

A sense of desperation and panic gripped him and he fought the urge to shout for help. To be found here in a green tunic with the corpse of a legionary from the Twelfth? The consequences didn't even bear thinking about. Shaking slightly, pale and panicky, Cervianus leapt into the air and almost screamed as the man's fingers shot out and grasped the laces of his boot. The heap was alive!

Professional training immediately overcoming all else and filling his mind, he dropped to a crouch and peered closely at the man, lying there covered in blood and filth. His arms and legs seemed to all be lying at comfortable angles so if any limb were broken, it was at least only a minor fracture, which was a blessing. Anything else and he might have to be escorted straight back to Nicopolis.

Gently and with great care the capsarius turned the man over, cradling his head and arm so that he rolled slowly and calmly onto his back. Through a slick of black and red, the man coughed, blood spraying from his mouth and a large red bubble forming at the end of his nostril. One of his eyes had taken such a pounding that it had sealed shut and swelled. The jaw was likely fractured and the nose broken beyond hope of straightening.

Carefully, Cervianus grasped the neckline of the tunic, which was already torn in three places, and ripped downwards, revealing a torso that looked black, purple and red. The man had been beaten within an inch of Elysium.

Shaking his head at the stupidity of men, Cervianus

straightened. He had to get the man washed and tended, but there was no way he could do it alone.

With a nervous glance, he left the gurgling heap and ran out of the latrines. The nearest tent of the Twenty Second legion would be one of the last centuries of the Tenth cohort – men he didn't know, though they possibly knew him, at least by sight and reputation.

Trying desperately to decide, his gaze fell on movement. A man was sitting outside his tent further along the line, partially hidden between the rows. Nodding, Cervianus ran toward him. The man looked up in surprise, a small wine beaker in his hand.

"It's not what you think…"

Cervianus shook his head and stepped back as the man rose to his feet, pulling a face as his nose caught the drift of latrine from the newcomer.

"I don't give a damn what you're doing, friend, but I need your help, now!"

The man frowned.

"A soldier's been kicked half to death in the latrines. I need you to go to my tent." He paused, making a mental calculation. "Fourteen rows back from here and three in. Just inside the tent flap to the left is a leather bag. That's my medical bag and I need you to go and get it, alright?"

"What if someone catches me and thinks I'm stealing it?"

Cervianus shrugged.

"Knowing them, they'll probably help you or buy you a drink. Now run; a man's life's at stake."

The soldier, suddenly aware that this man must be a capsarius and therefore his nominal superior, saluted and, dropping his cup, ran around the corner and off toward the tent. Paying him no further heed, Cervianus turned and jogged back to the latrine.

The man had not moved, his bruised and bloodied chest heaving as he lay on his back in the filth. Clenching his jaw, the awful smell now going almost entirely unnoticed, Cervianus crouched and lifted first one arm and then the other, running his hands very gently up and down, probing as lightly as he could, checking for breaks. Clearly there were broken fingers and his wrist seemed to be fractured but, given the feel of them and the simple groans of general pain that issued from the soldier, it appeared there was no real damage between wrist and shoulder. Gently, he lifted the arms until they lay straight out from the shoulders. The groaning stayed the same. No extra strain there.

Cervianus glowered. He'd dealt with the aftermath of enough fistfights that he could see clearly how this one had gone. No breaks or serious damage to the arms and no stress on the shoulders meant that the man did not use his arms to protect himself from the blows; nor were they being restrained. This had been done by one or two men at most and they had taken their victim so by surprise that the flurry of beatings had rained down before the man even knew what was happening.

His irritation still building, Cervianus reached down and repeated the checking procedure on the legs. A sharp yelp from the barely conscious man announced a fracture on the left shin, probably the result of a last farewell kick from the assailant. He couldn't be dragged, then, for fear of extra damage to the wrist or shin.

Gently, he began probing the chest, testing for broken ribs and was dismayed at how often his tender prods caused a violent explosion of noise from the man. Seven broken ribs.

Seven! The man would be very lucky if he hadn't lost the use of a lung; in fact, he probably had, since five of the breaks were on one side. Leaning close and allowing the victim time to settle from his ordeal back into a gentle steady agony, he listened to the breathing. Shallow and rapid, with a crackling sound.

Leaning back, he nodded dismally. The man was working on one lung. The other likely had a shard of rib sticking through it. This man was for the medicus at best and probably medical discharge if he even recovered enough to dismiss.

Grinding his teeth, he crouched until he heard the sound of running footsteps approaching the latrines, and then stood. The other legionary entered, breathless, the leather bag held out in his hands. He turned and looked down at the wounded man, his hand going to his mouth and nose to try and block out the smell.

"He's from the Twelfth!"

"Yes," Cervianus nodded. "And he's lucky he's not dead."

The legionary stared at him.

"He's lucky we're not finishing the bloody job!"

The capsarius turned and glared at the younger man.

"Get over your petty rivalries, soldier. This is a human being and a legionary. He has been beaten almost to death and if he does die, someone else will join him for having done this. Help me."

As the man continued to stare, Cervianus took his medical bag and slung it over his shoulder before beginning to dismantle one section of latrine wall.

"I said help me!"

The soldier, startled, sidled toward him, his gaze still locked on the wounded soldier. Between the two men, the section of leather walling was quickly unfastened and lowered, the poles that supported it still attached at either side, forming a makeshift stretcher. Gently they lowered the leather to the ground next to the body and, under Cervianus' directions, they slowly and carefully moved the man onto the stretcher.

"Grab that end. We need to get him to the river upstream."

The soldier stood shaking his head.

"Do it!" the capsarius snapped and the soldier jumped again before grasping the poles and helping to lift the burden from the ground. The wounded legionary groaned in pain as he was jolted and moved between the walls of leather and out into the open air.

The freshness of the breeze was welcome, and the pair carried their burden, struggling to keep the man level and comfortable, thirty paces upstream.

"This should do it. We're above the latrine and far enough down from the next one that the effluent will have mainly flowed out into the centre with the current. It's as clean as any water we're going to get here."

The soldier gave him a baffled look but helped lower the stretcher to the ground by the water's edge. Undoing his bag, Cervianus retrieved sponges, gum, bindings and cuprinon paste.

"Help me lower him into the water. First thing is to try and clean off all the muck and blood so that I can see exactly what I'm dealing with."

"No."

Cervianus stared up at the legionary. "What? Help me!"

"No. I shouldn't have done *this*. He's a bastard from the Twelfth. We should have given him a couple more kicks and rolled him into the shitter."

The capsarius ground his teeth again angrily. "He is a human being who is close to being taken to Elysium. Now help me!"

"No. No more. Nothing to do with me."

As Cervianus spluttered angry protests and demands, the soldier turned and clambered up the gentle slope before running off into the night.

The capsarius glared after him for a moment and then concentrated on the man in his arms. Gingerly, and with some difficulty, he turned the stretcher so that it was tilted toward the river, giving him the angle and ability to slowly slide the patient down and into the water. Carefully, as the body slid into the dark, burbling flow feet first until he was submerged to the waist, Cervianus removed the man's tunic, freeing his battered torso.

The moments passed in darkness and silence as he ran a sponge over the man's legs and arms and then chest and stomach, being careful to apply as little pressure as possible. Finally, he cleaned the man's face, drawing a sharp breath with each gentle wipe as the full, horrific extent of the man's injuries became apparent.

Shaking his head in anger, the capsarius dipped a jar into the river and poured the water over the man's hair, repeating the gesture several times and running his fingers through the tousled locks in between torrents to remove the caked, matted blood. Further damage to the head above the hairline became slowly apparent and Cervianus' estimate of the man's recovery chances plummeted again. The last time he'd seen so many splits and cracks on a man's skull, he'd spent the rest of his days a drooling idiot and a beggar.

Sighing, he gave the body another quick look-over. The damage was definitely bad but there was still the possibility that the man would go on to lead a full and healthy life. Not a likelihood, true, but a possibility. Slowly, he hauled the man as gently as he could back up from the river and onto the stretcher.

As he crouched and began to apply the cuprinon to the worst of the wounds and salves to remove inflammation and lessen bruising over most of the skin, he thought through his next move.

The man would have to be seen by a medicus. There was nothing they could do that Cervianus couldn't, admittedly, but a legion's medicus had the authority to reclassify the man, assign him to the wounded cart, or even provide an escort to take him back to the fortress at Nicopolis: the only realistic option at this point.

The medicus would have to be the Twelfth's, on the assumption the man had travelled with them. It was no good taking the man to the Twenty Second's medicus, clearly.

After binding the wounds slowly and carefully, he took the blanket he habitually kept rolled up and fastened at the bottom of the bag, and draped it over the man.

For some time, he crouched in the heavier growth by the riverbank and gazed down at his patient. The man had managed just one day of what would likely be a six-month campaign or more. How many senseless attacks would there be between the two rival legions before they even reached the first sign of civilisation? The commanders would need to be informed and would need to work on instilling a little more sense and discipline in their men.

His mind flashed back to that night at the tribune's house in Nicopolis: the black eye and broken fingers; the shared looks of seething hatred. No. The commanders would be absolutely no use in healing the breach between their legions; indeed, they seemed to be helping to widen it. And once they reached Thebes and picked up members of the Third legion as well? What then? More attacks? Fresh waves of hate?

Sadly, he concluded that the only solution was war. Throw the three legions into a cauldron of combat and death and they would soon find brotherhood in their shared pride and in the face of the Kushite invaders. It was perhaps the first time in his life that Cervianus found himself eager for the fight, wishing the coming battles were already upon them. Better to stand as brothers and fight a dreadful enemy than to kick one another to death in the latrines, after all.

Taking a deep breath, he moved around to the end of the stretcher and, facing away from it, grabbed the poles and lifted slightly, walking half bent to keep his burden steady on the makeshift litter. Slowly and with infinite care, being watchful of bumps and dips in the ground, the capsarius dragged the wounded man up the slope and into the camp proper.

His back making argumentative noises, he staggered toward the tents of the Twelfth and suddenly became aware of people nearby. Glancing to his right, the body behind him bouncing and jiggling on the litter as he moved, Cervianus realised that a crowd of legionaries in green tunics had gathered – perhaps a score of them, watching him with sour expressions.

"Scum-lover!" someone shouted.

Cervianus ignored them and dragged the litter on. As the crowd edged closer, several of the legionaries spat at him, their aim off at this distance, so that the ground was peppered near his feet.

"Well done," he commended himself silently, as he shuffled forward dragging the wounded man, "you've actually contrived to make yourself even *less* popular."

Angling away from the angry group, the capsarius dragged his burden on toward the tents of the Twelfth, where men were emerging in russet tunics in response to the noise.

As he approached the line, Cervianus paused and looked up at the nearest man.

"Where's your medicus?"

The man stared at him, shaking his head slightly.

"Where is your *damn medicus*?"

Behind the man, another stepped out. His bearing, with hands clasped behind his back and chin high, suggested he was an officer of some variety – an optio perhaps, or a standard bearer?

"This way."

Without another word, the soldiers of the Twelfth parted and Cervianus dragged his litter between them in the wake of the man. Irritated that even now, among the Twelfth, with one of their own men wounded and in trouble, nobody offered to help lift the stretcher, the capsarius followed, grinding his teeth again, between the lines of tents, until the officer stopped outside a larger one near the main road.

"Leave him here with us."

Cervianus' brow furrowed. "I should make a report to the medicus. I've tended the wounds I can, but the man has broken ribs, a lung problem that—"

The man was waving his hand. "That's enough. Now go."

The capsarius stared at him in disbelief. Realising that a large crowd of glowering legionaries in red-brown tunics had gathered around him and suddenly acutely aware of the growing tension and resentment in the air, Cervianus gently lowered the stretcher to the ground and backed away between the tents, the legionaries of the Twelfth filling the path behind him and blocking sight of the wounded man as they flowed with him like a tide, washing him back out of their camp.

Backing out away from the tents into the open air, he shook his head in disbelief. This was getting ridiculous.

Turning, he realised that the crowd of men in green tunics had grown and now he was standing between two groups of angry legionaries. Biting his lip and taking a deep breath, he backed away to the waterline and, as soon as he clambered down the slope and lost sight of the two crowds, ran for his life.

The mutual enmity between the legions was the only thing that prevented them from following him and, as he ran for his tent, hoping that he would be granted the chance of a night's sleep without receiving a similar beating, he shook his head sadly. The worst thing of all during the last quarter of an hour had not been the treatment he received from either legion, or the way they put their dislike of him over the needs of a wounded man, but was rather the fact that, as he turned and ran, the last face he had seen among the legionaries in green had been that of Ulyxes, shaking his head sadly.

It had been a nervous night. Though there had been no overt moves by the men of his contubernium, Cervianus had felt eyes on him at several times during the night and had dozed for moments at best, aware of the very real possibility of not waking up at all should he fall deeply asleep. Evandros and Batronus had slept with their gladius at hand, prompting Cervianus to lie the same way, though devoid of blessed rest. The most worrying thing had been the strange way Ulyxes had simply gone to sleep and snored through as though nothing had happened. While he had not joined the others in any plan to beat him, he had shown no sign of solidarity with him either.

When morning came and the buccina call rang out, Cervianus was already dressed and ready, his kit packed, apart from the section of rampart he would be carrying onwards. The eight men had worked in silence, taking down the leather sections and stowing them for the journey, the capsarius trying as hard as possible to keep to himself and become effectively invisible.

It was difficult and troubling. He had never been popular, for certain, and had been shunned by most of the men, living the life of a recluse in the midst of an army of thousands, but he had generally been safe. Alone, but safe.

This was something else entirely. The soldiers who had seen him last night had had violence in their eyes at the end, their fears and hates stirred up by the ever-present bully Evandros. The thugs of his contubernium had perhaps spent the night wrestling with the matter of how to deal with him. An overt beating would end in serious repercussions for all involved, despite Batronus' threats. Likely their anger would be vented in other, pettier ways until the day came when opportunity presented itself.

He had never lived in real fear before and found suddenly that he was far more afraid of what his fellow legionaries might do than any force of Kushite warriors awaiting them to the south.

He stuffed the folded leather into the bag and attached it to his furca, irritably. All this because he had followed the ideals of Hippocrates and helped a man who *needed* that help.

Crouching by his kit and running a last moment check, he almost leapt out of his skin when a hand touched his shoulder.

"Hades, calm down!"

The capsarius, his heart racing in his chest, turned to see Ulyxes leaning over him. A quick glance thrown about him confirmed that the pair were as alone as it was possible to be in the busyness of breaking camp, the other six members of their unit having wandered off to make a last use of the latrines or perhaps find some bread and cheese before the march began. He shivered, though already the air was warm and cloying.

"You scared the life out of me. I thought you would be off with your new friends, planning where to hide my body?"

Ulyxes shook his head. "I'm not after you, Titus, though I wouldn't say the same for the rest. You're about as popular as a turd in a bathhouse right now. It'll all die down eventually, so long as you don't do anything stupid or draw attention to yourself."

Cervianus chewed on his cheek. "It's not that easy. I can leave everyone alone; I'm used to that. But by noon, the entire legion's going to know I saved a soldier from the Twelfth and want me dead. Evandros will be stirring up trouble even now, in the shitter. There's no justice in this, though. It's my reason for existence: to save lives. He was a legionary, after all."

A strange look passed across Ulyxes' eyes and the capsarius frowned, worrying suddenly that not everything was as simple and clear-cut as it seemed.

"What are you not telling me?"

His suspicions deepened as Ulyxes shuffled uncomfortably. Cervianus' gaze fell to the shuffling feet.

"Oh for the love of Venus!"

Despite the dust, the stains of excrement and blood on his friend's boots were all too obvious to a trained eye. As his eyes slowly came back level, he realised that Ulyxes was also wearing a brand-new tunic – one of those they had stolen from the supply building, probably. He wondered where the other, incriminating, blood-soaked green rag was now.

"Why, Ulyxes? Answer me that."

"Because he had it coming, Titus."

"*No* man deserves that. What did he do? Cheat you at dice?"

Ulyxes grasped him by the shoulders and pulled him close. "That bastard tried to smash my brains out in Nicopolis. You might remember the incident, funnily enough, since you lost a lot of pay over it, though, if I remember rightly, you were busy at the time being beaten with a plank."

Cervianus stared at him.

"This wasn't a random act of violence, Titus. This was retribution, served in the name of Nemesis. If it makes you feel any better, I intend to dedicate her an altar in thanks when we get back."

The capsarius railed. "Makes me *feel better*? That you're going to thank the gods for an opportunity to half kill a man? What makes you think that was him? Have you been following him since we left? Keeping an eye on him? Just waiting for the right time?"

Ulyxes' face hardened. "You know me, Titus. I'm still fairly new here, but you know me as well as any man. You know that if I see those men again, I'm going to recognise them."

Cervianus stopped. While he could only picture the men who had attacked them in terms of general size and shape, his friend would remember the look in their eye, every mark or dimple on their face, the cut of their hair. With his perfect recall, there was no chance he had the wrong man.

"You took it too far," he said in quiet exasperation. "You all but killed him. He'll probably be pensioned out within months. You know what that means!"

Ulyxes nodded. Medical discharge was never a good thing. If it happened, it meant the man was crippled, lame, or permanently deficient in some way. They would be unable to get another job that required full physical capabilities and their pension would be forfeit due to early dismissal. It was a one-way trip to the begging bowl. If the man couldn't be returned to full health, he would end his days in a gutter in Alexandria, shouting desperate pleas at the passers-by.

"You can say what you like. A man who plans to tear my head off deserves anything he gets. I'll not apologise for it."

Cervianus held his gaze for a moment and then looked away sadly.

"Are you intending to sell me out to the centurion?" Ulyxes asked quietly.

"Of course I'm not. What good would it do anyway? It wouldn't un-break the man's ribs, would it? No. You're safe… or at least you will be when you wash the blood and shit from your boots. Bit of a giveaway, that."

Ulyxes nodded. "I'll go wash them in the river. Thank you, Titus."

The capsarius replied with an exasperated gasp.

"I'll do what I can to keep you safe and divert any trouble," the heavy-set, smaller man said earnestly. "You know that."

Cervianus nodded. "But you'll have to stay away from me too. Else you'll just be putting yourself in danger for no reason."

Ulyxes looked troubled. "I don't like the idea. Good friends aren't easy to come by, I find."

The capsarius shrugged. "I'm used to being an outcast;

won't do me any harm. Just be careful, and if you're going to do anything like this again, come and talk to me first?"

The legionary gave him a wry grin. "So you can talk me out of it, you mean?"

"Precisely."

Cervianus stood watching as his friend patted him on the shoulder once more and then wandered off toward the river, conflicting emotions battering him. The sheer revulsion at what his friend had been capable of was somehow muted by the knowledge that it was he who had done it, and by the reasons behind the attack. The fact that he could almost justify it worried him almost as much as the act itself.

A sudden feeling made him look up to see Evandros, Batronus and Petrocorios standing by their packs a few paces away, their eyes locked on him. Hopefully Ulyxes had been right and this would eventually fade and just go away. The look in their eyes suggested otherwise.

Instinctively, he reached to his neck and he was irritated to realise he had grasped the crocodile-tooth pendant again. Letting go, he crouched once more, ripping the leather thong on which it hung from his neck. Grasping his purse, he opened it and jammed the pendant inside. He was about to close it, when the glint of silver caught his eye.

With a smile, he withdrew Ulyxes' "lucky coin" and spun it back and forth, examining it. Slightly worn and smooth, one side showed the Galatian eagle, symbol of King Deiotarus and of his army, standing majestic, its head turned to the west, the origin of the Galatian people. The inscription below it was worn, but made mention of Pompey and the king. The other side showed a winged Roman victory over a scene of battle.

If he was going to be superstitious and wear some symbol round his neck, why the tooth of a beast and not a symbol at least of his national pride and that of his army?

Nodding to himself, he placed the coin on the plain leather cover of his shield and drew the pugio dagger from his belt. Noting once again the irritating nick in the blade, he held it over the medal, dropping the point to the silver at the top of the coin. Slowly, he exerted more and more pressure, pressing down on the hilt until the sharp tip pushed a deep dent into the softer silver. Turning it over, relieved that the mark was not on the eagle's head, he repeated the act, forming a small hole at the top.

Smiling to himself, he undid and unthreaded the leather thong from the tooth and slid the coin onto it instead, tying that around his neck.

Sheathing his dagger and replacing his purse, he stood and tucked the lucky coin away beneath his tunic. Somehow it felt more reasonable and logical than its predecessor.

Ignoring the glares of his peers, he gathered his pack as the muster call blared out across the camp.

The first incident, when it came, was a surprise and was every bit as petty as Cervianus had dared to hope, though with far deeper-reaching consequences than the puerile assaulter could have guessed.

The army had marched throughout the morning, Ulyxes in his accustomed place beside the capsarius, carefully not meeting his eye at any point. Fuscus, to the far side, kept knocking him with his furca, sometimes harder than others, rarely enough to bruise. Petrocorios in the row in front managed somehow to keep standing on his toe – a miracle really, given how difficult it would be to achieve at marching pace without falling over. Even the man behind, who he didn't know, occasionally kicked him on the heel. The whole thing was so childish it would have made him laugh, had he not still held a deep fear that something much more brutal was in the works for him.

A halt was called late morning by the river not far from the edge of the city of Naucratis. Cervianus had wandered off on his own to the water's edge, away from the rest of the cohort, peering up at the great city.

While Hermopolis had been a reasonably populous town, Naucratis was a different affair entirely. A Greek trading settlement long before even Alexander had conquered Aegyptus, Naucratis was huge and seething with life, glorious monuments rising up among the streets, clustered around the great temple complex of the Hellenion, with its raised, walled enclosure.

Cervianus had been familiar enough with the city from descriptions in his Herodotus texts back on the trireme that he could even take an educated guess as to which temple was dedicated to which god, just from the vague hints of decoration visible above the city's roofline and from their positioning in relation to one another.

Naucratis had been the closest place to Alexandria that had been on the capsarius's list of fascinating sites to visit, and here he was within arm's reach of the place, but would have to march on past it in four hours without ever setting foot on its streets.

He had been slowly shaking his head at the unfairness of it all when the unseen assailant, who must have crept up behind him like a mischievous child, gave him a hearty shove on the back, sweeping him clean from his feet and launching him several paces out into the water.

Cervianus' world flurried in turbulent murk as he disappeared below the surface. Taken entirely by surprise, he had swallowed a large mouthful of the dark water as he fell and was suddenly among reeds and weeds at the bottom of the channel, choking and desperate, blinded by the absence of anything but brown river.

Papyrus reeds and other vegetation entangled his legs and the more he tried to kick and free himself, the worse his predicament became.

Aware that he was perhaps thirty heartbeats from drowning, he forced himself to become calm, pushing the panic down and out from himself. This was no time for hysterics. Thinking through the problem, he reached down to his belt and located in the Stygian gloom the hilt of his pugio. Drawing it with difficulty, he began to cut at the papyrus stalks and the other binding weeds that held him down until, with a sudden burst of activity, he found himself free.

Launching himself with all his might, he pushed for the surface, his lungs burning with the effort of holding in the wasted air.

Bursting through the slowly shifting surface like a leaping fish, Cervianus heaved in a desperate lungful of air as he fell back, treading water slowly, recovering his strength and blinking away the slimy water.

It was then he realised that he was not alone.

His heart lurched once again at the sight of the slitted, yellow eye regarding him coldly from the reeds. As the eye shifted slightly, he caught sight of the horned, ridged crown behind it and the raised snout. Then, suddenly, the eye closed and everything shifted. The fronds above at the tip of the papyrus plants shook slightly, and the beast was gone with the sound of a weight disappearing beneath water.

Ripples ran across the surface of the river, the only remaining sign of the suddenly invisible monster.

For a moment, Cervianus remained still, in shock, his feet pedalling the murky depths, until he realised what the disappearance of the beast very likely meant. In a sudden desperate flurry of movement he lunged for the shore, horribly aware out of the corner of his eye that the reeds nearby had just been forced apart by something large.

Floundering in the shallows, he threw himself forward onto the bank and scrabbled up it, grasping mud and grass in clenched, white hands as he sought distance between himself and the water, expecting at any moment the agony of jagged teeth sinking into his calf.

There was an ominous, earth-shaking thud, quickly followed by an unpleasant slithering noise and a splash behind him and he stumbled to his feet and ran as though Pluto himself were on his heel, ignoring his kit that sat in a pile close by.

A number of people had stopped what they were doing and looked up at the sudden commotion to see the tall, bedraggled figure backing toward them, away from the river, stained with silt and algae and shaking as though freezing to the bone.

Some of them immediately lost interest as they realised who it was. The rest displayed a variation of vile hatred and smug interest.

Cervianus stared down at the ripples that marked where the thing had just submerged once again. A line of mud and grooves on the bank showed quite clearly how far out of the water the creature had come in search of food, and just how close it must have come to ending the capsarius's career.

Shuddering wildly, he stepped gingerly forward to where his kit lay, grabbed it hurriedly and dragged it back far from the shore.

"Sh... shit," he announced to himself, breathing heavily.

Collapsing to his backside on the warm ground, he finally pulled himself together enough to take in his surroundings and the many legionaries watching him with varied, generally unfriendly, expressions. Of anyone lurking, standing out, or laughing at their own inventive and hilarious prank there was no sign.

The culprit had got away with it. Moreover, hoping to simply wet, embarrass and severely inconvenience the capsarius, they had almost claimed his life by total coincidence.

Crouching, he opened the pack on his furca and started digging around for his spare tunic, when his hand fell on the small purse.

With a frown, he pulled it from the pack and stared at it. His brow remaining furrowed, he took a deep breath, opened it, and withdrew the crocodile-tooth amulet from within.

Unfastening his neck-thong, he added the tooth to it and then retied it, feeling somehow happier as the coin and tooth tinkled together and settled against his soaked skin beneath the sodden tunic.

As he kept trying to explain to people: he preferred to believe that science and reason were the source of more of the world's wonders than were the will of gods, but that did not mean that he did not believe in the masters of Olympus at all.

Something beyond his ken was clearly happening in

Aegyptus and it had not been to Pythagoras or Herodotus that he had turned when that terrifying yellow eye had closed and marked the start of the attack.

It had been to Jupiter. Plain and simple.

V

MEMPHIS

Cervianus slumped. Days had passed in a blur of nervous exhaustion. Each night he had slept lightly, aware of the slightest sound or change in the environment. A retribution attack of some variety was coming, and he could feel the malice rising and thickening the atmosphere each day. The distant cry of a night bird or the sound of a cat on the prowl would be enough to force his eyes sharply open, backing him up against the leather of the tent, his gaze dancing around the dim interior, unable to relax even slightly until he was convinced the other occupants were asleep. Evandros and Batronus spent their time grinning maliciously, enjoying his continual discomfort as much as the promise of further fun.

Of course, his imagination and fears had amplified the situation during the march. The chances of the intolerant legionaries taking any action against him while en route, when nothing would go unnoticed, was small. Besides, Ulyxes would probably find a way to warn him. Still, a peaceful, uninterrupted night's sleep had been impossible.

Things had taken a turn for the worse today, though.

The legions had arrived at Memphis in the late afternoon, while the sun was large and low, and had begun to make camp outside the north wall of the city, digging their ditch and raising their rampart in standard form. Tonight it had been different, though. Repeatedly, during the sweaty strain of ditch-digging, he had been struck with shovelfuls of dirt, designed more to attract his attention than to annoy him. Each time he had looked up for the culprit, the legionaries, not just the two principal thugs in his contubernium, but even men he did not know, would make signs at him, slapping their fist into the palm of their hand, drawing a finger across their neck or some such.

His heart in his throat, he had caught Ulyxes' eyes as the man worked some ten paces down the line and the stocky legionary had paused to wipe his short brown moustache, shaking his head sadly and meaningfully at the medic.

Tonight would be it.

It had come as no surprise to find out that his contubernium had been posted right at the edge of the camp, close to both the latrines and a gate guarded by their own cohort. "Accidents" could so easily happen here; "accidents" could easily be covered up. The body might never even be found. His dismay had heightened when he discovered that not one senior officer would be in camp with them for the evening as they had been called to a meeting at the local military command building beyond those high walls. The few optios left in charge would be unlikely to lift a finger to prevent this kind of trouble.

Slumped against the completed rampart, aware that he was relatively safe here, alone, out in the open, he wondered whether he might possibly try and pass the night here. No, the optios or the men on guard duty would move him along like a vagrant. He would have to chance things in his tent and be alert and prepared to run when necessary.

His gaze rose from his position to look at the city beyond the camp.

Much like Naucratis, which they had passed days ago, Memphis was a name steeped in both history and mystery – a place he ached to explore and discover. And yet here he was stuck in camp, facing imminent demise. Though the army would be here for more than a day, the chances of him having the time to see the great once-capital of Aegyptus were minimal. If he survived the night, which was touch-and-go in itself, he would be called upon tomorrow to resupply along with the rest of the men.

The part of the city he could see from here would be the great palace complex of which he had read, the home of ancient kings. Its huge, featureless limestone walls presented an impressive façade. Within were many structures including, he had overheard an hour or more ago, the barracks of the army and the headquarters of the local military controller. It was there that the tribune and senior centurions of the Twelfth and Twenty Second were currently occupied.

Somewhere beyond the massive complex that stood on a high bluff and towered over the south rampart of the temporary camp lay the great city of Memphis itself, with its temple complexes so revered by the Macedonian conquerors, the bustling port that controlled all trade up and down the Nile, the warehouses and granaries, and the great monuments to a world rapidly slipping from memory.

His gaze darted to his right, where he could just make out the jutting points of the many pyramids on the hills to the west. Nothing spoke of exotic Aegyptus like the great tombs of the pharaohs. He would give a year's pay just for the opportunity to wander round them at leisure, soaking in their ancient atmosphere.

His eyes fell once more to the tents that lay between the great sights and himself. Somewhere in those tents, men were planning his downfall. Would it be swift? A knife between the ribs behind a tent and then a small group of men carrying him out of the gate and for a few hundred paces before unceremoniously tipping him in the Nile?

More likely he would be dragged, kicking and screaming, into the latrines, to re-enact the beating of the man he had saved. Would anyone come to his aid and deliver *him* to a medicus?

Warm night... relatively fresh latrines... ancient tombs.

With a snort and a start, he realised that he had been asleep, sitting hunched and hugging his knees on the rampart below the palisade. How long had he been unconscious? Not long, surely, or the guards who needed to pass would have kicked him irritably out of the way.

He was rapidly approaching the cut-off point. His exhaustion was so almost complete that he would be incapable of staying awake before long. Already this morning when he had examined himself in the bronze mirror he carried, his face had had an unnatural pallor and his eyes were sunken and stained pink, rimmed with deep black and purple, comically reminiscent of the make-up the people of this land applied to their face.

He would not last the night tonight without sleep.

And when he slept, he would probably die.

A sad way to end for a man of culture and learning.

Taking a deep breath, and after three abortive attempts, Cervianus pushed himself upright, swaying wearily for a moment as he regained his balance. He would have to do it. While the optios would hardly check the tents to make sure the men were present during the night, he would soon be found and sent in anyway if he loitered in the camp.

Staggering uncomfortably down the bank, sliding here and there, he steadied himself and strode toward the tent. There was no sign of light inside, which was a nerve-wracking sight. It was still evening, just past mealtime, and hardly late enough that the men would have given up socialising and gone to sleep. No movement.

He stopped and watched. Nothing. Cocking his head to one side, he concentrated. He could hear the low murmur of conversation, so low that the occupants were clearly whispering.

Clenching his teeth, he strode forward and threw open the flap.

Four white, intense eyes fixed on him from the depth of the tent. Something made him snap his head this way and that and he realised two more men lurked in the corners to either side, waiting for him to enter. Of Ulyxes there was no sign. Of course, they would get Ulyxes out of the way first as they would be unsure as to where his loyalties would lie. Four on one. His chances were impossible, especially given the sheer exhaustion he felt.

In a flurry of desperation and not knowing what he was going to do, he backed out, letting the tent flap fall and wishing as it closed that he'd had the foresight to grab his kit before backing out.

Sudden panic set in. His time had come. No officers around to stop it; no Ulyxes to leap into the fray and help. Just four men in the tent with murder on their minds: undoubtedly

Evandros and Batronus; probably Petrocorios, and one of the others.

A scrabbling noise inside, beyond the wall of leather, announced that they were coming for him now. Before he had even decided on a course of action, his legs had carried him around the corner and into the rows of tents. He was five or six tents away before he paused, wondering which way he had run in his blind panic.

As he listened, somewhere off to his left, he heard the barks of consternation as his "fellow" legionaries emerged from the tent, trying to locate him. Between these sounds and the gentle reek of the latrines on the breeze, he could pretty much pinpoint his position. He briefly considered calling for help, but the chances of attracting more enemies were higher than those of drawing the attention of anyone who might come to his aid.

He nodded at his own sudden mental decision and turned, running between the living quarters of his cohort, out toward the ramparts. The latrines were off to the right, stinking already, only a couple of hours into their usage. To the left: the main thoroughfare of the camp and another gate with torches burning and guards chatting away.

He was almost at the gate, his feet pounding on the packed earth, when the four men from his contubernium burst out of the line of tents.

"There he is!" Evandros bellowed and pointed as the others looked this way and that for their quarry.

Cervianus' speed increased in desperation as he closed on the bright torches of the gate. Of course, the gate was closed at this time of night and, while the men on guard there would be unlikely to help him, there would be an optio in charge and he could at least hope that that man would hold his rank in enough esteem to try and maintain order. He—

Panic exploded in him once more as he realised that the gate was guarded only by six legionaries and that two of them were the remaining soldiers from his tent: Vibius and Fuscus. No officer stood with them to prevent violence or murder.

Without even slowing, he slewed to the left, into the main road that led toward the headquarters. Out in the Via Principalis, men were sitting round small fires outside their tents, playing dice and drinking, munching on bread and meat. Briefly, Cervianus wondered whether he could call upon the help of strangers, but the simple truth was that he could rely on no one at this point. In his own legion there were more people that hated him than not, let alone among the Twelfth.

As his pursuers rounded the corner behind him at a run, he realised with dismay that their numbers had grown, picking up three more helpers from the gate.

Where were any of the optios? The centurions wouldn't be back in camp until late, but at least *some* of the optios should be around. Was he that unpopular that even the officers were deliberately staying out of the way?

In blind panic, he ducked left, disappearing once more into the rows of tents.

The important thing was not to get lost. Stay ahead of them to stay alive, of course, but if he got turned around somehow, he could find himself running directly into them instead of the other way.

Wishing he had Ulyxes' perfect memory, he jogged right by one line of tents and then ran forward past three of the leather structures. Another tent to the right and three more forward. Now three tents to the right and two forward.

He was acutely aware that he had no idea where he was and had forgotten already how many tents he had passed. The shouts of his pursuers were still reasonably close behind and he had no plan; no idea where he was going, beyond the need to stay out of their reach.

He suddenly panicked, wondering if he'd left his precious medical bag in the tent, but discovered with relief that it was still over his shoulder. The morning after that first incident, he had removed anything of value from his kit, including their ill-gotten gains from the storehouse, and handed them to Ulyxes to look after. Keeping his bag about his person at all times, he had left nothing but his standard kit to be rifled through by the others, an activity that he suspected had occurred a number of times.

"This way," a voice bellowed, disturbingly close.

Taking a deep breath, he ducked between two more tents on his right and ran forward desperately. An open space began to loom in front and he tried to decide whether open ground would be a blessing or a curse in this situation.

Before he could come to a decisive conclusion, he burst out into the Via Praetoria, another of the camp's main roads. Off to his right he could see the command tent and the officers' quarters. On the other side of the road stood the tents of the Twelfth, though he would find little solace there.

He glanced to his left in despair. The gates in every wall would be closed at this time and would open only with documentary proof of leave from an officer. By the time he'd argued, the others would be on him. Besides, the last visit to a gate had taught him he could hardly rely on the guard there for help.

His eyes took in the scene and a sudden surge of hope swelled in him. The heavy timber gates were swinging ponderously open even as he watched. A long line of men approached the portal, marching down the road with the clear intention of leaving the camp.

He frowned.

The men were clearly auxiliaries in plain, un-dyed linen tunics and chainmail, spears over their shoulders and flat, blue oval shields bearing the symbolic Aegyptian "Eye of Horus". Their bronze helmets gleamed in the torchlight as the group, perhaps thirty strong, marched on in perfect unison.

"He must be out on the Praetoria!"

There was nothing else for it. Taking a deep breath and offering up a prayer to Taranis, Lord of Thunder and patron of Galatia, he ducked across the street and ploughed into the side of the column of marching, white-garbed auxiliaries, pushing deep into their number, to the centre of the column.

There were barks of irritation in the unfamiliar local language as this interloper broke their ranks, but a shout from their commander at the front silenced them instantly and the men tried to fall back into step, making room for the man who had suddenly buried himself in their midst.

Cervianus crouched slightly, aware that he was considerably taller than the rest of them. Hands and fingers probed his shoulders and back and murmurs of disapproval surrounded him. A man that was clearly some sort of junior officer grasped him by the collar and yanked him forward.

He stared, frightened, at the man. Heavy-set and broad-shouldered, the man was plainly Aegyptian, his sun-darkened features heightened by a prominent nose, neat beard without a moustache, and brilliant white eyes and teeth that shone from the brown face like stars in the canopy of night.

"What... you?" the man asked quietly in broken Latin.

Cervianus panicked again as he heard the pursuers bursting out into the open behind the column. His chest heaving wildly, he gestured toward the noise with his thumb and then, meaningfully, drew it across his own throat, miming death.

The man grinned, highlighting the darkness of his features. With a deep rumble, he said something in his own language and there was a ripple of laughter from the men around him.

Cervianus tried to look as distressed and pleading as possible, clasping his hands in desperation. To his immense relief the man nodded and turned, the men around him falling into perfect marching unison despite the extra man in their midst who seemed to have trouble keeping time.

The shouts of futile anger back along the street suggested that the legionaries had instantly discounted the unit of auxiliaries from their search. Such was often the lot of auxiliaries: they were considered so disposable and inferior by the legions that they were almost invisible except during battle when they were of use.

The initial panic fading, Cervianus turned his attention instead to his immediate destination between the bobbing bronze helmets. The gate was wide open, half a dozen legionaries standing by to check the documents of this untrustworthy, irregular bunch. If they saw a hint of the legionary hiding among them with his relatively pale features and green tunic, everything would be for naught. He would be pulled out of line, the men following him would find him again easily and he would have earned the enmity of a group of auxiliaries who would be disciplined for the act.

He reached into his tunic and gripped Ulyxes' lucky coin so

hard he felt the edge biting into the palm of his hand. Closing his eyes, he prayed again, this time not just to Taranis, but also the Roman gods he'd become familiar with these past years.

Suddenly a hand grasped him and hauled him forward through the crowd.

Panicking, wild-eyed, Cervianus found himself passed quickly along the centre of the marching unit until he arrived at the front, the panorama of the open gate before him.

He made a strange, desperate squawk as he found himself on display. In panic, he tried to push his way back into the crowd, but the men behind shoved him forward again. The officer leading the column, wearing a skirt of leather pteruges beneath his mail shirt and carrying no spear, a blade slung at his side, turned slowly to face him as they marched.

"Shut up, stay still and agree with anything I say if you're asked."

In equal parts panicked and baffled, Cervianus simply nodded, falling into step. There was nothing he could do now but fall in line.

The unit approached the gates and came to a halt as the officer held up his arm.

"Authorisation," barked a legionary, stepping forward, though the look of sheer boredom on his face made it clear that this was a mere formality for him. He cared not where this rabble went, so long as it was away from him.

The officer handed over a roll of papyrus, which the guard unfurled, barely glancing at the contents before handing it back nonchalantly.

He straightened and frowned as he noticed the legionary among their group, out of armour in simple tunic and scarf. His frown deepened. The russet tunics of the guard and his men labelled them as men of the Twelfth. At least they might not be aware of who Cervianus was...

His arms by his side in formal stance, Cervianus wished he could grasp his lucky coin again.

The auxiliary officer gestured at him. "Medical personnel temporarily assigned to our unit."

Cervianus blinked in surprise, amazed that the man had spotted the bag for what it was. The legionary on duty glowered for only a moment and then shrugged and gestured to his companions.

"Don't forget to send him back when you're done with him," he sneered. "The Twenty Second need all the help they can get."

Cervianus ignored the jibe, just grateful that the man hadn't thought to question things further. The man leading the column barked a command in his strange, esoteric language and the column marched on through the gate, the capsarius struggling to fall into step again. Silently, the Aegyptian auxiliaries descended the gentle slope from the gate, making for a camp ahead that was similar, though smaller and with lower, less impressive defences.

As soon as they were out of what Cervianus judged was earshot of the gate, he cleared his throat.

"I don't know how to thank you, centurion."

The officer turned his head. He was short and wiry, dark-skinned even for an Aegyptian, and clean shaven. There was a twinkling spark of inquisitive intelligence in the man's brilliant eyes.

"Decurion."

"I'm sorry, sir?"

"I am not a centurion. I am a decurion; a cavalry decurion."

Cervianus nodded uncertainly.

"I would not expect you to know how our units work. Most of your legionaries see an auxiliary uniform and instantly forget we have ranks."

Cervianus swallowed. "You may very well have saved my life, sir."

The officer nodded. "Almost certainly, legionary Cervianus."

The capsarius blinked.

"Do not be surprised. I make it my business to know everything that goes on in an army I travel with. To be unaware of feuds and troubles is to be blind to potential dangers."

"I... I don't really know what to say, sir."

"You will not be safe in your camp at the moment. We shall make provision for you to join the cavalry of the Nome of Sapi-Res tonight. I shall send a man to your centurion to apprise him of the situation. I believe he is too strict a man to become involved in your predicament. Also to your friend, the troublemaker."

Cervianus let out a slow breath. "I don't know how to thank you, decurion. You speak exceptional Latin, if I may say?"

The man laughed again, a rich laugh, deep and heady, like the date wine his country produced. "I served under your Caesar and your Antonius. I have known the tongue of Rome for many years."

"And those of a few of your girls," a voice called out from behind, triggering a ripple of sniggering.

The decurion laughed aloud, surprising Cervianus. Such outspokenness in the legions would invite punishment duties at best. Centurion Draco had been known to beat men for less.

"Calm yourself, capsarius. You are so taut and jumpy you may do yourself an injury."

"Sorry, sir."

"I am Shenti, and my men here are the finest cavalry you will find in the kingdom."

"The province," corrected Cervianus and then bit his lip in irritation at his own stupid outspokenness.

"If you wish. Rome can call us what it wishes. To *us* this is Kemet, "the Black Land", home of the pharaoh, of Osiris the King and of Ra. Rome is an upstart child and will come and go like the others, but the kingdom will go on. Kemet is forever."

Cervianus frowned. "This is not *Aegyptus* to you?"

"Kemet," repeated the decurion. "Aegyptus is a name for Greeks."

The capsarius shook his head. "I spent weeks reading everything I could before we travelled. I wished to know everything about your land, and now it seems my research is lacking, after all."

Shenti raised an eyebrow. "Your books were written by Greeks and Romans. How can they tell you everything about us? Tonight you will drink my wine and I will teach you the truth about Kemet."

Cervianus grinned.

He had expected to meet death tonight.

Truly, this land was a place of marvels.

The capsarius awoke with a confused start and looked about. The surroundings were unfamiliar and it took a long moment to work through the fug of his newly wakened brain and remember what had brought him here.

The tent itself was a standard leather military affair, but the interior was far removed from its legionary counterparts.

Covered in hangings and rugs, it was comfortable and inviting. The bright early morning sun shone through the doorway and lit the interior.

Shenti, the cavalry decurion, sat cross-legged a few feet away, reading a text. The man looked up as he heard the movement and smiled. He wore only his linen tunic, soft, enclosed Aegyptian boots, and a belt that held a curved knife in a decorative sheath. His head was bare and the perfectly straight black hair was cropped short into an almost Roman style.

"Good morning, Titus Cervianus. I trust you slept well?"

The sound of military activity outside combined with the bright sunshine sent a wave of panic through Cervianus.

"What time is it? I'll be late for muster!"

Shenti merely continued to smile his pleasant smile and allowed the scroll he was holding to roll closed.

"Calm yourself. I allowed you to sleep late. You were close to collapsing point and needed the rest. I have spoken to your centurion. I must say, he seems an enigmatic fellow."

Cervianus stared. "Enigmatic" was hardly a word he would have applied to the miserable, grizzly veteran.

"He told me that so long as your kit was complete, you would be best to… 'stay out of his way for the rest of the day'. I gather your predicament has come to the attention of the more senior officers. You are in my care for the day, but I suspect you will be safe back in camp after today, with the watchful eye of your superiors expecting trouble."

The capsarius continued to stare at him, a feeling of welcome relief slowly seeping through him.

"I will help any way I can today, decurion, of course, but I know little of horses and the ways of cavalry."

Shenti let out a light laugh. "We do not need a complicated

supply session in the manner of your massive infantry force. We are ready to move at any time and so I have given my men the day to hunt and rest. Tonight we will eat well and take advantage of the chance to relax. From Memphis onwards, things will become much busier."

Cervianus frowned. "With respect, decurion, I do not remember much of last night after leaving the fort."

Again: that light, carefree laugh.

"You stumbled into my tent. You may have been asleep before you touched the ground. I covered you against the chill and let you rest. I hope I have not crossed some unseen boundary?"

Cervianus smiled weakly. "Hardly, sir. Thank you."

"You are welcome to stop referring to me by rank or title. I am not one of your superior officers."

"Very well… Shenti?"

The man smiled.

"How do you intend to pass the day?" Cervianus enquired, stretching.

"I will visit places while I am here and have the opportunity. I have spent my adult life as a soldier, first of Ptolemy Auletes and then of his children and of a succession of Roman generals, all in the Nome of Sapi-Res, but that is not my home. I am a child of the city of White Walls, Men-nefer: the place you call Memphis. You will come with me, as you say you wish to learn of Kemet… 'Aegyptus'," he rolled the name around his tongue distastefully.

Cervianus smiled and clambered to his knees. "I would be most grateful for the opportunity."

"Then come. I am tired of reading and crave the morning sun."

Shenti stepped out of the tent and into the streaming sunlight.

"Shall we go first to the city or the sacred cemeteries in the west?"

Cervianus, emerging behind him and blinking in the light as he adjusted his belt, shrugged. "I had wanted to see it all."

Shenti nodded. "Then we shall take a quick walk in the city itself. You will find, despite your belief that Kemet is exotic and strange, that a city is just a city, after all. Memphis may be the far end of the world to you, but the beggars will beg the same the world over, markets will still be noisy and the docks will still smell of dead fish."

Cervianus grinned. "But the great temple complex and the palaces?"

"The palace we may not visit. The entire precinct is undergoing rebuilding and reorganisation on the command of the new prefect; it will be a centre for one of the governor's military officials. The temple complex I will show you, however." He smiled. "Rome believes itself to be the master of the world – even the world of building. But I will show you that for countless lifetimes the people of the great river have constructed temples that soar and stop the heart with magnificence."

As the pair strode to the gate of the small cavalry camp, past the snorting horses in the stables and men carrying feed sacks, Cervianus cleared his throat. "You keep referring to me as though I were Roman. I am actually Galatian. My people came from far north of the borders of Rome and settled in the east. Only in these past few years has the republic claimed us."

Shenti nodded appreciatively. "Then perhaps you understand

us better than I expected. Your men often wear their hair long and in braids and bear moustaches. Is this from your culture and a form of identity that separates you from Rome?"

Cervianus nodded. "We are Galatian first, and then Roman."

"Then let me tell you of Kemet and the land you call Aegyptus, of the rise and fall of kings and of the gods that give us life through the Tears of Isis."

The pair strode out of the camp gates without being challenged – another difference between these provincial auxiliaries and the disciplined legions. The capsarius found, as they walked and talked, that he was beginning to relax for the first time in a week. He had not realised just how taut and nervous he had become until he felt it flow out of him.

They walked around the periphery of the huge legionary camp, where groups of soldiers were foraging, gathering goods and hunting birds in the flat land that led across to the river. As they strolled, Shenti began to tell Cervianus tales of the land that he loved, from the birth of gods, the jealousy and betrayal of Seth and the dismembering and reuniting of Osiris, to King Scorpion and his son who united the two Kingdoms, of the greatest of the pharaohs and the various transitory rules of foreign lands.

This last subject seemed to be of particular value to Shenti and he emphasised several times how these invaders had come and gone, each time leaving Aegyptus stronger and more independent. The land might be periodically conquered, but while its conquerors were lost to time, Kemet remained and never diminished.

The people he called the *heka khasewet* had come from the deserts and had ruled for only a few generations before the great warrior King Ahmose drove them out. At the time that Rome existed only as a simple village with grand dreams, the Kushites, the very same people the legions now marched south to chastise, had invaded and had ruled over the land of the lower Nile for a hundred years, only to be driven out by Assyrian invaders from the east. The Assyrians in turn only lasted a short time before Aegyptus became free once again.

Alexander, the great King of Macedon, had "conquered" Kemet, only to fall under its spell instead. He and his successors became one with the land, and Aegyptus had ruled Ptolemy and his successors rather than *they* ruling *it*. They had become "pharaoh" as sure as any ancient king. Now, however, there was no pharaoh and Rome claimed the land, but Shenti was sure of his world. Kemet endured and would be a power long after the "eternal" Rome fell.

Something about the notion and the way the decurion described it sent both a thrill and a shudder through Cervianus. To dismiss the greatest power in the world as transitory somehow changed his perspective.

By the time the pair had passed the great white walls of the palace compound and reached the city itself, entering its busy, smelly, noisy streets, Cervianus was enthralled.

"I can't say I truly understand the nature of a people who can view their king as some sort of god," he said after some time with pursed lips. "Gods are gods. Men are men. There is no blurring…"

He frowned.

"Unless you believe in Hercules and other Greek half-gods, but I have long considered them simple tales of old. How can you, who are clearly a clever and educated man, believe that your pharaohs have been divine?"

Shenti laughed. "The spirit of Horus fills the pharaoh while he rules and he becomes part of Osiris when he dies. He stops being simply a person when he becomes pharaoh, with the power of Horus guiding him. He is a vessel."

"I still cannot see it."

Shenti shook his head. "And I cannot understand a practitioner of medicine who does not understand the ka... the spirit, and how it moves and affects things. How can you heal without touching the ka?"

Cervianus sighed. "Anyway, what do the people do now, with no pharaoh? Surely, if pharaoh is divine, there is some sort of hole in the life of the people while there is only a Roman governor?"

Shenti's eyes darkened for a moment. "Truly. Some believe that your Octavian has already taken in the spirit of Horus and that he is now pharaoh. Others believe that pharaoh is dead and Horus lost. You will find groups of these all over the land now, clad in ash grey and predicting the end of all things as there is no pharaoh to lead us."

The two fell silent, the subject having killed the lively conversation.

Before them, the street opened out into a wide square and Cervianus' carefully worded retort on the subject of Aegyptian superstition died in his throat as his eyes took in the great temple complex of Ptah.

A wall of brilliant white ten times the height of a man rose before him, buttressed along its length and topped with decorative battlements, etched with countless images of ancient kings long gone and of animal-headed gods, scenes of offerings, of farming activities and of war. Carved men in grand crowns stood upon weathered chariots preparing to cast stony javelins at some unseen enemy.

His eyes straying along the wall, Cervianus saw the entrance to this, one of the foremost religious centres of the province. Eight statues, each painted with disturbingly life-like colour, stood, perhaps forty feet high, in a line, flanking the gate and its massive, breathtaking pylons that seemed so tall they might support the sky.

Cervianus realised that he was standing, mouth agape, while Shenti smiled knowingly at him.

"It…"

"I know," the cavalry officer replied. "It has that effect on many visitors. It is neither the grandest nor the tallest temple in Kemet, but there is something about it that fills me with awe. The statues are of the noble Ramses, perhaps the greatest of our kings."

"Galatia has nothing that could even reflect this, let alone match it."

Shenti nodded. "Come in. The temple complex is open to all, though many of the structures and shrines within are closed to all but priests. You will find the next place of interest, I am sure."

It took a little urging and nudging to get Cervianus moving again. He walked as though in a dream, his eyes staring up, marvelling at the sheer scale of the place as they moved ever closer. Craning his neck, he approached the huge open gateway and passed through, amazed at even the enormous lintel above the doorway that displayed a great eagle painted in bright colours against an indigo sky.

"Much as the Romans sometimes share their holy sites

between gods, this is the great temple of Ptah, but others have their places of worship here, for the ties that they share. See there the temple of Sekhmet and that of Hathor. Three on that side are all temples to Ptah himself. Aten is present, along with Amun. These are all places of great reverence, and you would not be admitted to them and must marvel from the outside."

Cervianus was doing just that, his mind reeling at the sheer effort and imagination that had gone into the place with its colonnades of enormous columns, shaped like papyrus stalks and painted with accuracy and care in bright hues. The huge, square buildings were as decorative and perfectly constructed as any he had seen anywhere in his travels. More so. His jaw refused to close.

"The Romans think our constructions crude. Without the use of an arch, the Romans consider most buildings crude. I suspect this is a simple display of jealousy in our new rulers."

Cervianus simply nodded as his attention was drawn to the left with a gesture.

"This, however, is what I wished to show you, Titus Cervianus, medicus and scientist."

A temple, smaller than the rest, though not much so, stood in the south-west corner of the complex, catching the brightest rays of the rising sun. Its colours seemed somehow more muted than the others; its decoration more sober; its construction more simple. Somehow, given the intricacy of the rest, this simplicity gave the building a significance that struck him instantly. To the side of the temple stood a smaller, more utilitarian-looking building, connected with the religious structure. Cervianus looked at his guide in incomprehension.

"This is the temple of Apis, the bull that is god; the sacred animal that is Ptah in our world."

For a moment a look of cynical disbelief rose in Cervianus' eyes, but he forced down the sardonic comments that leapt to mind. He would view this as a visitor and a man of reason without poking fun at his new friend's beliefs.

"Come. I will show you what I can. You may not enter the temple, but there are two things you must see."

Following Shenti, he strode around to the eastern side of the temple and was surprised to find something he had not seen in any of the temples in Aegyptus so far: an aperture.

"A window? I had read that your temples were always plunged into darkness to guard the secrets they contained?"

Shenti made a non-committal gesture with his hand. "That is an over-simplification and not entirely accurate. You are correct, however, that our temples do not have windows. This is the exception. Go, look."

Slowly, tentatively, not knowing what to expect, Cervianus shuffled closer to the window and, as he moved, the interior of the temple came into view. While the central chambers were likely dark and enclosed, here a large open room with no roof and a covered veranda around the perimeter came into view. The room was richly decorated with elaborate columns, but the floor was dust, sand and straw to suit its occupant.

The great black Apis bull stared out of the window at him, a large golden disc representing the sun anchored between the powerful curved horns on the creature's head. The beast was as well-groomed as any pet dog he had seen and was clearly well-fed and attended. Its back was covered with silks and linen in bright hues and with gilt tassels.

"This is a god?"

There was, surprising even himself, no sarcasm in the

question; it was a genuine enquiry. He was finding it difficult to look the bull directly in the eye. Something that smacked of an intelligence far beyond its species glittered in that brown orb. The capsarius had the unshakeable and very disturbing feeling that he was being asked something, or possibly demanded, by this supposedly simple creature.

"This is Apis which is Ptah," Shenti said quietly. "When he dies, he will join with Osiris in the same manner as the pharaoh. When that happens, a new Apis who is Ptah will be born and priests will scour the land for the signs and markings."

"And he is on display?" Cervianus simply could not wrap his mind around the concept of a beast of burden that was a god and that breathed, ate and defecated in a temple... and that was looking at him in that spine-tingling fashion, too.

"He is a living god. People must be able to worship him and give obeisance."

For the first time, the capsarius looked around and became aware that the decurion was half-bowed, making sacred gestures with his hands. Three other locals had joined them and were bowing, their baskets of offerings on the floor before them.

Unsure what he should do, he fumbled at his neck and fished the coin and tooth from his tunic.

"No. You need make no offering to Ptah. Save your charms. You will have times to make offerings and they will not be to this god. Apis understands."

Cervianus' brow furrowed. "You sound like a haruspex, casting divinations."

Shenti gestured away, toward the attached building. "Come. I know something of the gods and of science, both, and I suspect I understand you far better than you do I. My father was a *swnw*: a healer. He taught me a little of the herb and the spell. Your medici seem to only comprehend half of what healing is about. They understand the cut and the binding, the poultice and the potion. They can make a broken body well, but they pay no attention to the ka and the whole. You will not know the spells or practise the magic, and you will fail to save patients that my father could heal."

Somehow, despite the new friendship and Cervianus' speechlessness at the astounding sights he was being introduced to, this simple denial of his skill and beliefs cut deeply and annoyed him enough to pull him up straight.

"I appreciate your beliefs, Shenti, but you must understand that no amount of muttering sacred words and waving mystical sticks at a wound will remove infection, heal broken bones or halt the spread of disease. You mock me."

Shenti smiled enigmatically. "Not my intention, friend Titus. I merely wished to let you know that I understand the balance between science and magic."

"There is no balance."

Shenti simply smiled again. "If you believe that, the days to come will go hard on you. Surrender yourself to the ways of Kemet and your job will become easier."

The capsarius harrumphed and stopped. "What is this building, then? Another shrine?" he said petulantly.

"This is the place of embalming."

Once more, Cervianus frowned at him.

"Let me explain. You have read in your Greek texts, no doubt, of how our people are prepared for the next world?"

"You mean the mummification of the pharaohs? I have read in some detail. It is…" He stopped for a moment, aware of the pit trap he was about to walk into, but at this point unable to avoid doing so. "It is the most curious meeting of the science of medicine with the practice of religion."

Shenti simply nodded and Cervianus ground his teeth at his accidental consensus.

"This is where the Apis bull is embalmed after his death and before he is taken to rest in the western cemetery."

"You embalm and bury a *bull*?"

It sounded harsher than he had intended.

"Now you mock *us*, Cervianus the scientist."

The capsarius gave a small smile of surrender and held up his hands. "Not *my* intention, this time."

The two stood in silence.

"Would you like to look inside? You may visit the embalming house if you wish?"

Cervianus paused and finally shook his head. "Somehow it seems wrong to do so. What I would very much like to do now is to see the pyramids, if that is permissible?"

Shenti nodded. "There will be, as here, some buildings forbidden and barred to you, and the tombs are sealed, of course, but you will, I suspect, be fascinated by that which can be seen by the visitor. Come. We shall purchase fruit and water before we go. Then we will call back at the camp and I will collect my horse. Can you ride?"

Cervianus made a face. "I have ridden twice in my life and suffered three falls. The record is not good."

Shenti threw his head back and let out a loud laugh that attracted the attention of a number of local worshippers. "Then we shall travel by foot as the gods intended and save your rump from damage."

Cervianus followed the laughing decurion as he strode back toward the gate, but something was unsettling him deeply.

Shenti seemed to know a great deal about him, and had repeatedly dropped tantalising hints about what lay ahead for them, as though he had already been on the journey and was telling a tale of what had already passed.

He watched the back of the white-clad man as they walked.

With what could very well be the loss of Ulyxes to the company of thugs that was the Second century, he could very much use a new ally, and the auxiliaries were curiously far more accepting than any of the legion's personnel.

The sun had long passed its zenith, though the heat in the baking sands on the high ground to the west of Memphis remained sweltering.

Cervianus stood for a moment in the shadow cast by the immense pyramid that Shenti had told him had belonged to a king named Pepi. A cluster of smaller monuments rose immediately to the south – the burial places of queens and consorts, he had learned. To the east lay the great funerary complex of temples and passageways. Each pharaoh's tomb was similar. The cavalry officer had been at great pains to point out the differences and individuality of each pyramid and its ancillary buildings but, of the dozen they had walked around slowly and studied at great length throughout the heat of the day, the similarities far outweighed any imagined differences.

They were breathtaking and enigmatic, ancient and mysterious; but after the tenth one, they simply became "pyramids". It had come as something of a relief when, two hours ago, the cavalry officer had spotted a small, tented encampment out in the sandy dunes that appeared to belong to acquaintances of his. The chance to rest in the shade and drink fruit-flavoured beverages and hibiscus tea was most welcome. While the four traders they visited spoke not a word of Latin, they seemed genuinely friendly and flatly refused Cervianus' offers to pay them for their kindnesses.

As the sun began its descent, however, the capsarius had become conscious that he would have to return to his own camp tonight and prepare to march on in the morning. Shenti had stood to leave with him, but Cervianus waved him back down, telling him to make the most of the time with his friends. He would see the cavalry officer often enough during the long journey south.

Walking directly east from the tent, he had aimed between the great peaks of Pepi's tomb and that of his son, each on a high rocky bluff, and then closed on the left-hand monument to make the most of the shade. Just beyond them the sandy slope descended to the fertile river valley, packed with fields, drainage channels, palm trees and papyrus beds. Raised dusty paths cut between them and on toward the city of Memphis beside the Nile, where boats and barges were mooring for the night, the traffic on the great waterway dying away with the sinking of the golden disc above.

The route back was plain and simple: direct west would take him to the city walls. He would be back perhaps half an hour before the sun touched the horizon, in plenty of time to enter camp with a simple password, before the gates were shut and officers became involved.

Cutting to the right of the enormous pyramidal bulk, Cervianus entered the long, shady area of sand that lay between the perimeter wall that surrounded the tomb of the king and the resting places of his wives. In the blistering heat of the necropolis, this was one of the few places with respite from the ever-present sun. Sighing with relief, he walked on, running his fingers along the lowest slanting level of limestone of one of the queens' pyramids, the smooth surface buffed to an almost glassy sheen by the gusts of sandy wind over the many centuries.

He tried hard to remember some of the names Shenti had told him. Ininik-something-or-other; Merry-titties or something of the sort. Wives of a long-dead king. Ulyxes, for all the fact that he had as much academic ambition as a palm tree, would have been able to remember the whole list. The distribution of brains and talent in the world seemed so unfair at times.

And the pyramid at the far end would be some sort of small, false pyramid. This had been another point of contention between the two wanderers as Cervianus had been informed that, while the king's mummified body went to rest in the main pyramid, his ka, or "essence", needed its own, independent tomb.

What manner of belief could...?

Cervianus' heart lurched as a figure stepped quietly and menacingly out from behind one of the smaller queens' pyramids on the right. The thug Batronus was gripping a furca pole, his face a mask of grinning brutality. Another man stepped out behind him, also wearing the green tunic of a legionary from the Twenty Second, a man he didn't even know. This one, however, was brandishing his gladius, the sun gleaming dazzlingly from the polished blade.

Desperately, he turned, only to discover that two more of his "comrades" had entered the passageway behind him, hefting tools and weapons. Batronus, presumably sent by the cruel Evandros, had brought other lawless thugs from the legion with him.

Nowhere to go.

Desperately, he glanced left, wondering whether he could make it over the precinct wall. It was a death sentence to do so if he was caught, being in the sacred area of a pyramid, but then it was a death sentence staying where he was, too. A lingering glance, however, confirmed the impossibility of the plan. The blocks from which the wall was constructed were each the size of a man, fitted together so flush that there was no visible handhold. The wall was at least twelve feet high. He might possibly get over it, but not before they could get to him, drag him down and send him to Elysium.

The other side of the passage...

A quick glance and he realised that the recess between two of the smaller pyramids opposite was more than a mere narrow courtyard, but rather led to another passageway that ran parallel with this one behind the nearest small tombs.

With no other option, he turned and ran into the shadowy recess, panic overtaking him.

Where had they come from? They must have been shadowing him and Shenti all day to have found him now. Probably they had been waiting for the cavalry officer to be out of the way. While murdering Cervianus would be a difficult business, for all their dislike of the auxilia, the death of a decurion would mean an investigation pursued doggedly until the four of them ended hanging from a crucifix in the desert sands.

Indeed, if what Shenti had said was true and the officers of the Twenty Second had been made aware of the problem, out here would be the only safe place for the thugs to deal with him. His body would end covered in a mound of sand, desiccated and left forever to the desert, or possibly chewed over by scavengers.

Unless he could find a way out of this maze of monuments and get back to safety. Shenti and his friends were a good quarter-hour's run at full speed. He might just as well try and make for camp, if he could only get—

His thoughts became a whirl of spinning panic as his running foot hit a huge stone half buried in the sand, tripping him and sending him face first onto the gritty ground.

Now truly beginning to panic, his mind unable to focus on anything except a disturbing prophetic image of himself being carved open on the desert sand, he floundered, trying to make his limbs respond in good order.

Finally, with great strength of will drawn from the urge to survive, he managed to clamber to all fours, dust in his eyes largely blinding him.

Urgently, he reached up and brushed away the dust, spluttering at the sand in his mouth, when the heavy marching-pole his pursuer wielded swept his feet from under him and he collapsed once more, face first onto the sand, the sound of Batronus' guttural laughter surrounding him as it echoed back and forth among the ancient walls.

This was it. Four on one left him no chance.

The first dozen blows were not too bad, testing his mettle, and there was a pause as the two men who were already here tried to roll him over with their feet so they could get to his chest and face. His arms wrapped around his head for protection, his legs came up, knees touching his chest, trying to prevent too much damage, curled in a foetal ball. It would all be academic once the first sword blow landed. He could block the worst blows of a fist, but a gladius would signal the last moment of his life, if he was lucky.

Peering out desperately between his folded arms, he could see back along the passageway, out to the great pyramid itself. The remaining two men were sauntering along toward him as though they had not a care in the world, weapons out and ready for action.

Desperation lent him a sudden burst of energy and Cervianus rolled onto his front, bunching the muscles in his legs as they remained tightly curled beneath him. In a speedy, yet fluid motion that would not have looked out of place on the starting blocks of Olympia, his arms shot out, hands finding purchase instantly in the sand. His tensed thigh muscles pushed, launching him forward, out of the flurry of blows that bruised his back.

The move was smooth, though far from graceful. Rather than come up running, which had been his initial hope, he had frog-leaped forward a full body length and landed on his hands and knees in the sand.

Ignoring the pain from the many bruises and marks that had already been inflicted in such a short time, he pushed himself painfully to his feet and ran blindly forward to the next passageway, the men behind him barking in irritation at the sudden delay in their fun.

No longer cogitating enough to formulate a plan, he turned right into the next passageway with its own shadows cast by the tombs of ancient queens, purely because it was that knee that buckled and automatically turned him.

Struggling, he ran on and immediately found himself tripped once more, hurtling through the air to land with a thud on the sand, the breath knocked from his aching body.

Aware vaguely of the noises of his pursuers rounding the corner, Cervianus spun his head to see what it was that he had fallen over and registered surprise, even in his current state, to see that it was a stack of three shields, their battered, scratched surfaces showing golden thunderbolts radiating from the bronze boss across the peeling red background.

The Twelfth.

His mind reeling, he blinked away sweat and dust to see half a dozen heavy-set veterans sitting in a rough circle ahead, a mat between them covered in tantalising-smelling food and three small jars of drink. One of the men was holding his hands together and shaking them. Cervianus stared in confusion until the man opened his hands and the dice rolled out across the mat.

The men suddenly became aware they had company. Though their helmets and shields were stacked in two piles out of reach, each man had his sword and dagger to hand.

Standing slowly, they peered at Cervianus, floundering on his knees and trying to stand.

As he watched, their eyes rose from him, looking above and past the fallen medic. He realised the four pursuers had rounded the corner behind him.

"What in the name of shapely Minerva's arse is going on here?" one of the men laughed.

"Looks like the Twenty Second are getting impatient. They're going to kill each other first before we even get to Syene."

Cervianus tried to speak, but his mouth was full of sand and his throat as dry as it had ever been. Desperately he spat repeatedly on the ground and tried to scrape the detritus from his tongue.

"I know him," one of the men said.

"What?"

"He's that capsarius that got thrown in the slammer back in Nicopolis. You remember?"

Batronus' voice from behind growled, "You lot stay out of this. This is a matter for Galatians."

"Screw Galatia. Screw you."

The dynamic in the passageway shifted and Cervianus was acutely aware that he had suddenly disappeared from the picture almost entirely. The two groups of legionaries eyed each other warily.

"Back away and we won't have to beat you to death, old man. We just want the boy."

"Old man?" The veteran from the Twelfth's fingers danced across the pommel of the sword at his side. Cervianus watched through a veil of sand-induced tears as the veteran rose to his full height, the gladius sliding from his scabbard with an unpleasant rasping noise.

The capsarius tried to scramble to one side, but the first of his pursuers had reached him and stamped down hard on his leg as he moved, pinning him to the ground with excruciating pain and hobnailed boots. Cervianus whimpered as the pressure was released and blood started to flow from the seven or eight puncture wounds on his calf and the attacker kicked his leg away nonchalantly.

Staggering, he fell to his side and backed away, dragging the painful leg.

There was a chorus of metallic rasping noises as swords and daggers were drawn.

For a moment, he wondered whether to try and intervene; whether to attempt to stop the sort of madness that would result in legionaries dead from their own arrogance before they even met the enemy. Whether it was simple expediency or plain selfishness, he couldn't say, but in the end he remained quiet, clamping down his teeth against the pain of his bruises and his damaged leg.

The four soldiers who had pursued him clearly had the advantage of both size and youth. They were brutal-looking men, heavy-set and muscular, in the prime of their military career. The six men from the Twelfth were considerably older, each past retirement age, but they had the advantage of both numbers and experience.

Neither side looked worried. Batronus cast aside his furca and drew his blade from the sheath by his side. The challenge had already been thrown down and now this was no simple brawl or scuffle. At least four men would die in the sand between these pyramids.

For some irritating reason, a pang of guilt ran through Cervianus for having landed the half-dozen innocent veterans with this bunch of psychopaths. He shook it off as the four Galatian soldiers slowly stalked forward toward the six veterans, who stood calm and easy as though waiting to be served in a bar.

The men stalked past him, the one who had trodden on his leg sparing him a glance and motioning him to stay exactly where he was.

As the man turned his head away, Cervianus instantly ignored the threat and scrambled away across the sand. His leg was excruciatingly painful. Apart from the small wounds and the damaged muscle, his earlier attempt to move and the hefty kick delivered by the man seemed to have caused some tendon damage around his knee. As he tried to climb to his feet, the leg gave way uselessly, forcing him to collapse, floundering, on the sand once more.

He would never outrun them. It was perhaps an hour's walk at normal pace to reach the camp gate, but now he would be lucky to make it unaided before they called muster the next morning. Glancing back briefly at the two groups closing on each other, he scrambled as fast as he could in the other direction.

The desire to be far from this bloodthirsty act drove him on and, faster than he expected, he reached the corner of the nearest pyramid, pulling himself up onto it.

Turning, he realised that the ten men had engaged. The sudden bellows of rage and clanks and scrapes of fighting echoed around the mud-brick and stone structures, eerie in a place of the dead.

Cervianus bit his lip.

This whole mess was his fault. *He* had caused it. Now men would die.

But at least he might not be one of them.

His head peered around the corner, back past the stone that had first tripped him, and to the great pyramid of Pepi and the promise of escape.

Something drew his eyes back along the side corridor to the scene of escalating violence. Two men lay in the sand already, one of each colour. The man in the green tunic lay perfectly still, while the one in rusty red clutched his side and rolled back and forth, grunting.

Guilt.

Plainly it was guilt that had turned his head.

He had started this whole thing and now he was running away.

Shaking his head, irritated both at himself and at the fact that he was irritated at all, he turned round, staggering back toward the melee, his hand on the stonework helping guide and support him.

He had spent the day in just his tunic with his medical bag, the one item he never let out of his sight now; he was unarmed.

Shuffling across the sand, he passed the scuff marks and footprints and the small, crimson droplets where he had been wounded, and fell to a crouch. His fingers closed on the furca that Batronus had cast aside in favour of a gladius. The stout Y-shaped yoke, formed of inch-thick oak, was heavy and it took considerable effort with bruises, pulled muscles and a leg that hardly held his weight, but with gritted teeth Cervianus made it to a standing position, grasping the makeshift weapon.

Staggering, he moved slowly forward.

As he watched, another of the green-tunic legionaries disappeared in a spray of blood, collapsing to the ground as one of the veterans from the Twelfth ripped upwards with his gladius, carrying chunks of the man's chest and neck with it.

The casualties were instantly evened though as, while that man still fought to bring his gladius back down into the fray, one of the men from the Twenty Second thrust his own sword into the legionary's chest, driving it home to the hilt.

Gritting his teeth and ignoring the considerable discomfort, Cervianus picked up his pace, staggering forward until he judged he was within distance.

With every ounce of available strength, he raised the oak pole and brought it down on the head of the very brute who had carried the tool here from the camp, a sense of deep satisfaction coming with the blow. The dull thump confirmed nothing, but Cervianus was sure he heard a distinct crack, and the slight mist of blood from the blow showed how accurate his strike had been.

Batronus spun around, carried by the blow, his eyes rolling up into his head, and collapsed to the sand, his sword falling from loose fingers.

The remaining Galatian legionary suddenly realised that he was surrounded by four veterans in red and turned to see Cervianus behind him. His lip rose in a sneer but his eyes widened suddenly and he looked down with apparent casual interest at the tip of the gladius that protruded from his chest.

The veteran soldier behind him withdrew the blade, accompanied by a wet, sucking sound, and the man, dead from a single blow, toppled forward to the ground.

"Well timed. For a moment I thought you were going to run."

The man raised an eyebrow knowingly.

Cervianus swallowed nervously. "For a moment, I was. I don't know why."

"'Course you do. A wounded man who doesn't put his own life first is an idiot. Brave, but an idiot. I'm glad you came back, though."

The capsarius staggered forwards. "Perhaps I can save some of them. At least him," he gestured to the man on the ground in the russet tunic, gripping his side, "and maybe even Batronus... I didn't hit him that hard."

The veteran frowned as he followed Cervianus' pointing finger to the unconscious thug in green.

"*Him?*"

Cervianus nodded. "Hippocrates set the rules for medici. We do no deliberate harm. We have to bend those rules as soldiers, of course, but this man's not even one of the enemy."

The veteran shook his head disbelievingly. "Just how do you define 'enemy'?"

Reaching down to the unconscious Batronus, the veteran in red casually gripped him by the hair and drew his gladius across the man's throat, hard, cutting through flesh, cartilage and bone. The man who had held a threat of violence over Cervianus for weeks expired with a strange wheeze as the air escaped his severed throat amid the spray of crimson that soaked the sand. Cervianus stared in horror.

"Can you heal that?" the veteran asked with casual cruelty.

Still staring, Cervianus began to shake his head.

"Come on, medic. Sort my friend out and then we'll dump these bastards in a dark corner and leave them for the jackals. They come at night; there'll be nothing but bones in the morning."

As the capsarius staggered, clutching his leather bag, over toward the man with the deep gash in his side, a sword wound that had scraped along his ribs, he stared out at the fallen soldiers around him.

His fault. And yet here he was, wounded but eminently alive. Once again, he reached up and gripped the small silver coin on the thong around his neck. Ulyxes must be missing his lucky charm.

Cervianus went to work, professional as always, as the other men around him dragged bodies away and cast them into a pile in a dingy corner, throwing their swords and equipment in with them.

Around him, as he worked, Cervianus tried not to take in the huge sprays and pools of darkening, burgundy-coloured lifeblood seeping into the sand. Finally, two of them hoisted their dead comrade onto a shoulder. Cervianus frowned.

"What will you do? How will you explain it?"

The man who had first spoken to him, a man he had met

in a cistern in Nicopolis one week and a whole lifetime ago, shrugged.

"Men die. It's the way of the army. We'll sort it out. Don't worry, we won't involve you."

Cervianus blinked. "I don't care if you do."

And it was true. These men had saved his life today. Men from another legion had saved him from his own countrymen.

Sighing, he went back to work.

VI

THEBES

A whole week had passed since the incident by the pyramid. Seven days of aching recovery and nervous attention. Though he knew very well what injuries he had suffered during the fight, the medicus for the Twenty Second was still sent to look him over, confirming every diagnosis his patient had made. "Nothing critical" was the upshot; *unlike the poor bastards back across the river*, he thought. None of the scrapes, bruises or even tendon damage would cause any permanent trouble.

And so, when the legions had moved off south again the next morning, Cervianus had been assigned to the wounded cart that bounced along uncomfortably at the rear of the column with the supply wagons and artillery.

Initially, the very thought of the wagon lurching and jumping on the stony ground was enough to set his teeth on edge but, thinking more on the situation, it occurred to him that not only was he being spared the discomfort of marching along the endless dusty paths carrying a heavy yoke with all his worldly goods attached, but he was also being saved the distinct possibility that someone might just have another go at him while they travelled.

Evandros had not taken the disappearance of his pet thug

well, making veiled threats at every given opportunity. The fact that he and his small party of would-be assassins had simply vanished in the necropolis of Memphis had both worried and angered the man who had spent the past two years poisoning the men of the Twenty Second against him. Not only could he not prove that Cervianus was in any way responsible, he could hardly bring the matter to the attention of the officers, given the fact that they had had no business being out of camp and in the necropolis in the first place. And so Evandros had ground his teeth irritably as his sidekick had been labelled a deserter along with the three "heavies" they had borrowed from the Third cohort.

And yet the tide of opinion was beginning to shift. Without the support of Batronus' huge ham fists, Evandros was beginning to sound more and more like a petulant child. According to Ulyxes, the men of their contubernium seemed to have lightened somewhat in their attitude, Petrocorios even asking after the capsarius's health.

Oh, he still received bitter and glowering looks from some of the others, clear indication that the danger to him remained in the background, but somehow the threat to life and limb seemed less immediate without Batronus around.

And so for seven days he had travelled in the cart, his jaw firm to prevent biting his lip or tongue with every jolt. Seven nights he had stayed in the medical section with the rest of the wounded. He knew it wouldn't last. His leg injury was already, after a few days, so paltry he could realistically walk on it a little. Another few days and the medicus would pronounce him healthy enough to march, though he might yet be spared carrying his kit. He made the most of the opportunity.

The journey from Memphis to Thebes would take a little

LEGION XXII – THE CAPSARIUS

over two weeks, even at what seemed like a breakneck pace
for the support column, keeping to the fertile valley of the Nile
and following her bends and loops. A straight march would be
quicker but considerably less comfortable. It was *possible* the
capsarius could stretch out his recuperation until they reached
the great southern city; he would certainly try.

And then the world changed for Cervianus.

Ulyxes visited him the fourth morning after the attack,
grinning like an idiot. When the capsarius had questioned his
lunatic friend, Ulyxes had explained to him that Evandros had
been making overtures to some of the less savoury brutes in
the First cohort, but must have put the wrong word in the
wrong ear.

Cervianus had frowned as Ulyxes told him how Evandros
had gone out late the night before to meet with a particularly
nasty bunch of folk and had simply not returned. Questions
were being asked but the optio, knowing how close Evandros
had been with the men who had deserted a few days before,
had quickly called the matter to a close, adding a new name
to his list.

Cervianus had listened intently, scarcely believing his ears.
As he pondered the dangers inherent in proposing criminal
activities to dangerous men, a disturbing thought occurred
to him. Narrowing his eyes suspiciously, he glanced down at
Ulyxes' boots. No blood and shit this time. They were pristine
clean, as though they had just been carefully and thoroughly
washed. Cervianus pursed his lips and prepared to pose the
accusatory question, but changed his mind at the last moment
and sat back, allowing the matter to drop.

The threat to his well-being seemed to have gone, dealt with
by the helpful hands of a bunch of men from the Twelfth whose

names he didn't even know and by... well by an "unknown assailant". He'd leave it at that.

It was for Ulyxes to wrestle with his own conscience, after all.

Shenti had also made several visits over the days. As an officer, he found it considerably easier to make time to visit than the common legionary. The slight, dark-skinned officer seemed to have taken it very personally that he had not been there to help when Cervianus really needed him and had made a number of vows before a variety of deities not to let the same thing happen again.

But the week had been exactly what Cervianus had needed. Seven whole days that had involved no marching, digging, constructing or drilling. Seven whole days of feeling secure and not looking nervously over his shoulder every few moments. Seven whole nights of solid, uninterrupted sleep. And apparently time for the grudge against him to begin to lose its edge among the rest of the men, too.

Sighing with relief, Cervianus clambered down from the cart. It had been a stupefyingly dull hour, sitting among the other wounded, motionless and ignored while the healthy legionaries constructed the ward and medical tent, along with the latrines for the wounded. While there were little more than a dozen such men, the medicus of the Twenty Second, in a fit of reasonableness and compassion that surprised Cervianus, had insisted that the best facilities possible be made available at the end of each day's march, and so an hour's work had produced a full medical compound ready for the fourteen men as they climbed down from the three carts.

"Ward tent, bed three," the orderly said as he grasped Cervianus and helped him down from the cart. "The medicus will be round in one hour to check you, and then evening meal will be brought."

Cervianus nodded and smiled as his bad leg touched the ground, giving him a twinge in the knee for a moment and causing him to lurch before regaining his balance. Almost hopping until the sharp pain faded, he settled into a hobble and made for the tent. He was halfway there when he spotted the medical supplies being unloaded.

The position of capsarius was a strange one within the legion. The field medic was neither entirely physician nor full soldier. His medical abilities and duties spared him some of the more onerous tasks generally given to a legionary and granted him higher pay and a slight rank advantage over his fellows. And yet he was not part of the medical staff attached to the legion in any way and, as such, was entirely outside their organisation and command structure.

Professional interest got the better of him and as the other wounded or sick men were helped to their bunks, he limped forward in the late afternoon warmth, the sun now hovering tantalisingly over the rocky horizon to the west, and made for the medical stores.

Legionaries were still carrying the bags and boxes from the cart and stacking them in the centre of the compound, prior to their distribution and storage, and no one paid any attention to the wounded man standing beside them.

Frowning, he noted a number of items that he'd managed to glean from the stores during his night raid, though of a far better quality and much fresher. The medical staff was clearly higher priority for the stores than the capsarii. Trying to look as nonchalant as possible, his hand darted out to the pile and his fingers closed around a jar.

"Amagdalinum oil, lily root and Cypriot rose wax." The label was neatly lettered. As he tipped the jar, the oily substance inside slid down the glass surface, leaving a smooth slick that slowly sank toward the new level of the contents. He sighed. His own jar of this classic remedy for sunburn was so old and low-quality that when subjected to this treatment, it left lines of sediment on the glass.

Taking a deep breath, he thrust the jar inside his medical bag, through the narrow opening at the top, not labouring to undo the straps first.

"I hope that's going to be replaced."

Cervianus' heart lurched. Slowly, his face colouring embarrassingly, he turned.

The chief medicus of the Twenty Second stood half a dozen paces behind him, arms folded and foot tapping impatiently on the ground.

He sighed. Encounters with the legion's surgeon had rarely gone well. Albinus, like many of the officers of the Twenty Second Deiotariana, had been assigned to the legion by the senate and had come directly from Rome less than a year ago, his vision blinkered by Roman medical ideals and distrust of any form of innovative thought. The man, tall, thin and so pale that he could easily have been mistaken for one of his less successful patients, had receding, wispy hair and rheumy eyes that spent most of their time glaring from beneath furrowed brows.

Cervianus held an intense dislike of the man – a dislike that he knew was mutual. Sadly, while he was aware he had more medical skill in his left foot than Albinus had accrued during twenty years of practising with the legions, the man held an equivalent centurion commission and outranked him by such a margin he could barely see up to the man's level.

"Apologies, medicus. I merely wished to compare the mixture with the one that I have in my kit. It appears to be made to a different recipe. I assure you that you would not find the stores lacking later."

"Yes," the man said flatly. "I can imagine you will take every opportunity to replace it with the inferior rubbish you carry in that wreck of a bag. You are here under sufferance, legionary. I do not consider your leg strong enough to cope with a twenty- or thirty-mile march, but I might be tempted to amend my diagnosis if I find you interfering with the running of my valetudinarium."

Cervianus shifted uneasily. The man was as sharp as a shit-sponge, but had seen through his flimsy excuse with no difficulty. Sighing, he dug around in the bag, through the narrow hole at the top, until his fingers closed on the elongated jar. Briefly, he considered withdrawing his own inferior one to replace, calling the man's bluff, but the medicus was far too intent and irritable to take such a chance now.

Reaching out, he placed the jar back in the gap on the pile as two more legionaries dropped a heavy wooden box on the floor next to him. Albinus' head snapped toward them.

"Watch what you're doing, you ruffians. The contents of that box are irreplaceable out here!"

The legionaries nodded sheepishly and ran off toward the cart for the next load.

Cervianus was just considering slinking out of sight, when Albinus turned back to him.

"If there is anything you are missing from your kit, you may attempt to replace it tomorrow – with your own money, of course."

Of course, thought Cervianus, though even the *opportunity* was a rare one.

"There's somewhere around here to purchase supplies?" he said, frowning.

"Tomorrow night we will be camping before the walls of Oxyrhynchus. I am led to believe the markets there are some of the finest stocked south of Alexandria. I will *personally* sign your leave to go into the city and purchase goods if it will stop you rifling through my supplies and stealing the best."

Cervianus nodded thoughtfully. Oxyrhynchus was one of the largest cities in the province, a trade centre that stood at a major meeting point for caravans across the desert, from the sea to the east, oases hidden among the endless dunes, and even Kush, the land of their impending enemy. If herbs and salves were to be found in Upper Aegyptus, Oxyrhynchus would be the place to look.

"Thank you, medicus. I would appreciate the opportunity. I have no wish to cause trouble in your hospital. In fact, I wish I could be of assistance."

"That won't be necessary, legionary. I'm not offering this in the spirit of camaraderie. Just keep yourself out of my way."

Cervianus tried not to glare at Albinus as he turned his back.

"Help!"

The medic's head snapped round at the sudden shout to see a legionary carrying a body, staggering under the weight, blood splashed all across his mail shirt and tunic and running in rivulets down his legs.

The argument instantly forgotten, Cervianus turned and

hobbled speedily toward the two men. Albinus passed him a moment later and half a dozen orderlies and assigned legionaries rushed to join the sudden excitement.

"What happened?" the medicus barked as he reached the pair.

"Crocodile, sir. He was washing the latrine sponge for our contubernium in the river and the great big bastard thing just appeared from nowhere and got 'im."

Cervianus' heart lurched and he reached up and grasped the amulet round his neck.

"Did you see it?" he asked breathlessly.

"Aye. Three of us. Saw it and stabbed the bloody thing until it stopped moving. It's a big one."

His eyes roving across the wounded man, Cervianus joined the crowd of medical personnel, but his thoughts were elsewhere. Two crocodile attacks on the same column so close together seemed too coincidental. Unbidden, images flashed into his head of the strange old priest giving his blessing in the forum of Alexandria, and of the merchant at Nicopolis with his pendant: "*I not ask you want charm. I say you need charm. This charm.*"

He had seemed so curiously insistent.

He realised that, despite the warmth of the evening sun, he was shivering.

"Can you describe it?" he asked quietly.

"What? It's a bloody crocodile. Long and angry and with a million teeth!"

The medicus was shaking his head. "He's going to lose the arm. Lucky you were there, though. Just an arm; could have been a lot worse."

Cervianus frowned. "Let me see."

Albinus shot him a furious look, but Cervianus muscled his way through the orderlies and examined the patient. The bite had occurred just above the man's elbow, severing the muscle and removing a sizeable chunk of the flesh. He nodded quietly to himself as one of the orderlies applied a tourniquet and a temporary binding, trying to staunch the blood flow.

"I can save it."

"No you can't," Albinus said coldly. "There's too much damage; too much missing flesh. Hades, man, the muscle's torn apart!"

Cervianus shook his head again. "The joint itself escaped the bite and the bone is almost intact. Just a couple of tooth marks. The arm can be saved. Reattach the muscle and draw the flesh together. He might lose some mobility and it'll take a long time to heal, but it's salvageable."

He almost lost his footing as the chief medicus grasped his tunic at the shoulder and yanked him to one side, away from the crowd. Three steps away, Albinus rounded on him as though they were out of earshot of the small crowd who were, in fact, silent and watching intently, the blood still seeping to the ground beneath them.

"Listen, you: I will not be gainsaid by a common soldier. I know that you think you're the new Hippocrates and that those of us who have spent our life working to save lives and *not* with our nose in a book are little more than savages, but this is *my* hospital and *my* jurisdiction. Back off, or you'll find yourself back with your 'friends' before sunrise – possibly with disciplinary charges!"

Cervianus drew himself up, haughtily. "With all respect due to your rank, sir, I am not trying to gainsay you. I merely believe that the arm can be saved, and to not even contemplate doing so is to consign the man to the waste heap without even trying."

Albinus turned, aware that the wounded man, clearly in a pain- and shock-induced daze, along with all his attendants, was watching the pair with wide eyes. The medicus growled, angered at being put on the spot in public.

"You are quite right, *legionary* Cervianus," he announced loudly, stressing the rank. "The arm *could* be saved. It *is* possible. But before you get this man's hopes up and make me look like an uncaring butcher, would you like to inform the injured party of the inherent risks, or shall I?"

Cervianus swallowed nervously, aware of how more than a dozen eyes had just shifted apprehensively from Albinus to him.

"Well…" he began weakly. Clearing his throat, he found his voice, emboldened by the anger rising within him at the medicus. "There are inherent risks in *all* operations. If I were to repair the arm and it took infection, which is quite possible given the mess, there is the chance that the infection will spread. The arm will go bad, infect the blood, the humours will become out of balance and, in the end, it could possibly have fatal consequences. Certainly, the arm may have to come off eventually anyway."

He turned to the group.

"But they are risks; chances; possibilities. If we just remove the arm now, you save yourself the worst risks, admittedly, but you *know* what it would mean."

The men nodded silently. Limbless veterans formed a sizeable portion of the begging rabble that lined the streets of any city across the Roman world.

Albinus glared at him. "He may have to beg, but at least he'd be *alive* to do it."

Cervianus nodded. "I can't say it's without risk, but I consider the risk minimal and certainly worthwhile."

The medicus looked back and forth between the capsarius and the wounded man with his entourage. They were all looking nervous and expectant.

"What say we give the injured man the choice, then?" The medicus stepped back to the group and leaned toward the blood-soaked, deathly pale man. "Can you hear me? Are you lucid?"

The man nodded, a low moan escaping his lips.

"Legionary Cervianus has expanded your choice of treatment. Either I give you something for the pain and take the arm, clean and quick, or you can allow him to try and tie you back together, with all the inherent risks. Your choice: dangerous procedure by an upstart field-dressing applicator, or a clean quick safe job by your own medical section."

There was a tense silence.

"Save my arm," the man asked plaintively, his voice weak and quiet.

Cervianus turned and caught the anger in the medicus's eye before it glazed over with a professional hauteur.

"Very well," Albinus snapped, a suddenly aloof look to him, "I have better things to attend to than displays of false hope and breathtaking arrogance. I have a ward full of patients to look after. Minus one, of course." He turned his cold gaze on the capsarius. "He is *your* responsibility. You use *your* facilities and *your* equipment and *you* provide the aftercare. I relieve myself of all and any responsibility."

"Thank you," Cervianus replied. "Bring him with me." Turning and paying no further attention to the medicus, he strode off away from the medical section toward the carts that had finally been unloaded.

"Get that sheet of leather." Cervianus gestured down at a tent segment lying forlornly in the dust. "Wash it off and spread it on the cart."

The orderlies had gone, leaving only three legionaries and the victim. The men were staring at him.

"What?" he snapped irritably. The last quarter-hour had ruined a perfectly good day.

"I'm not going dipping things in the river after what just happened!" one man replied with feeling.

Cervianus sighed. "Then go to the water barrels on the supply cart and wash it there. The water should be clean anyway, not from the river."

One of the legionaries picked up the folded leather and ran along the carts to the water wagon. The capsarius regarded the other two men and their wounded companion. The patient was barely conscious, his head lolling.

"Hold him very steady."

Unfastening his medical bag, he withdrew several phials, handing them to the remaining unoccupied legionary, who took them with confused interest. Grasping the first phial, Cervianus undid the temporary dressing and tipped the contents liberally over the wound. Despite his mental fug, the man shrieked as the oil ran into the open wound and soaked flesh, blood and gristle. The legionary still holding the man, sweating and grunting with the strain, gave the capsarius a questioning look.

"It's ephedron. Very expensive. The amount I just used was probably a month's pay."

The soldier with the phials took the used bottle when proffered, his eyes wide at the value of such a small container.

"It will help staunch the blood flow and create clotting. I

haven't time to deal with each blood vessel, stitching them. We need to get the muscle reattached, clean the wound and close and bind as fast as possible to prevent too much chance of infection."

The two men just stared at him blankly, while the patient continued to loll. Behind him, the third legionary returned with the clean leather sheet and spread it on the cart. With great care, the two of them manoeuvred the barely conscious man onto the sheet.

Retrieving the second phial from his helper, Cervianus unstoppered it and leaned over the man, muttering to himself. "Six drops for a small incision or procedure; ten for a bad wound." With a shrug, he tipped a healthy quantity of the mixture into the man's mouth, closing it and smoothing the throat to make him swallow.

"I thought we were in a hurry?" one of the watching legionaries asked breathlessly.

"We are, but this is henbane, mandragora and cinnamon. It'll numb the pain, and we need to wait a moment for it to start working. We're about to drill holes in his bone and essentially tie the muscle through it. Would *you* want to be conscious for that?"

Cervianus cast a sidelong glance at the man who had spoken, the one who had fetched the leather flap. He had gone extremely pale and his skin had taken on a waxy sheen.

"If you don't need me, sir, I really ought to—"

"But I *do* need you, soldier. This is very delicate work and I will need him held very still, as well as needing things passing to me and taken away. I will also require an extra pair of hands at times."

The telltale noise of the man's gorge rising made him turn and cast a withering look at the helper.

"You're a *legionary*. Get a grip on yourself."

The man nodded, swallowing down the bile and trying to look at the wound without picturing drilling holes in the arm. He paled further, but stood straight.

"Good. I'll need all three of you. In a moment he'll be out, and the ephedron has already begun to arrest the blood flow. Who has the steadiest hands?"

The man holding the jars shrugged. "Probably me, sir. I'm a clerk in the fifth cohort. Good, close writing."

"Very well. You'll be doing the drilling."

The man paled to join his companion.

"Don't worry. I'll guide you, but I need to work on the muscle while you drill." He leaned forward, using a little water from his canteen to wash blood out of the wound.

"Two holes: here and here. Be careful not to slip when you start drilling, or you'll just create more work."

"Should *you* not be doing this, sir?" the man asked, quivering gently, and starting to wish they'd taken the medicus's offer of a clean amputation.

Cervianus smiled. "I would, but time is of the essence. As I said, I will guide you. Now fetch the tin in the bottom of my bag and I'll show you how the drill works." He turned back to the cart and nodded. "He's totally out. Time to begin."

Time had passed and with it Cervianus had watched subtle changes occur around him. Like a slow tide, the pall of distrust that had been directed at him for almost a fortnight had begun to recede – partially due to the absence of the poisonous Evandros, but also due to the slow recovery of the wounded legionary.

The operation at the supply carts had, thankfully, gone well. There had been a few hiccups and breath-stopping moments, but he'd managed to keep his worry at those times nicely hidden and, as far as the three men with him had been concerned, everything had gone precisely as planned. The muscle had tied neatly and had left enough slack that, with plenty of post-convalescence exercise, the man should be able to wield a sword again and his military career could continue. The flesh would take a long time to fully heal, of course, but there would only be a small reduction in flexibility. He would never straighten his arm fully again, but that was hardly a failure, given the circumstances.

Cervianus had spent most of his remaining pay on new supplies at Oxyrhynchus, finding, among other astounding things, a supplier of quality ephedron, somehow miraculously imported in from an unnamed location in the north of Aegyptus at almost half the price he'd paid back in Galatia. The sudden swelling of high-quality components among the capsarius's supplies had made the treatment of his patient considerably easier and more promising.

Regular applications of salves and oils and changing of dressings would hopefully keep away infection and pus. Shenti had tried to persuade him to a regular course of enemas, citing it as a critical part of staving off infection, gleaned from his father's clearly peculiar medical knowledge, but Cervianus had been saved having to order that indignity due to the lack of adequate clean water supplies.

He had prudently avoided the medicus after that dreadful episode, aware of how his standing with the medical corps of the Twenty Second had fallen even further now. Albinus had, according to the gossip, spent the two following days in an atrocious mood. Certainly, he'd signed off Cervianus that same day without a word, orderlies ejecting him and his gear roughly from the ward. He had returned, limping, with some trepidation to his own century, only to find that the tide had already turned.

News of his deeds had spread quickly from the three legionaries who had aided him, and, while there were still many glowering looks of dislike or distrust, some now openly smiled at him or nodded greetings. He was still an outcast in his own way as ever, but the hanging air of menace and danger that had accompanied him for weeks seemed to have evaporated.

Even Draco, never the most understanding or sympathetic man, had put him back on the excused-duty roster, allowing him to travel on the artillery carts and granting him leave to enter Oxyrhynchus for resupply, since Albinus had flatly refused even to see him, let alone sign his permission chitty.

It had made Cervianus smile to see the three helpers from that touch-and-go operation. They spoke of little else for the first few days, bursting with pride over their part in the saving of a fellow legionary and having performed surgery in the field. Imperceptibly and quietly, the legion's respect for their capsarii was rising; a fellow field medic from the Fourth cohort had stopped by to buy him a drink.

The wounded man, whose name he had since discovered was Sentius, had been delivered back to the camp with him, and the officers had authorised one of the spare tents for their use. Cervianus, along with those three men from the Fifth cohort, had moved into the new tent to care for Sentius, who first regained consciousness early the next morning.

The wound was still agonising and would be so for a long time yet. Sentius spent most of the days that followed in a haze of drug-controlled bliss, fed with a spoon and watched continually. Since Albinus still refused to have him in the wounded wagons, the man travelled, laid flat in the artillery carts, along with Cervianus. Each morning, he and the three legionaries with him drew lots for the dubious honour of being Sentius' latrine helper for the day. Both Shenti and Ulyxes continued to stop by socially as their duties allowed, though they were noticeable by their absence at latrine lot-drawing time.

Every day of the next week's travel he had examined the wound both morning and night, applying his salves and changing the dressing, and every morning there was marked improvement. Toward the end of the third day, however, he saw telltale signs and began to worry about pus in the wound. Without reopening, which he was loathe to do, he would have to wait and see if the sores erupted or whether there was just a slight imbalance in the humours. Regardless, he treated it as the latter, tending to bloodletting and application of unguents, sending fervent prayers to Asklepios.

But now, seven days on, as the Roman column approached the great sprawl of Thebes, there had been as yet no distinct sign of corruption in the wound and the man's lucid spells were becoming more frequent and made more sense. He began to sit up and feed himself a little and, to the great relief of all concerned, took over some of his own toilet duties.

The distant huddle of buildings that was Thebes, the ancient city known to the Aegyptians as "Waset", clustered around the massive pylons and courtyards of a great temple, yet even that immense and breathtaking structure seemed paltry and insignificant behind the great and famous complex of Amun that stood before the now-halted column, the fortress of the Third seeming dwarfed before it.

"Bet you can't wait to see Thebes."

Cervianus turned in his seat on the wagon, surprised at the voice by his ear. Ulyxes stood by the cart, grinning, his kit resting by his feet.

"How did you get out of formation without a beating from the optio?"

"Surveying duty. I've been sent out with the engineers to mark out the latrines, ditches, ramparts and so on. They won't miss me for a few moments. It seems like a year since I've had any time to see you."

The capsarius smiled. "Busy life, the military one. And in answer to your question, the answer is: yes. I've read a great deal about this place, and Shenti's told me more. Makes me twitchy to get in there and look at the temple of Amun."

Ulyxes' eyes took on a distrustful look. Though he and the Aegyptian cavalry officer had met while visiting Cervianus and exchanged words a few times, it was clear that Ulyxes was a long way from ready to place his faith in the auxiliary decurion.

Cervianus sighed. "And it'll be nice to stay in one place for a day or two. We're getting a lot closer to the action, I know, but I'm getting quite sick of bouncing along on a rickety cart every day."

"Try carrying half a storeroom on a stick and tramping through dust," his friend grumbled.

"Tried it. I'll no doubt try it again, too. Draco's being

unusually accommodating at the moment, but we both know that won't last. How's it going with him, by the way?"

Ulyxes' face fell into a miserable slump. "*One day* in the past seven I've not dug the shit trench. I was working it out this morning. If I keep this up all campaign, I could probably have tunnelled my way back to Galatia. If I ever catch that bastard out of uniform and in the dark, I'll jam my foot so far up his arse he'll be able to taste my bunion."

Cervianus laughed. "Dangerous talk. Keep it down."

"I mean it."

"I'm sure you do, but keep it down anyway."

"I did a little calculation yesterday morning. I've dug two thousand, five hundred and ninety-two feet of latrine trench since leaving Nicopolis. How much crap can one army produce?"

Cervianus grinned. The amazing thing was that he no longer even questioned the stocky legionary. With that memory of his, facts and figures were easily taken at face value.

"I can't believe you totted it up down to the last foot."

His friend nodded and stepped back, stretching. "If your charge can manage without his personal medic for a while tonight, we're having a few games of dice and a drink. I think it's safe to say the danger's subsided among the Twenty Second, so come and join us."

Cervianus nodded. "Perhaps. First I have to get things sorted for Sentius. The Third legion has been quartered in Thebes for quite a while and I think they have a proper valetudinarium. I'm going to take Sentius and try and get him a bed there, and ask their medicus to confirm that all's going well with him. It's nice to have a second opinion, even when you know you're right, and I'm never going to get one from Albinus now."

Ulyxes smiled as he hoisted his kit onto his shoulder again. "I hear they have everything on-site there. Even a few taverns and shops. I doubt we'll be allowed in, though. Hopefully they're not a bunch of pricks like the Twelfth."

"Oh I don't know. I've found some of the Twelfth quite affable."

"Sod off."

The capsarius grinned at his friend as he turned and wandered off to find the engineers and begin laying out the camp for the next few nights. Turning, Cervianus cast a professional eye over his patient, lying in the bottom of the cart.

"Think you can walk to the hospital of the Third, Sentius?"

The legionary pulled himself upright, slowly, being careful of the arm splinted with palm bark and slung from his shoulder. "If it means a comfy bed in a nice room, I'd get there on my knees!"

Nodding, Cervianus turned away and scanned the ranks of the Twenty Second who stood at ease, recovering from the march and taking a quarter-hour rest before unpacking their tools and getting to work. Centurion Draco was nowhere to be seen, though the optio stood nearby, overseeing apparently nothing, but with an intent concentration.

The capsarius hobbled across to him.

"Excuse me, sir. Could I have permission to take Sentius up to the fortress of the Third and see if we can get him into their hospital? He could do with the quiet rest and it would be useful to have their medicus look over him."

The optio frowned at him for a moment, his gaze rising to take in the wounded man slipping with difficulty from the artillery wagon. His staff tapped rhythmically on his greaves.

"Alright. Once he's in, though, you come back to the Twenty Second. If he's under their care, he doesn't need you."

The capsarius nodded gladly. While Sentius was pleasant enough company, Cervianus had been trying to think of a way to get out of the constant supervision at Thebes. There would be so much to visit in the city that he would be unable to see if accompanied by the wounded legionary.

He took Sentius' good arm to help, and the two men moved slowly out of the line and hobbled and shuffled along the ranks of the Twenty Second. The tribune cast them a brief glance as they reached the head of the column and passed the mounted officers, and then turned back to his conversation without acknowledgement.

The massive walled complex of Amun, along with its ancillary compounds, was everything Cervianus could ever have imagined, though the public approach had apparently declined since its heyday. A white, paved pathway ran up to the great pylons that flanked the main gate, twin rows of sphinx-like rams marching alongside it, creating a noble avenue for visitors to the enormous religious complex, visitors that had once disembarked on an elaborate wharf.

The wharf was now several paces inland, silted up and overgrown as the course of the Nile had shifted with time, while vessels were moored among the reeds that had grown up at the new waterfront. A faint, very regular depression in the ground inland suggested that once there had been some sort of harbour here.

Unlike the temples he had seen so far while journeying south along the great river, the enormous pylons of the Amun complex appeared to be incomplete. One side rose higher and more elaborate than the other, while the surface remained bare stone; in the deep shadows cast by the morning sun, he could see no carving or decoration. Somehow the lack of images made the entrance more sombre and meaningful.

How the Aegyptians, with their extremely religion-motivated culture, felt about the home base of the Third Cyrenaica legion sprawling at the base of the walls close by was a question that rose unbidden in Cervianus' mind.

Abutting the great temple's enclosure wall, the fortress of the Third had been constructed in the crook of a corner, where the ramparts of the precinct turned a right angle, and overlooked the new arrivals as they planned their camp between it and the river.

The Third legion had been raised in Cyrenaica by Marcus Antonius some ten years ago, but had prudently given their allegiance to Octavian before their former commander's fall. Six years now they had controlled Aegyptus along with the Twelfth. Six years spent almost entirely at Thebes.

Those six years had allowed them to construct a fortress under the authority of their tribune, using the only readily available local materials. The fortress was of mud-brick and nestled in against the enclosure walls of what Cervianus knew to be the temples of Amun and Montu. The colours of the legion, red and gold, rose above the gate. Just this side of both it and the sphinx avenue, a second structure was rising, Roman legionaries in dusty russet tunics clambering about on scaffolding. Presumably a bathhouse separated from the fort, perhaps for hygiene?

"Come on. Let's skirt round by the great avenue on the way."

As the two men approached the great complex of Thebes, Cervianus became aware of a low whistle from between Sentius' teeth.

"That's a big bloody temple," the injured legionary said as they made for the complex's elaborate approach.

"Enormous," Cervianus replied. "It's about the size of the fortress they're building at Nicopolis, but that's without all the ceremonial roads and ancillary complexes, of which there are several." He counted off his fingers. "Those of Montu, which is the one behind the fortress, and Mut and Khons. Each has temples of several gods within too…"

He realised that he'd drifted off for a moment within his own reverie, mentally picturing the various structures from their descriptions in his books. He looked around at Sentius, who was staring at him in befuddlement.

"Yes?"

"What's an 'ann-sillery'?"

Cervianus grinned. "I think it's something to do with bulls. Come on."

Leading the way, yet slowly due to his bad leg, Cervianus kept silent, watching the vast complex as he approached and trying to blot out the rising scaffolding of the new Roman structure that would stand defiantly before the walls. He could just manage a tantalising view of the rooflines of enormous temples within the complex, as well as the chiselled tips of huge obelisks rising toward the sky. Later, he would find a way to spare time to visit these places.

Later.

They walked slowly across the scrub ground between the river and the temple, blissfully aware that they were in no hurry. Neither man would be expected for camp duties and they had the optio's permission to be here. They would not be missed for an hour or more.

A few moments later, the two soldiers reached the great

avenue leading to the complex of Amun and paused to stare along the avenue of perfectly still, stony-eyed ovine guardians. Through the great, open gate they could see a wide, brightly lit courtyard, occupied by only a scattering of people, behind which loomed a huge building, whose brightly painted interior seemed to be constructed of myriad columns, lit by flickering braziers.

"You know all about this stuff, don't you?" Sentius asked quietly.

"I've read a lot on the subject, and a friend of mine in the auxilia has been rounding off my education when we have time."

"The cavalry decurion?"

"Yes. I didn't realise you'd seen him."

"Here and there, mostly through a blur, I'll admit. Why are you so bothered about it? Sooner or later all this will be pulled down or changed to look like a Roman temple anyway. They've done that all over Galatia."

Cervianus frowned at the thought.

"I seriously hope you're wrong there, Sentius. These temples pre-date anything Rome can boast. Romulus and Remus weren't even born when parts of this place were already ancient. As to why I'm bothered about it…"

He paused. It had begun as something akin to the interest of the keen traveller, but somehow it had become more. There was little room in Cervianus' life for superstition. Superstition was a grey area, and grey areas had no place in the world. To the capsarius, the world was largely built upon science and the decisions of men. There was a place for gods, but it was more ethereal – somehow withdrawn and separate. To mix the ideas of gods and of reason seemed such a ridiculous notion, and yet the longer he spent in this place, the more he was seeing the lines blur. Aegyptian life seemed to be constructed from a balanced mix. Of course, *they* believed it was *all* down to the gods, but that was a peculiarity of the Aegyptian mind – half of their superstition seemed to be clear science to him.

Certainly he had never in all his days placed his faith in trinkets and charms, yet now for weeks he had borne two of them and found himself clutching them with irritating and increasing regularity. The land of Aegyptus got under the skin.

"It fascinates me. I can't say why, but it does. It's so unlike Galatia or the world of the Greek peoples or the Romans. Somehow the differences between all the cultures on the other side of the sea are almost non-existent when compared to this place."

He fell silent, his eyes drinking in every detail of the temple complex's façade and the beautiful yet austere rams before it. Sentius turned to look at the building once again, nodding slowly to himself, presumably over Cervianus' words.

"Come on," the capsarius said eventually, and the pair turned away from the sphinx avenue and the great temple pylon toward the Roman fortress.

The home of the Third Cyrenaica had been constructed for convenience rather than defence. No traditional ditch system surrounded it, yet the fortress was protected well by thick, brown walls on two sides and the enclosure of the great temple on the other two. The gatehouse, as they approached, stood open, guards standing to attention within, beside and above.

An air of curiosity seemed to wash over the guards as they saw the two legionaries in their dusty green tunics hobbling toward the gate. By the time Cervianus was close enough to see the long street of mud-brick and timber barracks through the gate, a dozen guards and a tired-looking optio had assembled just outside the entrance.

"Halt there and announce yourselves."

Cervianus and Sentius tried their best to achieve a military stance, but the result seemed to be comical enough to make the legionaries of the Third grin.

"Legionary Cervianus, sir. Capsarius in the Twenty Second Deiotariana legion. Our commanders are surveying for our temporary camp, but this man, legionary Sentius, is injured and in my care and I was hoping to get permission to see your medicus with him."

The optio frowned. "What's wrong with your own medicus, soldier?"

"Our medicus is occupied and won't see us, sir. It's peculiar, I know."

The officer laughed. "All medici are peculiar. It goes with the job. What in Hades *happened* to you both? You've only been in Aegyptus a few weeks, haven't you? How'd you get into such a bad fight?"

Cervianus sighed and nodded. "Slight disagreement with a couple of drunken soldiers, sir. Me, that is. Sentius here was attacked by a crocodile downriver."

The atmosphere outside the gate changed instantly, the laughter cut short and the grins replaced by wide-eyed… what? Anger?

A chill ran up Cervianus' spine for no explicable reason. "Sir?"

"Get him away from my fort, soldier."

"But sir?"

"He'll bring the wrath of Sobek down on the whole damn legion! Get away with you!"

Cervianus stared at them. "He's alright, sir. He's going to be fine and the crocodile's dead. His companions took its head off."

The legionaries began making signs to ward off evil. One dropped his pilum in the process and the optio didn't even glance at him. "Jupiter! Are you *mad*?" the officer snapped. "The crocodile god claims him and you don't just *save him*, you kill the croc *as well*?"

Again, Cervianus could only stare in disbelief. The optio grasped him by the shoulder in a most un-officer-like fashion, and pointed into the gateway. "Who do you think that is?"

Cervianus squinted into the shadowy recesses of the gatehouse. Half a dozen altars stood in recesses, used by the common soldiers to crave boons of the gods. He couldn't see the carved inscriptions from this distance, but the centre one was all too familiar. A statue of a human figure in mid-stride with a staff in one hand and the head of a crocodile rose from the top of the altar, cemented on to the crown of the block.

"You can't be serious?"

The optio growled. "Sobek is the warrior god of this country. He watches over us. Occasionally he decides to take a sacrifice. We don't give him them... he likes to take them himself, and they're not always animals. You don't want to be a sacrifice, you don't go near the river. The locals allow us to stay here without any trouble, even in their holiest places, because we honour Sobek and their other gods. Believe me, you don't want to cross the crocodile god. Now take that cursed bastard away from my fortress and get him across the river. Camp there. If the locals find out what happened and that he's still here, they'll go *loopy*!"

Cervianus shook his head. "Sir, can I see the medicus first?"

"No you bloody can't. If I tell him what's happened, he'll be the first to throw you out. Now piss off."

As Cervianus stood staring blankly at the officer, the man turned to his guards and gestured with his free hand.

"You three: take this pair back to their unit and explain the situation to their centurion. Then get them a boat and make sure they're nowhere near Thebes by nightfall."

The three legionaries strode forward, one of them grabbing Sentius roughly, causing him to wince, and turned the pair, marching them away from the gate. The capsarius followed, his mind reeling. What was wrong with this place?

Draco stood beside the optio and frowned. "Run that by me again?"

The legionary nodded, still standing to attention. "It's for the good of everyone, sir. My commander is busy making the stores ready for your resupply, and provisions will be made for you and your men to use our bathhouse, but he graciously requests that the man marked by Sobek stay on the far side of the river."

The centurion turned and raised an eyebrow at his optio, who simply shrugged. Cervianus and his patient stood a little apart from the group, their expressions wandering back and forth between anger and disbelief.

"Alright," Draco said finally. "Seems damn stupid to me, but this is his command. I'll attend to it. Run along and report back."

The legionary dithered, looking distinctly uncomfortable.

"Problem?"

"My centurion told me to get them on a boat and make sure they go."

A low growl issued from somewhere in Draco's throat. "Don't test my patience, soldier. Go and report. I will deal with this."

There was an air of finality to his voice that brooked no argument. The legionary saluted and turned, gratefully, marching off with his two companions toward the fortress. Draco shook his head in disbelief and Cervianus cleared his throat, ready to take a chance.

"Sir? This is ridiculous."

The optio's head snapped round and his vine staff came up in warning, but Draco nodded solemnly. "For once I agree with you. Sheer idiocy."

Cervianus sighed with relief, but Draco shook his head.

"Still, this is the Third's territory. They know the land and the people better than us; we're just guests here. We'll commandeer a couple of those little fishing boats down there."

Cervianus stared. "Sir?"

"I'm not about to defy the local garrison. You'd best stay across the river until we're ready to move on the day after tomorrow. I'll have supplies sent over periodically."

The capsarius shook his head. "Sir, there's no defences over there, no latrines or baths. We can't resupply or *anything*." The sudden looming likelihood that cult city of Thebes would be added to the list of great sights of Aegyptus that he would be forced to walk past without seeing plunged his mood deep into the earth.

"We'll make all arrangements necessary." The centurion turned back to the construction work being undertaken on the

LEGION XXII – THE CAPSARIUS

temporary camp. "Cervianus' contubernium," he bellowed, "get your kit and report to me."

The capsarius watched in dismay as the remaining five men in his unit hoisted their tools, wiping the sweat and dirt from their brows, and collected their yokes and shields. In just moments they were standing to attention before the officer.

"This wounded man is required by the local garrison commander to remain on the far bank while we stay in Thebes. Since legionary Cervianus is currently dealing with him, that means *he* is also going, which means I'm sending the rest of you across so there's enough of you to set sentries. I know you're below strength without your two deserters, but we'll reassign someone and send them over to join you."

Two of the legionaries glowered at Cervianus, but said nothing. Ulyxes smiled.

"Take one or two of those fishing boats down there and set up somewhere across the river. Have a fire going for signalling. If you need to report or request anything, one or two of you can come back across but not Cervianus or the wounded man. Got that?"

A mumbled chorus of affirmation rippled through the unit.

"Now go."

The seven men turned, two of them supporting each other, and made their way down toward the bank of the Nile, an area of the shore having been cleared of the interminable reeds here for the mooring of small fishing boats.

"Bloody typical. No living it up for us, just 'cause of him," Fuscus grumbled loudly as soon as they were away from the officers.

Ulyxes punched him lightly on the arm and laughed.

"You daft sod. You've just got out of hours of camp construction and then trench digging and everything. Plus you won't have to do camp guard duty. There won't be any officers over there with us, either. I've got dice and..."

He glanced over his shoulder to make sure the centurion was paying them no attention and then rifled in his kit and peeled back the bag to show the stoppered top of two wine jars inside.

"I think we'll have a better night than most of that lot eh?"

The mood among the group lightened noticeably at that and by the time they had chosen two of the unmanned boats and loaded their gear, the men were laughing and making plans for the night.

Cervianus was almost relaxed as he dropped his battered leather bag into the small vessel, and then he caught sight of Sentius. The wounded man stood back from the bank, rubbing his splinted arm rhythmically and staring out into the water with wide eyes. He was shaking slightly. One of the legionaries in the other boat, using an oar to push off from the bank, laughed.

"Come on you knob. Get in the boat. It's only water."

Taranis, but I hope that's true, Cervianus thought to himself.

"Come on. There's nothing here," he said to Sentius, yet his eyes roved around the bank and out across the water as he spoke. There were no reeds and the bank was solid and steep here. Logically it would be an unlikely place to find a crocodile, but recent events had led some of the men to become a great deal more wary about the great life-giving waters of Aegyptus.

Hesitantly, the wounded man made his way down to the boat, his eyes darting back and forth constantly. Even in the boat, as he sat, his shuddering was felt by the other occupants as a vibration in the wood. Slowly, carefully, Ulyxes grasped the oars and pushed away from the bank. The other boat was already a way out and, following their example, Ulyxes angled the vessel upstream and rowed into the current to stop them drifting too far off course in the strong waters.

It was a nervous trip for at least two of the passengers, but some quarter of an hour later the boats were on the west bank and being tied to wooden posts among the reeds. Cervianus had become more and more nervous as they approached the mass of green at the river's edge, and Sentius had begun to let out a series of low moans, his eyes wide and apprehensive. It had taken a supreme effort for Cervianus to bite down and control his own fears long enough to smile confidently and help Sentius onto dry land.

And so the seven men clambered ashore and stomped up through the soft silty earth until they stood together on the western bank, looking across the wide waterway to the great sprawl of Thebes with its temples and fortress. Cervianus gave the city a longing glance and then, sighing with regret, turned away and followed the laughing, unconcerned legionaries as they moved away from the river. Sentius walked fast, desperate to be away from the reeds.

"Let's get back far enough from the water to be safe and set up," Cervianus said, pointing ahead.

Sentius shook his head. "Back to the rocks. For safety."

"That's got to be a mile and a half away!"

"No," Ulyxes said flatly. "We need to be close enough to the bank for anyone from the legion to find us quickly, and any further back than this and our fire won't be seen; it's flat as a fart right back to those cliffs."

Sentius continued shaking his head, but the others downed their kit. Cervianus turned to the wounded legionary, trying to put on a confident voice, though their proximity to the water was having an effect on his own nerves.

"Nothing will come close when we have the fire going. Besides, we'll put up a small fence and rampart and set a sentry."

"Great," one of the others complained. "I thought we'd got out of digging and building."

Ulyxes laughed and grasped his trenching tool.

"Come on. It's only got to be fifteen feet across. We can fortify the place in about quarter of an hour."

Cervianus reached down for a dolabra, but Ulyxes shook his head and pointed.

"We can do this. You look after him."

The two wounded men stood in the late afternoon sunlight as their companions hastily constructed the defences of their tiny camp and then put up the large leather tent and started the small fire that would provide warmth, food and a method of staying in contact with the rest of the legion.

Time passed for the exiled unit, the sun slowly descending behind the cliffs to the west. The setup was, he had to admit, quite cosy. There was something relaxing about being the masters of their own camp, running their own schedule and setting their own watch with no officers around to bully them and no stink of the latrine trench. There would still be Vibius and his notorious wind to deal with later, but the entire contubernium was used to that. Might come as a surprise to Sentius though. Cervianus smiled.

Dinner had been early, quick and easy, supplemented with a few vegetables they had found growing in a small garden area in the corner of the next field while searching for wood. As soon as the meal was done and the sun made its last farewells before falling into the western desert, Ulyxes produced his wine flasks and dice. Cervianus noted with a grin that the flasks were stamped as the property of a man called Facilis from the Second cohort.

Bowing gracefully out of the dice game, Cervianus had agreed to take first watch. For over an hour he had moved around gradually, viewing the inky landscape from the four corners of the small rampart in turn.

The landscape was impressive. Flat and lush, green fields extended up and down the valley as far as he could see, as well as a mile or so each side of the river before giving way to brooding, buff-coloured cliffs and peaks, spotted with regular angles that spoke of human constructions.

Cervianus sighed. Oh to be able to visit Thebes.

He almost fell over his pilum when the figure of a man in a white robe drifted silently out from behind a dark stand of trees nearby like one of the *lares*, the spirits the legion's priest had them honour on feast days and special occasions.

"Halt. Give the password!"

Damn it. Forgot to challenge with who they were first.

A familiar, velvety voice replied, "Veniunt porci." There was a light laugh. "And your camp prefect apparently has a sense of humour, given his choice."

Cervianus relaxed and lowered his hastily raised weapon and shield. "Shenti? What in Hades are you doing here?"

The decurion approached the gap in the defences that served as a gate and the capsarius moved the sudis stakes that formed a temporary barrier, allowing his friend access.

The cavalry officer entered the circle of firelight and smiled at the noises of revelry from the tent beyond the dancing flames. He was clad only in his white tunic, scarf and cloak, the curved knife at his belt his only equipment.

"We just returned from a sweep of the surrounding area and as soon as I heard the news I decided to wander over and see you. My men are occupied sorting out gear with the extra auxiliary units we're collecting here so I left them to it."

Cervianus smiled. "Can't say I'm not glad. This lot are good enough company I suppose, but there are times I long for a more involved conversation than what Vibius would like to do to a young woman he met in Nicopolis or how Fuscus' feet smell."

The officer laughed and sank to a crouch by the fire. "So I hear you're the victim of superstition?"

The capsarius joined his friend, frowning. "You mean you don't share their sentiments?"

Again, his friend laughed. "Gods, no. But then I am from the low country and things are different this far upriver. We of the delta respect and fear Sobek, of course, but he is as much a curse as a blessing. Where I come from, dangerous crocodiles are killed to prevent them taking people and animals. You're near Ambo here, though, and that's the very centre of the crocodile god's cult."

"Great."

Shenti grinned. "I'm sure you'll be pleased to hear that they keep sacred crocodiles there. The whole precinct, the town around it and the entire bank nearby are crawling with them."

Cervianus shuddered. "I'd best keep my nervous new friend far away from there, then."

"Sadly, no." Shenti's face took on a serious cast. "While I do not share these peoples' voracity in their worship, it would still be best to seek Sobek's blessing at Ambo. An offering from you both would go a long way to redeeming you in the eyes of even the most superstitious local."

"But it won't matter when we leave here. No one else will know."

"Do not forget," the auxiliary officer reminded him, "that we are taking two cohorts of the Third with us from here, as well as several local auxiliary units. It would be as well if they were willing to work alongside you rather than seeing you as a problem."

Cervianus sighed. "Every time I think I'm starting to get to grips with this land, it throws me again. Will you come with us to this Ambo? Should we go tomorrow?"

Shenti shook his head and laughed.

"We will pass the temple in three or four days' time. It lies between here and Syene. I may join you, if duties allow; we will be joining battle soon after, and it is worth seeking the Crocodile Lord's blessing before then. I have already made my offerings to Maahes and Sekhmet at a temple perhaps a mile from here."

Cervianus slumped slightly. "I was dearly hoping to see the great complex of Amun and others while we were in Thebes, but it seems that is yet another place I shall miss."

The decurion nodded thoughtfully. "You may be forbidden from crossing the water here, but there is much I can show you on the west bank. You will be astounded by some of the things here, I am sure: the temple of the queen who was a king, for instance? Or the twin statues of Amenophis the Third at his temple near here? That is where you can give offerings to Sekhmet if you wish. Ask her to turn her arrows of flame upon the Kushites and aid our cause?"

The capsarius pulled himself a little further upright, his smile slowly returning. "There's enough to see here to fill a free day?"

Shenti laughed. "There are wonders and marvels on this side of the river that would fill a lifetime for you. Tomorrow I will return and take you to them. For now, I must return to the east bank. I have yet to use the baths and, while I'm sure you would love nothing more, I have been in close and sweaty contact with a horse for the past week and am in greater need."

Cervianus laughed. "Go on then, my friend, and I shall await you in the morning."

Shenti nodded and stood, stretching, before turning and pushing his way through the defences to disappear off in the night. Cervianus watched him go, weighing the decurion up in his head. He was an insightful and intelligent man, prone to some dubious superstition, but clearly more reasoned than many of his countrymen.

A cough from behind startled him and he swung around to the tent.

"Who was that?" asked Ulyxes, frowning.

"Shenti. Stopped in for a visit."

"Oh," came the unemotional response.

Cervianus stretched. "I've done my hour and a half. Your turn on watch now."

Ulyxes' face fell, but he shrugged resignedly. "They're starting to resent my luck anyway. Go get some wine and play some dice. Your patient's bloody awful at it. You could get rich."

Cervianus laughed. "Actually, I just want to sleep. For some reason I'm absolutely knackered."

Ulyxes stood and leaned on his pilum. "Good night. Dream of slippery women."

Cervianus laughed as he disappeared into the tent.

Mist billowed through the night-shrouded vegetation – a warm mist, as though the sun had boiled the great Nile dry and wafted it across the land.

It was a dream. Cervianus was curiously aware that it was a dream, although he appeared to be too invested in it to wake – not even sure he would wish to if he could.

He was alone in the field this time. No hilarious japes with Ulyxes leaping out of the bushes and urinating himself. The statue stood as it had in his waking memory, at a slight lean, half hidden by foliage, the piercing eyes boring into his above that long, curved beak.

Like most of the statues he had seen, Thoth was portrayed with one foot forward, as though striding from his plinth, one hand stretched out before him, holding an ankh that had long ago been stolen or destroyed.

Although…

As he watched, the grey basalt began to crack, hairline fractures appearing, expanding and meeting up all across the smooth exterior. He tried to step back, but his feet were as heavy as lead and he felt somehow weighed down as though with the kit of a thousand soldiers; of ten thousand soldiers.

His eyes widened as the cracks spread and shards of basalt dropped to the ground. The surface was moving, twisting, rippling like living flesh. The ankh long gone, grey fingers closed into a fist and then opened once more, palm up, hand stretched out forward.

And now he could suddenly move. He wanted to shout in alarm, but for some reason it seemed impossible to do so. He stepped back, not knowing where to go. The god was stepping forward toward him without moving. Curious. A trick of perspective?

A flitting movement caught his attention at the periphery of his vision and his eyes swivelled in panic. A great crocodile-headed god of some black stone reached out with a grasping hand, drawing, taking...

No. Not now! To his left, another: a goddess with shapely figure and full breasts, surmounted by the head of a vicious lion, roaring defiance at the night, fangs of granite glistening wetly as the surface rippled and cracked. She reached.

Behind the three, other animal-headed gods loomed in the darkness, their hands raised.

Cervianus felt his heart stop.

He awoke with a start, running with feverish sweat, shaking uncontrollably. The interior of the tent was dark. The sounds of sleeping men and gentle flatulence mobbed his ears. A gentle golden glow on the leather confirmed the watch fire was still burning outside, and he could just hear a low voice humming an old soldiers' tune out by the rampart.

Lying in the dark, desperately trying in his panicked, confused mind to draw a definite line between the world of dream and that of reality, he was sure of one thing: a thing that confused and worried him and yet somehow made him feel better about the whole experience.

The gods had not been clawing or lunging or grasping.

They were reaching out desperately in supplication.

Closing his eyes and lying back, quivering, Cervianus failed entirely to return to sleep.

VII

AMBO TO SYENE

"Is that Ambo?"

Shenti nodded, his horse dancing slightly, impatient to move faster. Cervianus squinted into the bright, dust-filled air. He was in equal parts anxious and pleased at having finally reached this place, even if that put them only twenty-four more hours away from action.

Three days on from Thebes and with yet more soldiers, both legionary and auxiliary, the column marched in a stolid silence, each man introspective and contemplating their mortality and the danger of the coming days.

The dream Cervianus had experienced on the west bank four nights ago had continued to colour his waking hours ever since. The next morning, Shenti had led him on a tour around the temples of long-dead pharaohs, the huge three-tiered complex of Hatshepsut, colossal statues that howled eerily at the morning sun, and more – endless breathtaking marvels.

Sights most citizens of Rome would never see.

Sights that a month ago would have made Cervianus twitch with anticipation.

Somehow, though, walking around those enormous structures had merely brought constant jarring recollections of the dream; echoes that threatened to overwhelm him. He had found that he had trouble meeting the blank, glassy stares of the various gods that stood silent witness to his passing in those great buildings. He had been uneasy around the temples and had not enjoyed the day in the slightest.

The army had resupplied and taken the chance to use the bathhouse and visit the city. Cervianus and his charge had not. Ulyxes had stayed in the small encampment with Sentius during Shenti's visit and tour, citing a bad head from the previous night and the need to sleep late and relax.

The next night the capsarius had lain down on his blankets with no small amount of trepidation, fearing what the night might hold for him but, despite his nerves and the added influence of the temples on Thebes' west bank, he had slept early, long, and peacefully. Still, though he took some solace in his dream-free night, his solid belief in reason had been repeatedly assailed by undeniable strangeness for weeks, and this place had left him feeling jumpy and uncertain. He had been almost glad to move on the next day as the army mustered for the march.

Draco had, perhaps shrewdly, sent him and Sentius to travel with the auxiliaries, keeping the pair of them away from the superstitious men of the Third, and for three days up the river, the two legionaries had bounced along in the support carts for Shenti's cavalry. Sentius seemed as relaxed as a legionary on campaign could hope to be, smiling happily in the wagon as they travelled. Shenti was his usual calm and enigmatic self.

Cervianus, on the other hand, was becoming prey to nerves and tension, the intensity increasing as they neared their destination. Syene would introduce them to their enemy: the Kushite invader. He had been on enough campaigns with the

Twenty Second that he knew this one would be extraordinarily unlikely to end at Syene, but that would certainly be where it would begin.

Tomorrow.

And he couldn't escape the feeling that his dreams were trying to tell him something, and that whatever that was, it was both important and imminent.

"Shenti?"

"Yes, my friend."

"What do you know of the Kushites?"

Shenti narrowed his eyes. "You wish to prepare yourself for your enemy." It was not a question.

Cervianus made a non-committal face. "Perhaps."

Shenti nodded thoughtfully. "The Kushites stole the essence of Kemet for themselves."

"Sorry?"

"In the beginning," the cavalry decurion said, settling into his tale as the column wound slowly up the hill toward the settlement of Ambo, "perhaps fifty generations ago, the pharaohs ruled the lands to the south of what you now call Aegyptus. It was ruled in the same way that Rome rules its provinces, I would say. Then, in a time of dynastic trouble, pharaoh lost control of Kush and it became independent."

His face took on a disapproving look. "They took with them our architecture, our gods and our culture entire. Then, centuries later, during a time of weakness, the Kushites returned with their own pharaoh, seeking revenge on their masters. For a hundred years, the kings of Kush imposed their will upon Kemet, yet they were but a shadow of *our* ancient pharaohs. They were a replica; the *children* of Kemet, if you like. Finally, the people of the Black Land rose up and drove the Kushites south once more, back into the sands beyond the second cataract."

Cervianus nodded patiently. The look in his friend's eye was a familiar one, one he had seen many times in the eyes of the people of Galatia when speaking of their Roman masters: bitterness and wistfulness coloured with a touch of pride.

"So they are much like your people, really?"

Shenti shook his head vehemently. "They may follow our gods and mimic our ways, but they are not like us. They are a hard people with no culture or learning except that which they have stolen. Their kings are no longer called pharaoh, but 'Kore', and they lead their kingdom as warriors. But there is no Kore even now, and Kush is ruled by its 'Kandake', the warrior queens." He turned to Cervianus with a dark expression. "They are without compassion or mercy and the only thing they respect is strength."

"And the gods, presumably?" Cervianus added.

"And the gods, but only after their queen."

Cervianus frowned. "They follow the gods of Aegyptus, though?"

"Yes."

"And you believe it is important that we pray to these gods... Sobek, and the Lion goddess, so that they will protect us in the coming battle?"

"Yes."

"Even though we go to fight their worshippers?"

Shenti gave him a peculiar look as though he couldn't understand what the capsarius was saying. "But they are our gods, so of course we pray to them. They are the gods of Kemet. If the Kushites had started worshipping Jupiter, do you think your legions would stop praying to him to help against them?"

Cervianus fell silent. It was not a subject he felt inclined to indulge at this point.

"They will be a hard enemy to fight," Shenti said with an air of finality.

The capsarius turned back to face the slow-moving column, deep in thought. The notion had formed somewhere deep within him that all these strange encounters and dreams were connected with the nature of their enemy. Either the gods were truly interfering in the world of men and trying to... what? To stop him going to war against their Kushite worshippers? No; that was an idiotic thought. If the gods were going to speak to someone to prevent the coming massacre it would be someone in power, not a lowly field medic. What could he do? No. The other possibility, of course, was that he himself was uneasy with their task and that his mind, steeped in the local culture as it currently was, was putting a solid face on his fears.

And yet, as he looked up at the one great monument that stood on the bluff at Ambo, he found it much easier to lay the blame for these fears at the feet of the gods.

The column marched on past the great temple and the surrounding settlement. There were still hours of daylight left yet and the army would camp for the night closer to Syene in order to be fresh and prepared when they arrived at their destination. Cervianus looked up, from their position toward the rear of the travelling army, over the low-lying town and regarded the great temple with trepidation.

"You need to go, my friend." Shenti nodded at the great building. "You and Sentius can both ride. Take two of the horses and rejoin us when you have finished. We will not have moved far."

Cervianus paused, on the verge of argument, and squinted at the building, the nerves growing with every closing pace. "I'm not sure this is really necessary. We can travel with you the rest of the way."

Shenti shook his head. "Go and make your offering and receive the blessing of the god."

With a last pleading look that fell flat in the face of the decurion's expression, Cervianus turned to the convalescing legionary beside him. "Come on, then. Faster we get this over with, the faster we can rejoin the column."

Sentius shrugged. The notion of visiting the temple of Ambo apparently filled him with as much ambivalence as it did with foreboding for the capsarius. Being careful of their injuries, the pair clambered down from the slowly moving cart and reached out to grasp the reins being handed to them by one of the auxiliaries.

"Hurry back," Shenti said, his lip curled in a half smile. Cervianus glared at him and then, turning, led his horse away from the column that marched along the bank of the great river in front of the town. The two men angled their mounts toward the wavering path that led away from the bank, up between the low, mud-brick buildings and to the temple.

Ambo's religious centre stood above the town on a bluff that overlooked the Nile, the road along which the legions travelled passing between them. The temple's precinct wall, a low, wide and heavy mud-brick structure, afforded a reasonable view of the upper reaches of the buildings within. The great pylon gate that faced the Nile stood much the same as others Cervianus had seen, but there were subtle differences that he began to note as they approached the entrance.

The left tower of the pylon bore the familiar shape of the

crocodile-headed god, here looking powerful and imperious – more so than anywhere else. The sight of the image sent a tingle of nerves up Cervianus' spine that was only muted by his curiosity. The tower opposite, forming the far side of the gate, showed a different image entirely. A falcon-headed god faced Sobek, apparently on equal terms. The capsarius frowned.

"What's up?"

He glanced across in surprise at Sentius.

"Two different gods," he noted, pointing at the pylons.

"So?"

"Two gods in one temple? Even the Capitoline triad don't share a temple; a complex maybe, but not a single temple. Seems strange."

"This whole *province* is strange, Titus."

The capsarius shrugged and smiled. It was a view he'd heard numerous times in the past few weeks and, like it or not, it was a difficult view to gainsay. "Come on. Let's go in."

The precinct behind the gateway was not as busy as he'd expected, but held surprises. Priests and local people went about their business, apparently unconcerned with the ever-present danger posed by the low, man-made pool that lay off to their right, home to dozens of young crocodiles and hatchlings. Sentius, wandering on toward the temple entrance before them, had yet to notice the swarm of small crocodiles, watching, as he was, some sort of ceremony going on at a deep well off to the left.

Before the wounded man could lay eyes on the young crocs, Cervianus pointed at the double entrance to the main sacred structure to distract him. Sentius still suffered nightmares after the attack and watched the river intently and nervously.

"That's where we want," the capsarius said brightly.

A young boy ran up to them and Cervianus glanced down at him in surprise.

"Yes?"

"Hold horse?"

Cervianus looked at Sentius and the soldier shrugged.

"Why not?" The capsarius smiled. "Look after them for now and we'll make it worth your while before we leave."

The boy grinned and took the reins from the two men.

"Will he not just run away and sell the horses?" Sentius frowned.

"I don't think so; not in a temple. They're a very superstitious people."

Satisfied of their security and continually aware of the need to keep his companion's eyes from straying over to the right and the pool of unrestrained beasts, Cervianus grabbed the man's good elbow and urged him forward.

"Two entrances," he mused as he looked up. The temple appeared to have been designed so perfectly symmetrically along an invisible central line that even the decoration in the doorways to either side matched. A suspicion began to fall over the capsarius and he tapped a local on the shoulder as they reached the frontage.

"Excuse me. This is the temple of the crocodile god, yes?"

The local shrugged, looking confused.

"Doesn't even speak basic Latin," Sentius said with a snort.

Cervianus frowned at the man, pointed to the temple and said, "Sobek?"

The man nodded and smiled. "Sobek. Har-Wer."

"Har-Wer?"

"Har-Wer."

The capsarius turned his perplexed expression on his companion. "What?" Sentius said blankly.

"I'm not sure about Har-Wer, but I think it's the local name for Haroeris, the falcon god. Saw his image on the gate opposite Sobek, and I think this is some sort of combined temple. Seems exceedingly strange, though. Sobek is a violent god, but Haroeris is… well, he's sort of my patron. A lord of healing."

Again, a shudder ran up his spine. The fact of his repeated contact with the crocodile god while being himself a healer and coming across a temple devoted to these two seemingly opposed facets was just too much for him to pass off as simple coincidence. For all his protestations of the superstitious nature of the Aegyptian people, he was finding it hard to deny that something powerful seemed to be at work in this strange land, and that it had set its eyes on him specifically.

"You have a weird look on your face," Sentius said.

"I have this horrible feeling that your attack was in some way just part of a strange conspiracy to get me to this place."

"Nothing like a healthy ego, is there? Come on. Let's get in and make an offering so we can piss off and get away from this creepy place."

Cervianus found himself nodding as he followed his friend through the heavy portal and into the temple. A constant tingle bothered his spine and the hairs on the back of his neck stood up as they entered, but "creepy" was not a word he would apply. The strange double temple seemed somehow curiously right and welcoming; somehow expectant, waiting for him.

The wide hall into which they walked was dark and surprisingly chilly. Twin rows of heavy, decorative columns supported the slabbed roof; the walls were carved and painted with beautiful designs and endless rows of the ancient pictorial writing of the Aegyptians.

Strangely, the other doorway, to their right, led into exactly the same room. Twin doorways continued on from this hall into another, deeper within, lit by guttering lamps.

"Vultures circling," Sentius said quietly, his voice hoarse.

"What?"

"Look up."

Cervianus did as he was bade and noted with surprise the painted images of dozens of vultures across the ceiling. Perhaps the image held some strange cult significance for the local worshippers. For Sentius it meant something else, and the capsarius nodded strangely. Vultures circled over them in the hallway of the warrior god of Upper Aegyptus. There was definitely something happening here that he did not entirely understand.

"Let's get inside."

The second room was similar, smaller and more intense than the first, the guttering flames giving it a strange glow. The pair shivered, and not due to cold. A priest of some sort with a shaven head and a strange, shiny fake beard, strode toward them, his painted eyes slightly glazed, a smoking censer in his hand, swinging slowly back and forth, dangerously close to the white linen skirt he wore.

"Excuse me," Cervianus said very quietly to him, aware of how easily sound intruded in silent, sacred places.

The priest turned to him and raised one eyebrow, creating a strange shape in the elaborate painting around his eye.

"Where do we go to make offerings to the Crocodile Lord?"

The priest looked the two soldiers up and down and pursed his lips. In quiet, broken Latin, he spoke as he gestured to another smaller doorway ahead. "Go next room. Find flat stone offering."

Cervianus nodded his thanks and the pair walked through the dim columned hall and into the yet smaller corridor beyond. This narrow hall had matching doorways on the far side, though these were blocked with heavy wooden doors. Low plinths stood in the hallway, and Sentius turned to the medic.

"It's not occurred to me before... I brought a libation for offering. What about you, though? You've brought nothing."

The capsarius shrugged. "In a Roman temple we'd give anything. Whatever was of value. I imagine it's the same here."

Closing his eyes, he lowered his head. "Sobek..." He paused, unsure of how to go about this. "Lord of warriors. Please accept an offering and watch over us with your powerful gaze as we go into battle."

Silently, he added *and relinquish any claim on this man*.

A thought struck him and, suddenly sure of what he should do, he reached into his tunic and undid the leather thong around his neck, sliding the crocodile-tooth amulet from it. Taking a deep breath, he placed the tooth on the plinth and stepped back. It felt right, and he found himself smiling as he retied the thong and tucked Ulyxes' lucky coin into his tunic once more.

Sentius looked from the capsarius to the amulet and back. He shrugged again, a movement that caused him discomfort but a habit that he seemed unable to break. Leaning forward, he poured his wine, a high-quality brew in a small jar purchased at great expense back in Nicopolis, onto one of the plinths.

"I hope this works, Sobek," Sentius muttered. "Roman

altars often have a bowl to collect it. Please accept the wine and…" His voice tailed off and he looked helplessly at his companion.

"I expect he knows what you mean," Cervianus smiled.

"Let's get out of here," Sentius shuddered.

The capsarius's smile broke into a grin. "Alright. Let's hope Sobek's happy with us now. But before we go, I think I ought to pay my respects to Haroeris, since he's the 'Good Physician'."

With the uneasy Sentius by his side, he wandered along the corridor to the opposite side of the temple, seemingly identical but for the imagery that centred more on the falcon-headed god than the Crocodile Lord. Scouring the walls, the medic locked on an image of Haroeris looking regal and impressive and strode across to it, inclining his head as he stood before the wall.

"Thank you for my skills; for the ability and the desire to heal, without which I would not be a worthy person."

He stood for a moment in silent contemplation, the darkened hall quiet and deserted apart from the pair of them, and almost jumped and yelped as the wooden door to the inner sanctuary opened next to his elbow and a man appeared in the space.

"Crap!" Cervianus snapped reflexively, and then shrank back, aware of where he was and how unseemly the outburst had been.

The man in the doorway, holding the wooden portal so that the interior remained hidden from the capsarius's view, furrowed his brow and peered at the medic in the dim light.

"Yes, yes. You."

Cervianus blinked and stared at the priest, who shuffled slightly, his leopard-skin covering settling over his white linen tunic and skirt, the beads and bangles tinkling and clattering.

"Pray to Har-Wer with all your heart, but make Syene your end."

Cervianus shook his head. "I don't understand."

"Rome's world ends at the second cataract. To go beyond is to invite death and worse for you and your army. Beyond the second cataract fear, pain and death await. Beyond the second cataract, Sobek will not protect you. Beyond the second cataract, Horus cannot save you. Scourge your enemy at Syene and avenge yourselves there, but go no further."

Cervianus stepped back, the cold shiver returning to his spine. Once again, the hairs on his neck stood erect.

"I am just a capsarius. It is not my decision."

The priest said nothing; he simply retreated back into the shadows of the inner chambers and allowed the door to close behind him. Cervianus spent some time staring at the closed door before he felt Sentius tug at his tunic, causing him to jump yet again.

"This place is putting the shits up me," the wounded soldier said earnestly. "Let's get back to the column."

Nodding, Cervianus allowed himself to be led from the temple, the priest's words ringing in his ears: *make Syene your end.*

The frown of worry and confusion remained with him as they collected their horses from the eager boy, paid him handsomely and, once mounted, rode out of the temple precinct and slowly down the slope toward the rear of the Roman column, visible mostly as a cloud of dust perhaps a mile from the temple.

Make Syene your end.

The army had travelled a further ten miles or so beyond Ambo before making camp for the night. Shenti had looked up once with interest as the two men had rejoined the column, but something he saw in Cervianus' eyes had deterred him from asking questions, for which the capsarius was extremely grateful.

The night in camp had been a traditional pre-battle scene. The men coped with the impending danger in several ways, some getting drunk and gambling, even indulging in fisticuffs here and there; others lay silently in their blankets, contemplating their own mortality. Some prayed. Some sought the company of their friends.

Word had spread that the medic and his charge had presented offerings at the temple of Ambo and, though nobody had officially cleared them of their fresh ostracism, the pair had rejoined the legion without incident, Cervianus falling in alongside Ulyxes in his allotted place, Sentius returning to his own century. Ulyxes had greeted him warmly and talked and drank for a short while before wandering out into the dark, full of tension and anticipation, looking for someone to punch.

This morning had begun subdued and quiet until the legions had settled into the march for the remaining ten miles to Syene. Not long into the journey, an enterprising soldier from the Third started shouting out a bawdy song about a Jewish whore in Alexandria with apparent extreme flexibility and endless endurance. The rest of the Third quickly joined in and by the fourth verse the Twelfth had picked up the chorus. Without knowing the song, the Twenty Second remained silent for a few moments, but the lyrics were simple and colourful and the chorus hilarious, and soon all three legions were belting out the tune.

The atmosphere lightened, the previously lacking camaraderie between the legions growing in the face of mutual peril, until suddenly a cornu sounded as the sun began to climb higher.

The legions came to a halt at the call. Peering out along the line of men, Cervianus could see one of the local mounted scouts deep in conversation with the senior officers.

"Looks like we're here," he muttered quietly to Ulyxes, standing beside him.

"Shut up and stand still," snapped the optio behind him. "It's been so easy and peaceful the past few days without you lurching around and chattering, Cervianus."

The medic grinned. Things seemed finally to have returned to normal. A cloud passed over his thoughts briefly and he deliberately ignored the memory of the priest's warning that surfaced, threatening to destroy his sudden optimism.

It was certainly nice, despite the marching and lack of wagon seat, to be back near the front of the column, only one century back from the vanguard. The dust cloud was smaller and less bothersome here.

With the advantage of his height, Cervianus moved his head only very slightly so as not to attract the optio's attention again, and peered between the helmets of his comrades. The primus pilus of the Twelfth, along with that of the Third, was in deep discussion with tribune Vitalis.

Though Vitalis outranked the pair on a direct level, with the two senior centurions in effective command of the detachments from the other legions, they acted with the full authority of a tribune and held an equal share in the command of the army. It took only a quick glance at Vitalis' face since they had picked up the Third to see what *he* thought of this situation, being outnumbered by junior officers acting as his equals and questioning his decisions. Vitalis was not the most forgiving of men.

Another call rang out and was picked up by the musicians of the First cohort. The centurions and optios barked out orders and the First and Second centuries stomped forward in response, coming to a halt ahead of the column and close to the van. A century from each of the other legions came forward to join them, creating a separate force of some three hundred men altogether. As they stood, tense, waiting for orders, the tribune and his counterparts from the other legions strode over to join them.

The four centuries looked up expectantly as Vitalis took centre stage, the expressions on the commanders of the Third and Twelfth unreadable. He cleared his throat.

"Our scouts inform us that the Kushites will be unlikely to meet us on the field of battle, cowards that they are. This means we will likely be forced to fight them on their own terms within the bounds of the city." He straightened and clasped his hands behind his back. "As such, we will make one swift foray to the edge of the city to gauge the situation before drawing up plans and committing the entire force. These four centuries will accompany the staff while we examine the city. Centurions, be prepared for any trouble and if we encounter anything other than a few hapless barbarians, we will pull back to the army in good order and redeploy. Until we return, all you men will down packs and bear combat equipment only."

The tribune turned and nodded to the musicians and signifers next to him and the calls went out. Cervianus, along with the rest, unshouldered his yoke and dropped his kit off to one side, keeping his medical bag on his person.

Draco, centurion of the Second century, stepped out alongside the column, a twinkle in his eye that only appeared with the promise of battle.

"Shield covers off!" he bellowed.

This was it.

Cervianus caught the anticipatory grin from Ulyxes as he began to untie the thongs on his bulky leather covering. Tradition among the Twenty Second held that, with the exception of maintenance and cleaning in the privacy of their barracks, when the shields of the Deiotariana were uncovered, there would be battle. To a man, pride swelling the legion, the soldiers of the Twenty Second tucked the empty shield covers in with their travelling kit on the ground and stood, proudly displaying their scuta.

The heavy, oval shield of the Twelfth with its battered and dulled red surface emblazoned with lightning bolts was an image steeped in the symbolism of Rome. That of the Third, a similar red with the legion's number and the horned goat image was also a typical symbol of Rome's military.

The heavy shields of the Twenty Second, larger than their counterparts and almost rectangular, exhibited a deep, lush green colour, emblazoned with the golden eagle image of King Deiotarus of Galatia, its razor-sharp talons gripping the lightning bolt of Taranis while its wings spread wide and powerful, its noble face turned to the left, ever watchful. It was a symbol as powerful as the ancient roots of the legion and, between the eagle itself, which was a different, more aggressive shape than the legions' standard, almost staid bird, and the brilliant colours, nothing could possibly have announced the non-Roman origin of the legion and the pride in their heritage more than this.

Not a scratch or dent marked the pristine and bright, glorious shields of the Twenty Second. The spectacle caused the battered and dirty soldiers of the other two legions to draw breath and stare.

There was a pause as the legions shuffled into precise formation once more, ready to move off. Vitalis wanted to show off his legion in as much pomp and splendour as possible and was drawing out the moment. Eventually, the horn called again and the army began to move. Cervianus marched along with a curious mix of nervous anticipation and glowing pride. There was something about the unveiling of the shields that brought out the pride in even the most nervous or cynical man of the Twenty Second, and it almost, though not quite, overcame the tension raised in him by the memory of the priest at Ambo.

Make Syene your end.

And here they were, cresting a low rise and laying eyes on their destination for the first time. The capsarius had been expecting something different, something grand and impressive, like the great cities of Aegyptus he had seen on their journey.

What he saw instead failed to elicit the kind of emotion for which he was prepared. Syene sat in a low dip, surrounded by rocky inclines. The far side of the river rose straight from the bank into a steep hill. The city itself had no walls and resembled a cluster of broken and impoverished homes, not unlike the hovels outside the walls of Alexandria.

A few public buildings lay dotted around within, including a few temples that were on a much smaller and more basic scale than those great monuments of Memphis, Ambo and Thebes, barely even rising above the mud-brick housing. An open area with a colonnade appeared to be a recent addition somewhere in the centre and probably marked a partially constructed forum endowed by the Roman governors.

The one impressive structure in Syene that did draw the eye was the island. Here, the Nile ran wide and impressive, reed banks at both sides broken only by deliberate quays and jetties. However, in the very centre of the widest part, an island rose like a huge turtle shell, ancient walls proclaiming its status as a military stronghold. It occurred instantly to Cervianus, as it would have to the others also, that while clearing Syene's streets and housing of any occupying force would be a difficult and dangerous task, the bulk of the Kushite forces were likely entrenched on the fortified island, and that would be a fight that no general would relish undertaking.

Trying not to imagine ahead of time what was coming, Cervianus instead turned his attention back to the mud-brick structures of Syene's town that they were rapidly approaching.

The horns of the legion blared out, fanfares echoing around the river valley.

"There goes any hope of surprise." Ulyxes shook his head.

"Three hundred men in green and red are hardly capable of surprise," Cervianus replied drily and grinned until the optio's staff whacked him on the shoulder, smarting even through the mail shirt.

"Eyes front and shut up."

The army marched on down toward the edge of the town, the houses poor and damaged from the recent attacks. In fact, now they were closer, the damage to many of the buildings was evident, but the most telling statement of the recent troubles was the emptiness and silence.

Nothing moved in the streets of Syene; no children played, no merchants traded. No one moved. It was a chilling picture.

"Where are the people?" Cervianus whispered.

Ulyxes shrugged. "Dead? Gone? Who knows?"

The words of the priest at Ambo came back unbidden and filled Cervianus' thoughts:

Scourge your enemy at Syene and avenge yourselves there, but go no further.

But the man had not prophesied death and destruction *here*. Syene was not the problem, the capsarius repeated to himself. It was *beyond* Syene the trouble lay...

Not *every* house was empty.

In response to the horns, figures appeared from a few of the structures on the edge of the settlement – running figures, silent and menacing.

"They're coming out. Maybe they'll fight us in the open after all?"

Hope filled Cervianus. While a pitched battle in the open field would very likely be a bloodbath with heavy casualties on both sides, it was by far the preferable option to a dangerous siege of an island fortress.

"No," Ulyxes relied sharply. "No... they're Roman. Look!"

This time it was the shorter legionary who received the warning thwack with the optio's stick and the frown, but Cervianus squinted over the heads of the dozen or so rows of men in front.

Ulyxes was right!

The men scurrying from the buildings and rushing along the street toward them were wearing the brown tunics of Roman auxiliaries, chain armour on their torsos, some heads covered with bronze helms, others bare or wrapped in scarves. Spears and swords gripped tightly, the men converged from half a dozen streets and raced up toward the legions atop the slope.

A bellow in a deep, strange tongue sounded like an alarm from the town behind them and within moments a dozen dark-skinned men in white appeared on rooftops, bows stretched tight, visible even from this distance. Another sound from the cornu halted the column and the newly arrived legionaries watched with dread anticipation, silently urging the scattered Romans on as the enemy began sighting along their arrows.

There were perhaps forty of the auxiliaries, all told, as they gathered into a group, still running. The first few shots from the town behind them fell wonderfully, happily, short, and the legions heaved a collective sigh of relief.

Then, with dread certainty, the Kushite bowmen began to find their range and the first hit took one of the rearmost Roman runners through the calf. The man screamed and tried to struggle upright to run on. Other archers had now found the range, though, and three more arrows pierced the man's back as he clambered to his feet, throwing him forward once more onto his face in the dirt, dead as he landed.

Four other men disappeared to the ground with cries of agony before the fleeing auxiliaries managed to leave the range of the frighteningly accurate Kushite archers. Staggering, struggling for breath and in a state of deprived starvation, the soldiers rushed up and came to a halt before the officers of the legions, off to the side of the column. Cervianus stared at them and then turned to the optio.

"Sir?"

The optio glanced across at the auxiliaries and nodded.

Running out away from the column, Cervianus started unfastening his bag. The officers glanced across at the sudden activity and, realising it was a medic fumbling in his bag, paid no further attention, turning back to the ragged auxiliaries.

It was clear immediately to Cervianus that not only were these soldiers starving and suffering from extreme exhaustion, some were still prey to horrible, festering wounds that they had received in the initial assault or during the Kushite occupation.

He passed his water flask to the nearest soldier, who took it gratefully and silently, raising it to chapped, torn lips and drinking deeply before passing it to his friend.

As the capsarius began to clean off a leg wound that was already coated with pus and infection, he glanced around among the others. Broken arms, arrow wounds, neat cuts hastily stitched closed by an amateur, missing eyes and digits, sickness, infection and sores affected almost every man.

He shook his head in sadness and examined the wound. It was all straightforward work, though he would have no time to sedate or soothe the patients and the worst would have to wait until the temporary hospital was set up. This had to be quick for now.

Some he would not be able to help at all. Infection had run its course so deep in some of the men that Cervianus was amazed they'd had the life left in them to run up the slope. His experience and skills allowing him to fall into an almost automatic series of tasks, the capsarius allowed his attention to wander while he worked.

A man with a torc, an honour won for some great military act years earlier, stepped out from the crowd and saluted Vitalis and the two chief centurions.

"Report," the tribune snapped, displaying little in the way of sympathy.

"Sir. Hazael, sir. Optio of the Second Cohort of Itureans. What's left of it, anyway, sir."

Vitalis sagged slightly. "Five hundred men... the garrison of Syene. All gone?"

The man nodded with exhaustion. "Apart from us, sir, yes. The Kushites took a few prisoners, mind. Perhaps a dozen or so, but they've been nailing them to the outer walls on the island so we can watch them die, so I doubt there are any left now."

Vitalis shook his head incredulously. "There are... what... thirty of you left? And you've been hiding in the city all this time?"

Hazael nodded. "Yessir. We tried to withdraw so we could return to Thebes and the legion there, but every time we tried to leave the shelter of the streets, their damned archers started on us. Once we got out of range and decided to make a run for it, but their cavalry chased us down and we had to turn and run back into town. Frankly, sir, it's been a bitch of a time and we're bloody glad to see you."

The tribune's head snapped up angrily. "You stow that tongue, Optio, before I have it sawn off. Who do you think you're talking to?"

The man fell silent, a look of astonishment on his face, as Vitalis scratched his chin, deep in thought. The tribune turned and muttered with the two chief centurions for a moment and then turned back and addressed the battered optio.

"Very well. Tell us about what's happened here, the disposition of the Kushite troops, anything you know about their commanders and anything else helpful."

The optio saluted. "Sir. Well, there are a few of them among the streets, mostly cavalry and archers in small bands. The archers are essentially your first obstacle. They're all over the periphery of the town and they can be in position and reacting pretty quickly, as you saw. The cavalry are based in the forum, where they can use the three main roads to get out into the open and skirmish in moments. It's well thought-out sir."

Vitalis nodded, making a "harrumph" noise.

"Well, sir. The main infantry force is on the island, along with a few more archers. They're just a garrison though, sir. Maybe a thousand or so under some minor commander. The queen and her vicious bastard of a general led most of the army back south once they'd flattened the place."

The tribune frowned, unable to wrap his mind around the notion of invading a country and not settling in it with a strong occupation force. "Why did they leave, soldier? Why abandon this fortress with just a small caretaker garrison? Are they coming back, perhaps to make a move on Thebes?"

The man shrugged. "I don't think so, sir. I think they just did it for the gain and the combat. They're a bloodthirsty lot, sir. I think they just enjoy inflicting pain as much as stealing the goods."

"You said they 'did it for the gain'?"

"Yessir. They took the entire healthy population of Syene for slaves and then executed the rest: the old, the young and the injured. They marched thousands of locals off back up the Nile all roped together like cattle. And cartload after cartload of loot, too. There's nothing worth more than a sestertius left in the whole town. They even took the three bronze statues of the Princeps Octavian that were raised last year. I'd guess they'll melt them down and sell the bronze on to the Arabian traders."

A look of intense anger and hatred crossed the tribune's face and Cervianus' heart lurched as he realised what was coming next. Concentrating on the wound, he listened with a sinking feeling.

"They not only invaded Roman lands, but took citizens as slaves and looted the Princeps's statues?"

"Yes, sir."

Vitalis turned to the two senior centurions of the Third and Twelfth. Both wore looks of outrage and indignation. "We'd best get the legions deployed, gentlemen. I want this commander alive when we take the island. I want to put my boot on his neck and hear him beg for mercy." The two men nodded their agreement. "Can the Third and the Twelfth handle Syene? The archers and cavalry? I'll take the Twenty Second across by boat and we'll take the island?"

There was a pause. The island was the toughest choice, by far, but was also where the glory would be found. No awards would be won by the men clearing Syene's streets of ragged bands of archers.

The two chief centurions huddled briefly, but turned back nodding. Glory notwithstanding, there were only two cohorts of each of the Third and Twelfth present, while all ten cohorts of Vitalis' legion stood ready. The decision was purely down to numbers in the end.

"Very well," the tribune said, drawing a deep breath. "Let's get Syene under control so we can chase this bitch queen down and retrieve our people and goods."

And there it was. Cervianus' heart slowed as he acknowledged the simple truth: Vitalis would no more stop at Syene than he would abandon the whole campaign and walk away now. And the priest's warning would come true. Death and pain would await them.

Unless Cervianus could stop it somehow.

Why else would the priest tell *him*?

Finishing the binding on the man's leg, the soldier smiling gratefully at him, he moved on to the next wound: a badly broken arm held in a sling that was strapped to the man's torso.

"Back to the army," Vitalis shouted.

The Twenty Second Deiotariana, glittering like the scales of a massive fish, moved slowly down the hill toward the town. Cervianus had hardly had time to ready his weapons before the column moved off, having just returned from the medical cart where the auxiliary garrison's survivors were being assigned to treatment or, with casual efficiency, written off and sat somewhere cool to wait for Elysium to claim them.

Half an hour or so they'd paused, allowing plenty of time for the rest of the army to begin its task. The three auxiliary cavalry units were each allocated a section of the city's perimeter to patrol, preventing the enemy from escaping should they feel so inclined, or from launching any kind of offensive against the support wagons and supplies. Several units of auxiliary infantry had been assigned to bolster the numbers of the Third and Twelfth, with only one unit of archers joining Vitalis' legion on their potentially brutal assault.

The Twenty Second had then been granted a short break before their part in the attack began, while the cohorts from the other two legions along with their auxiliary support moved into the streets of Syene and began to clear them.

The chief centurion of the Third had concentrated the bulk of his men in clearing the edge of the city nearest the waiting legion, by the riverbank, which would then allow the Twenty

Second safe passage and room to move in and make a play for the island fortress.

The men of the Deiotariana legion had watched the action unfold from their vantage point on the slope. The enemy were fascinating to watch, at least from a safe distance.

As the legionaries of the Third approached the city, they split into separate centuries, each centurion taking his men into battle independent of any grand plan. With complex street warfare, an overall strategy was almost impossible to maintain, after all. The centurions of the Third were veterans with a great deal of experience and knowledge, though, and for all the dirty, ragged appearance of the men they had seen at Thebes and on the march since, the cohorts that had been sent with the army represented the best that legion had to offer, not the recent intake of cutthroats, thieves and slaves that made up the numbers since the disaster in Arabia.

As the soldiers approached the walls, defenders began to appear here and there. Many of the centurions were already prepared, and even those who had not fully anticipated the speed of enemy reactions quickly joined their colleagues in ordering defensive formations.

With practised ease and precision, the centuries of the Third legion fell into the testudo formation, creating an outer wall of shields, each man interlocking his own with those of the men to either side, while the legionaries in the centre of the formation raised theirs to form a solid roof. It was achieved with the minimum of fuss and command and was a beautiful thing to watch from above.

The enemy, though, appeared almost as if they had suddenly flashed into existence in front of the Romans. One moment the rooftop of a building was a rough dust colour with piles of reeds prepared for creating a shelter; the next moment there were three men on that roof, two with bows, stretching back and releasing their dark missiles at the oncoming force, while the third stood with a long spear, waiting to jab down from the rooftop and defend his companions.

Despite the efficiency and speed of the centurions in bellowing their orders and that of the legionaries under their command in following them, not every man managed to fall into position before the swift, strange enemy loosed their first shots and, inevitably, scattered men fell prey to the arrows, falling out of formation with missiles protruding from heads, chests and legs.

They had, however, fared better than the auxiliary infantry, not trained in such tactics and bearing unsuitable shields. The auxilia managed passable impressions of the testudo, but gaps here and there left them open to the brutal attacks of the Kushite archers, who proved to be excellent shots.

Regardless, a short time into the attack, the waiting legionaries watched their counterparts from the Third, along with the auxiliary support units, begin moving into the streets, the Twelfth's attack at the far side of town not visible at this distance. The skilled, dark-skinned bowmen on the rooftops continued to find gaps in the formations as the centuries moved below them in the streets, and an intermittent scattering of bodies lay in the avenues and around the edge of town, mute testament to the brutal efficiency of the enemy.

The result was, however, inevitable.

Once the centuries were in the streets, commands were shouted and, with a roar, each unit split into the individual contubernia, groups of eight who fought, ate, and lived together. Each eight-man force made for the door of a house that harboured archers. There would then be a pause of a few heartbeats before glittering steel and russet linen would appear on the white, dusty roof, moving in on the defenders for the kill.

The spearmen who had been desperately jabbing down at the soldiers in the street as they made for the door turned desperately at the new threat from their own level, thrusting out to keep the legionaries at bay while the archers turned and loosed urgently at point blank range. The tactic was surprisingly effective and legionaries were dying even at the moment of victory as they charged across the rooftops, shields held high protectively as arrows punctured legs or sword arms, spears glancing off shields and entering chests.

It was a brutal and grisly business. The army of Rome was a perfect machine, unstoppable by even the greatest or most determined forces in the open field, but far less suited to the sort of warfare the Kushites were driving them to.

Yet despite the losses, the men of the Third were clearly making inroads and the rooftop archers were gradually silenced as the centuries moved inward, leaving the dead of both forces lying on the flat roofs to deal with later. Shenti's cavalry made a swift run along the edge of the town below the waiting legion, catching a few bright Kushite archers or spearmen who had evaded the wall of Roman steel moving through the town like a wave, and were making for the hills and freedom.

The cavalry were every bit as efficient as the legion in their own fashion. Riding down the archers, they stabbed downward with their spears, almost universally killing their enemy with the first blow. Others, wary of riding down spearmen who were well equipped to defend against horses, instead reversed the grip on their weapons as they rode, using them as javelins to pick off the fleeing spearmen and then drawing swords in preparation for the next move.

As the noise of battle began to be muted by distance and the buildings that lay between, and as Cervianus hurried back from the wounded carts where he had observed the attack while patching up auxiliaries, the cornu sounded and the Twenty Second received its orders to move.

The capsarius shifted his shield slightly and watched, with some trepidation, as the outskirts of the town drew nearer. There were no guarantees that the Third had managed to clear out every defender and, since Draco and the other officers of the Deiotariana had not ordered testudo formation, any stray archer could do massive damage before he was caught.

Moreover, Cervianus was still uneasy in himself, the warnings of the priest of Haroeris ringing in the back of his mind, interspersed with the image of the outraged tribune Vitalis stating his intention to hunt down the Kushite queen wherever she went.

Would *he* really have any say in that? A simple medic? It seemed incredulous, and yet in Aegyptus the gods seemed to take a much more personal interest in the day-to-day life of their people than those across the sea to the north.

As the army moved into the town, the damage from the war and occupation became disturbingly clear. Houses showed signs of destruction from bombardment, leading him to wonder what sort of horrific machines of war the Kushites might have invented. Brown, fading bloodstains on the mud-brick walls told horrible stories of how the Roman defenders and even the innocent local citizens of Syene had died here.

A huge, dried splash of blood, combined with a crumbling

hole in the brickwork, spoke with dreadful clarity of the person who had been impaled here with a spear driven through their torso and deep into the wall, left pinned to bleed out. Other doorways and windows were blackened with fire damage, the shutters broken where the attackers had thrown their torches through, burning the buildings with the occupants still inside.

It had been carnage of the worst kind. No pitched battle between armies here, but the simple slaughter and enslavement of a people by a brutal and uncaring invader. The parallels that could be drawn with the campaigns of Pompey, Caesar, Antonius and Scipio were disturbing, and Cervianus put such comparisons from his mind only with great effort. Rome might conquer and take slaves, but even the harshest of tribunes and generals would think twice before committing *this* kind of atrocity.

His fears of lurking defenders waiting to take the second wave of Romans by surprise proved to be unfounded, and the men of the Twenty Second moved into the dead streets of Syene without molestation. The sounds of fighting drifted back periodically from deeper in the settlement, muted by buildings but echoing eerily along the streets, sending a shiver up the spines of the men.

Within moments, trying not to pay too much attention to the grisly sights around them, the Twenty Second left the narrow street and filed out onto a wide dock area. Even here the fighting and looting had been extreme and horrific.

Smashed boxes and amphorae littered the ground, making walking difficult. Goods that were not worth taking had been strewn across the dusty ground and left to rot and crumble. The river, freed of reeds for ease of shipping, flowed slowly – the grave of many. The glittering surface was punctured in numerous places by the wooden bones and ribs of scuttled boats and merchant vessels, rising forlorn and ghostly toward the sky.

Total destruction.

The Kushites had not just come here to loot. The auxiliary optio seemed to have been right. The Kushites came here also for the sheer love of killing. The damage was so absolute that it had clearly been wreaked with the intention of leaving nothing of use or interest for Rome. The city might as well be pulled down now.

Cervianus shook his head, taking in the scene as the cohorts filed into formation and came to a halt near the dockside. His eyes fell on a heap at the far end of the small square and he squinted and frowned. With a surge of bile he realised that it was a pile of decomposing bodies, scavengers picking at the remains, white splashes over the stony ground mute evidence of the many vultures that had taken their fill here when the square was devoid of activity.

Sickened, he turned away and cast his eyes forward, to their destination. Though there were several reed-swamped masses in the river at Syene, the central one stood out proudly. The island was large – much longer than he had originally estimated from the hillside. Perhaps a mile in length and a quarter as far across, it was shaped like a giant trireme partially submerged in the Nile. The near end was the lower part, while the far end rose with steep banks to form a perfectly defensible hill. That end was surrounded at the base by smooth, strange rocks, while the part closest to the Twenty Second was low and green, perfect for docking boats.

The island had been walled since ancient times and, while much of that circuit had, in the past century or more, been allowed to fall into disrepair or even built over, the occupying Kushite garrison had reconstructed sections and hastily thrown up their own defences.

The legions had faced far stronger fortifications in their time, for sure, but rarely in such a perfect position, on an island in the centre of a river that was home to crocodiles and other dangers.

Boats were moored on jetties at the far side of the water, at the flattest part of the island. Of course, the defending garrison would need access to the banks when required.

His attention was drawn once more by the cornu blaring out.

Vitalis, along with his signifers, junior tribunes and eagle-bearer, stepped out ahead of the Twenty Second. He waited, a look of disapproval on his face, as the attached unit of Cretan archers shuffled late into position at the end of the legion. Once the entire force was assembled, he clasped his hands behind his back and nodded to himself.

"Men of the Twenty Second, salve!"

He paused for effect, not expecting a response; no soldier would dare speak without their centurions and optios taking up a call first.

"To us falls the honour of the main fight here in Syene. I am told that this island is Abu, which means 'elephant', and we all know how ineffective elephants are when faced with an immovable legion of Romans. I am also told that the island is defensible in three tiers, rising with the terrain from this end to the other. Landing by boat is only feasible at this end, so you will see that we have a daunting and massive task ahead of us today." He smiled unpleasantly. "That being said, I expect to be standing at that great temple building on the summit before

SIMON TURNEY

sunset today. This fight is an assault, not a siege. We will move swiftly, heedless of the danger and discounting any womanly worries over the casualty rate."

A few indrawn breaths followed the statement. Vitalis' reputation as a commander who could achieve impressive victories was solidly founded in his unwillingness to temper his assaults for the sake of his men. Victory was all. Cost was irrelevant. Cervianus shivered and cast a sidelong glance to that horrible pile of bodies at the far end of the dock.

"We will move," Vitalis went on, "by cohort."

He gestured to the small boats at the dockside, not one capable of holding more than twenty men at the most. Tiny private boats were all the Kushites had left intact, and even then only for their own use.

"The First cohort will fit into these boats, I believe. They will simply have to. Crowd together and stand if you must, but I want a flotilla in the water in a hundred heartbeats with the entire First cohort on board. The First cohort will land, secure the jetties and begin to form a defensive bridgehead, holding the low ground around the jetties while designated men are sent back with as many boats as we can gather to bring the rest of the army across."

He unclasped his hands and took a deep breath.

"I will cross with the First and two of the other tribunes, but we will not move on the defences until the entire legion and the support unit are across, as well as the scorpions." With a slap, he smacked a balled fist into his cupped palm. "Then we will take the island by storm and plant Rome's eagle on the high ground once again. I want prisoners, but only the officers and commanders. Be sparing with your mercy, but bring me their leader. Are you with me?"

The centurions and optios bellowed their agreement, the soldiers under their command dutifully taking up the shout.

"Good." He straightened and drew his sword theatrically. "For the senate and the people of Rome!"

This time the roar was not prompted. The men loved a show and Vitalis knew it.

As the tribune and his company stepped aside and began the serious task of planning the assault, the centurions and optios bellowed out the orders to their men, nine of the cohorts stepping back to allow room for the First to work. The six centuries of the First cohort moved to the dock under the coordinated instructions of their officers, spreading out along the waterfront and securing the vessels moored there. Cervianus was grateful when his century, the Second, was allocated the boats at the southern end of the dock, far from the pile of grisly remains and its stench.

In moments, with the practised ease of a legion under veteran officers, the First cohort was bobbing around in a multitude of vessels, bumping into one another by the dock, while men found oars or worked the small, triangular sails on the boats. Men stood by with the ropes that secured them to the dock, awaiting the order.

"Release!"

With grunts of effort, men heaved on oars and poles, shifted sails and manoeuvred their boats out into the ponderous waters of the Nile. Perhaps forty vessels in all, of varying styles and sizes, pushed out into the current.

Cervianus looked around his own small fishing vessel. Only large enough to hold his contubernium, the eight men sat cramped, their shields ready to use if they encountered trouble at the far side of the channel. Ulyxes had volunteered to take position on the oars, perhaps to take his mind off the coming fight. *No, probably not*, thought the capsarius. Ulyxes was rarely daunted by danger, and seemed to have an almost suicidal attraction to combat. Cervianus had to smile at the man. He was probably the longest-lasting friend the medic had made since joining the legion.

He made a mental note to get together with both Ulyxes and Shenti when the fight was over and to ask their advice on the matter of the priest's warning. Assuming the three of them survived, of course.

That was not a cheery thought and the capsarius pushed it far from his mind.

Like some sort of pleasure fleet, the flotilla of small, mismatched boats made their way out across the water, some vessels maintaining a good, steady course, others with no experienced sailor on board drifting alarmingly downstream, desperately trying to hook up with other boats using thrown ropes or rowing madly against the powerful current. The surface of the water might have looked slow and lazy, but the flow, once out away from the edge, threatened to carry them away toward Thebes in mere moments.

Slowly and with great effort, a few mishaps and a lot of sweat, the boats closed on the jetties of Abu Island. Taking a moment to glance back toward the shore and then ahead to the bank of the fortress isle, Cervianus' heart skipped a beat.

Long, brown shapes slithered into the water among the reeds on the island with quiet, subdued splashes. More crocodiles were observing them from the city side, past the end of the dock where the reeds began, yellow eyes just above the surface of the water blinking and then submerging worryingly.

"Crocodiles," he said quietly, pointing at the V-shaped wake that followed the beasts as they kept pace remarkably well with the boats, at a distance that was still far too close for Cervianus' liking.

"Shit loads of them ahead, near the jetty," another man said nervously.

Ulyxes laughed. "You think they'll stick around to take on several hundred men? Don't be stupid. They're just curious."

Vibius, the eldest of their unit, nodded, frowning. "The problem is that they might be curious as to what we taste like!"

"I made offerings. The crocodile god's watching over us." Even Cervianus himself had to admit that he didn't entirely sound convinced. "And other gods, too."

"I hope so. We're going to have to fortify near that lot and wait for the rest of the army!"

"What in the name of Artemis' balls is that?"

They spun around at Vibius' outburst to see him pointing at a huge shape that had burst out of the water by the island shore, causing a fountain of foam. Grey and enormous, it let out a roar like a lion with a chest infection and splashed back down to the surface, baring enormous tusk-like teeth at them.

"It's what they call a "hippopotamos". I've seen them displayed and killed in the arena at Rome."

They turned to the speaker in surprise. Suro rarely said anything of interest, and the fact that he had even *visited* the great city was news to them.

Cervianus frowned, running the Greek words round his mind. "Water horse?" he said incredulously. "Whoever looked at *that* thing and thought of a horse needed his eyesight testing."

There was a chorus of nervous laughs as all eyes remained on the huge beast.

"Is it dangerous?"

Suro shrugged. "Killed two gladiators before they took it down. Can smash a man to bits with those jaws."

The laughter died away as each man stared at the beast.

"Ulyxes? Steer away to the right a bit, eh? Let's try and land a few hundred paces downstream of that thing."

The shorter legionary grinned. "Way ahead of you there, and I think everyone else had the same idea."

They glanced out across the water and smiled. Boats that had been making straight and true for the shore were now allowing themselves to drift downstream a little, despite that bringing them ever closer to the watching crocodiles. Somehow this new beast seemed to have muted the men's fear of the reptiles.

There was a whirring noise and Cervianus looked up sharply as an arrow disappeared into the water a few paces ahead of the boat with a plop.

Vibius straightened and placed his shield on the boat's edge, granting as much protection as possible for the passengers.

"Nearly in their range, lads."

Following suit, the other six free men put their shields in place, forming a shield wall around the prow of the boat while Ulyxes picked up the pace, closing on the shore.

"This is it," the stocky rower grinned. "Get ready, boys. It's arse-kicking time!"

VIII

ABU ISLAND

Chaos ensued from the moment the Kushite archers found their range. Cervianus held his shield over the edge of the boat and gritted his teeth as the air all around him was filled with the whirr and hiss of arrows, countless black-fletched shafts zipping over his head and falling into the water behind the small vessel, others disappearing with a dull thud into the side of the boat below.

Most of the shots, however, were frighteningly accurate, and he lost count of the thuds as the missiles buried themselves in his heavy shield, defacing the beautiful Galatian eagle. Certainly four of the sharp, deadly points hit with such force that they drove themselves through the shield, the tips protruding from the inside. One even punched through, leaving the whole head visible behind. All the capsarius could think of as he stared down at it, listening to the *"thunks"*, was how lucky he was that it didn't hit where his arm was.

Suddenly among the terror, the deafening noise and the lurching chaos, the boat hit a jetty, steered and propelled surprisingly expertly by Ulyxes. The seven men at the rail clutched one another and the side of the boat to prevent going over. To fall now and drop the defensive shields would be unquestionably fatal, given the constant zip and whine of missiles.

Here and there, through the noise, cries and shrieks rang out as shafts found their target. A man simply had to close his ears to the dying, or the fear could become too strong and win out.

"Do we wait for the horns, or go now?" Cervianus asked, shouting over the noise.

"Go now. Moving targets are harder to hit!"

It was, of course, good advice. Ulyxes grasped his own shield now and pulled it up to join the others as the contubernium peered out between cracks in the small shield wall. Other boats were pulling up at the jetties in a similar fashion. Among the flotilla there were small vessels dotted around that had failed to cross, arrows finding their entire crew, leaving six or seven or even ten men at a time dead, lolling over the hulls' sides or bobbing face down in the water.

Streaks of crimson ran downstream in the Nile, mingling with the river and dissipating not far from the island's tip. The metallic tang of blood in both air and water was attracting an unhealthy interest from the crocodiles that loitered just on the edge of the scene, occasionally finding a body that had washed far enough downstream to claim as theirs. Fights were breaking out among the beasts as several tore and snapped at one body, each trying to claim the prize.

The ground beyond the jetties, of which there appeared to be five functioning and two broken and burned, was flat and easy, heavy cyclopean walls looming above it where the land began to rise slightly toward the south.

"What do we do about the bridgehead?" one of the others shouted.

290

"That!" bellowed Ulyxes, pointing out toward the jetty to their right and quickly retracting his arm before it was pierced by an errant missile. Another quick glance at the wall told them that the dozens of archers above were not about to let up their deadly hail. The others peered across to the next jetty where Ulyxes had gestured. Men from the first two boats that had docked there, the first two to reach land in fact, had disembarked and formed a proper shield wall, a row of six men straddling the jetty, crouching behind their shields, while a second row of six formed an angled second tier of shields. The arrows were making no headway penetrating the defence and, at a shout from an optio among them, the strange two-tier shield wall moved a few steps forward, drawing a tremendous amount of enemy missiles.

Behind them, four other men worked with knives and swords, smashing at the end of the jetty.

"What in Hades are they doing?" Cervianus asked, frowning.

Ulyxes shrugged. "What else would you need timber for in a fight?"

The capsarius frowned. Vitalis had launched his assault without due consideration of the situation. He might have all sorts of grand plans he had discussed with the other tribunes but, since he was still somewhere back in the flotilla, it had come down to the first men who landed to decide on their course of action, and an enterprising optio had hit on the solution.

Without having brought entrenching tools or sudis stakes or any such equipment they were in a poor position to put up any kind of defensive screen. Now, a small party was busy severing ropes and gathering planks almost ten feet in length from the jetty's surface. Used properly they would create an adequate palisade to protect them from the enemy archers while the rest of the legion crossed.

"Let's get to it, lads," Ulyxes shouted, launching himself fearlessly from the boat onto the creaky timber of the jetty, leaving the small vessel rocking sickeningly behind him. With a roar, the others leapt up and followed suit, falling in behind their comrade and locking shields.

"Shit!"

They crouched desperately behind their shields, listening to the regular punching of arrows against the surface, and peered along at the source of the expletive. Fuscus was staring at his arm. One of the deadly shafts had managed to slip between the shields as they ran and had caught their comrade in the upper arm, fortunately driving on past and leaving a deep rent along the flesh rather than embedding itself.

"It's only a minor wound," Cervianus shouted. "I'll sort it later."

Fuscus nodded and gave a last look at his rapidly numbing arm and the blood soaking down from it, turning his green tunic black and dripping from his knuckles. Turning his attention to the situation, he gritted his teeth and ignored the pain. The eight men could only just fit across the jetty and both Fuscus and Cervianus shuffled back behind and raised their shields for a second tier, mimicking their counterparts on the next jetty. A second boat pulled alongside behind them and the men clambered out onto the timber walkway, running up to join in, four more shields adding to the second tier while half a dozen other legionaries crouched in the protective shadow of the shield wall and hacked at ropes to free the timbers. The last man from the boat disappeared into the torrent with a squawk as an arrow found a gap beneath his shield and punched through his shin, sweeping him from his feet.

Cervianus watched in dismay as the man, wounded, but very much alive, floundered in the water, the current sweeping him away and under the next jetty where a huge set of serrated jaws appeared as if from nowhere and smashed down on him, both figures disappearing beneath the surface with a strange "gloop" noise. The capsarius turned away.

"Careful where you stand or fall. There are crocodiles under the jetties too!"

The news was greeted with groans from the others. As if the assault itself wasn't bad enough.

The moments passed by like hours, filled with the thud and zip of arrows and the occasional screams of unlucky men. Cervianus, positioned in the middle of the defensive line and with the advantage of height, regularly surveyed the landing zone as they held. More and more boats arrived at the jetties, most men managing to disembark without too much trouble, others unfortunately finding the wrecked and broken jetties and struggling to get ashore without falling prey to either the missiles of the defenders or the opportunistic animals in the shallows. Now, the jetties being full of moored boats, others were being forced to land among the perilous reeds.

"It's going to be damn dangerous for others to land if we've ripped up all the jetties," he noted.

"Screw 'em. Worry about yourself," shouted someone from another contubernium, gritting his teeth against the regular thumps on his shield. And the shield walls held, the defensive line on the shore of the island gradually taking shape. The boats that landed in the reeds spewed out their occupants who formed their own shield walls, gradually linking up until each jetty contained the same system, a line of single shields strung across the shore between them. Within moments the water-end of the jetties were a mere skeletal shape, legionaries carrying piles of planking forward.

A cornu sounded on the next pier and the beleaguered defenders, almost to a man, turned to look, the sudden distraction causing a number of fatalities as men accidentally left small gaps that were exploited by the horribly accurate enemy archers.

On the walkway to their right a boat had moored, bearing Vitalis and his staff, with signifers struggling to lift the heavy standards as they clambered onto the jetty, and fellow legionaries protecting them with their large shields.

"Move forward and form a palisade twenty paces from the shore. I want it the length of the landing site!" the tribune bellowed.

There was a brief shuffle among the staff and a senior centurion, along with one of the junior tribunes, fell into deep discussion with their commander. Already some troops were moving forward but others were watching the exchange with trepidation, noting the rising colour in Vitalis' face. The tribune was a man who looked unkindly on advice or argument. After a brief exchange, Vitalis straightened again, a snarl on his face.

"Belay those orders. Create a *small* bridgehead with a strong palisade, covering the central three piers. Get to it!"

A familiar voice called out from the other side and the men of Cervianus' contubernium snapped their heads around to look. Centurion Draco was standing shield-less, apparently unconcerned and invulnerable on one of the jetties, far away from the shelter of the shields, vine staff behind his back as arrows whirred past him into the water.

"Get those planks forward and start driving them into the ground. Any men not occupied, I want you into the reeds and killing those bloody crocodiles. We don't want them waiting for the next cohort landing. And make sure you stay away from that monster over there." He pointed at the "hippopotamos".

Under the expert instruction of the centurions and optios, the various units of the First cohort shuffled forward along the jetties or up the bank at the shoreline, their shield walls held steady, until they linked up beyond and consolidated into one huge line of double-tiered shields, men carrying the huge planks of wood running close behind them, making the most of the cover.

The arrows, which had begun to slow during the landings, the enemy presumably preserving their remaining ammunition, picked up in pace and intensity as the line of green eagle-emblazoned shields flowed slowly toward them, concentrating at the central jetties. The noise of shafts driving into the leather and wood of the shields was deafening once more, drowning out the orders of most of the officers.

In the tumult the cohort settled into three distinct groups. The men at the front maintained the shield wall; occasional fatalities were announced with a shriek, and the reserves stepped forward to fill the gaps. The second group, behind them, worked at driving the jetty planks into the ground, binding them together with lengths of cut rope and using helmets and shields to push piles of earth and gravel up to help support the palisade. The third, more unfortunate, group waded into the shallows among the reeds, their shields held over their shoulders, protecting their backs from the flying missiles, while they searched for the deadly animals that lurked beneath the surface of the water. The various shouts of victory, cries of alarm, and shrieks of pain declared their mission at best a qualified success.

Gradually, the defences began to take shape: a wide "U" of makeshift palisade marched up from the shallows, along the shore, leaving room to manoeuvre behind, and back into the water further downstream, enclosing the central three ruined, skeletal jetties.

Arrows continued to pound into the shields of the defenders as they pulled back through the final gaps in the palisade and joined their comrades in relative safety, while the workers pushed the last planking sections into place.

As the tall, wooden defence came to completion, a few soldiers, failing to take the full situation into account, lowered their shields, moving back toward the jetties only to fall prey to yet more arrows. The palisade protected only so far and men would still need to crouch behind shields from the moment they entered bow range of the walls until they were within perhaps ten paces of the palisade for safety.

The cornu sounded again and the officers rushed to counsel at the centre where Vitalis stood imperiously, nodding with satisfaction. Nearby grumbling legionaries hauled the dead and wounded to one side, clearing the approach for the next wave of men.

The constant thud of arrows into timber began to slow as the enemy realised they were simply wasting ammunition now, and the voices of the commanders rose above the noise of many labouring soldiers.

"First century: to the boats, two men to each vessel and row for the shore to collect the Second cohort. The rest of you help bolster those defences, clear out any more crocodiles, and start construction of raised platforms behind the wall for the scorpions when they arrive. Get moving!"

Centurions began to bellow orders to their individual units and the men of the First century made for the numerous small boats, shields held high to protect themselves as they ran.

Cervianus took a deep breath, eyeing the pile of dead and the small area where the wounded had been laid together in the lea of the defensive palisade. Dropping his shield, he fumbled for his leather bag and began to run across to the groaning men, unfastening the straps as he ran.

"What in Juno's name do you think you're doing?" Draco snapped, stepping in front of him and forcing him to stagger to a sudden stop.

"Seeing to the wounded, sir," Cervianus said with a confused frown.

"Back to work!"

"Sir?"

The centurion gave him a cuff around the back of the head and pointed at the palisade.

"We're a bridgehead for an invading force, under attack from the defenders, busy trying to remove crocodiles from our nice little camp and prepare for the push. You're a medic second; a legionary first. Now turn around, pick up that shield and start BUILDING AN ARTILLERY PLATFORM LIKE THE TRIBUNE ORDERED!"

Cervianus actually leaned back in the blast of halitosis and spittle from the centurion, his face going white.

"Yessir," was all he could manage in a small voice as he turned back, fastening his bag again and running for his discarded shield. Men all around had paused in their tasks to grin at him and he felt his pallid face suddenly colouring again.

Ulyxes chuckled as he approached. Behind them, Draco turned and swept his vine stick in an arc.

"Get back to work, the lot of you. The next man I see grinning like an idiot gets to do recon on his own."

Faces fell and expressions changed as the men got to work, piling up earth and stones and compacting it, adding timber to strengthen the platforms. Behind, the unhappy hunters had almost finished scouring the reeds for lurking dangers, their own numbers worryingly thinned in the process. The boats were already out in the water, one man rowing each like mad for the opposite shore while the second used two shields to keep them safe until they were out of range of the walls.

Dropping down behind the palisade, Cervianus began to help collect earth using his decorative shield as a shovel. Next to him, Ulyxes was, with a surprisingly dextrous talent, weaving reeds together to create some sort of wicker-type screen that would help solidify the platforms. Each raised podium would have to be six feet high to afford the artillerists a clear shot over the palisade at the walls and the defenders thereon. Theirs would be a dangerous task, being in sight of the Kushite archers while they launched the iron bolts from the small portable torsion weapons.

Gradually, as they worked, the platforms began to rise and take shape, each additional layer of stone, earth, wood and reeds being compacted by two legionaries with heavy pieces of fallen timber and driftwood gathered from the shore.

Such was the nature of the Roman legion and why it would never be beaten, the capsarius mused. Arriving on the island with nothing but pilum, sword and shield, in just less than half an hour they had cleared the landing zone of dangers, created a defensive palisade that protected them from enemy missiles, and constructed platforms ready for the siege weapons that would come across last, and all with just the resources that nature had provided them.

"Come on."

Cervianus looked up from his brief straying of concentration to see Ulyxes brandishing a newly woven mat of reeds and gesturing to the platform. Nodding, he pushed his shield through the damp silty earth once more and lifted it, laden, with a grunt, and climbed the small, low ramp behind his friend. At the apex, some five feet from ground, Ulyxes waited for the capsarius to dump the load of soil before placing his reed mat over the latest layer. The pair stepped back for a breather on the edge of the surface, which was some eight feet across, while two other legionaries tamped the mound down with a fallen sycamore branch, weathered and hardened over the years as it lay on the bank.

The two friends took in the bridgehead with quiet admiration. It was quite a work. Behind them the boats were almost all visible at the far bank, loading the Second cohort to bring them across. Within the hour the entire legion and their auxiliary archers would be drawn up behind the defence, the artillerists scattered among the scorpions making an effort to take out the first line of defenders before the push.

Sharp conversation in an imperious tone drew their attention. Vitalis and two other officers were descending from inspecting the next platform along, deep in conversation, and turning toward this one.

"Here we go," Ulyxes muttered in a voice hopefully quiet enough to escape the staff's attention. "Prepare to be pushed off the platform by a huge wave of ego and self-importance."

Cervianus gave his friend a sharp warning look but couldn't

help but smile at the accuracy of the description. The two came to attention in perfect military poise, covered in dust and dirt and devoid of weapons or shields, teetering near the edge of the mound, as the party of officers climbed the slope and reached the upper surface. Vitalis stepped out onto the mound, paying no attention to the men there. The two other legionaries saluted and stepped away with their log, back down the slope. Cervianus and Ulyxes remained where they were as the three officers examined the platform.

"Not as tall as the others. You're lagging behind in your work." Vitalis' face lacked anything but the most basic acknowledgement of their existence as he spoke.

One of the men with him, a centurion they vaguely recognised from the Sixth century, crouched down and touched the surface. He gestured to the other tribune, who crouched to join him. Vitalis looked at them in surprise, and the centurion glanced up at the pair of legionaries.

"It's not as tall as the others yet, sir," he agreed with Vitalis, while keeping a questioning gaze on the two men. "But," he added, "this is far more solid and stable than the others. We've had to set *them* extra men to tamp down the surface because you can feel it move under your feet. This doesn't, though. Feels solid as the ground. Is it this reed mat?"

Ulyxes nodded. "Old construction trick, sir. Build a wicker or reed weave into the mound at regular intervals and make sure the earth's damp enough and it becomes much more stable and solid."

The centurion nodded with satisfaction. "It's solid as rock, sir. Excellent work."

The senior tribune, standing erect, harrumphed with irritation. At every turn today people seemed to be gainsaying him or questioning his decisions. "I suppose that's helpful, but it still needs another foot raised as quickly as possible. I have other work lined up yet."

Cervianus ground his teeth at the unfairness of it and turned his head to look over the palisade, the top of which ran at an ordinary man's head height here, when standing on the platform, at least. He, of course, could see over the top clearly, with the advantage of his extra height.

The hail of missiles had all but stopped now, the enemy preserving their remaining shots. Only an occasional "thunk" announced sporadic opportunistic attempts.

The glint of sun on steel was the capsarius's only warning.

Cervianus' heart skipped a beat.

The arrow was flying straight and powerful, hurtling through the air almost directly at him. In a strange, drawn-out, slow motion moment, his head turned languidly in the direction of the arrow's true target, which had to be close.

There was only one other target possibly in the arrow's range. Ulyxes was too short and was covered entirely by the palisade. The two more junior officers were crouched, examining the platform's construction.

Vitalis, not a great deal shorter than the capsarius, stood proud and haughty, frowning with displeasure, his back to the palisade. He wore his helmet with its tall, green plume, ample evidence of his rank, and somehow, one of the planks in the palisade at this point must either be shorter than the others, or had been accidentally driven further into the ground.

The beautifully accurate shot had been one of pure opportunity.

Perhaps half a heartbeat passed in the world of the Twenty

Second legion, though a thousand years went by in Cervianus' head as he turned with agonising slowness.

Make Syene your end.

The words bounced around the inside of his head, echoing and amplifying until he could hear nothing but them and the whirr of the arrow.

Vitalis would take them to Kush. Into Hades. Vitalis would lead them to what even the gods of Aegyptus seemed to be telling him would be death and pain. It could all end in Syene. It *should* all end in Syene. The Kushites would be gone from Aegyptus and the borders could be reinstated. A violent war being taken into the heart of the southern lands, where no Roman had ever been? Had they learned nothing from the disastrous campaign to Arabia Felix last year: a campaign that had almost wiped out two legions, depleted vast amounts of resources and left Rome's most important province almost undefended?

Vitalis would never change his mind; he simply wasn't the sort of person who could even countenance going back on his decisions.

Vitalis would lead them to their deaths, despite the warnings Cervianus had received.

Vitalis had to die.

The whirring of the flying missile was so loud it blocked out every other sound from the capsarius's senses now, even the echoed, repeated words of the priest from Ambo.

The arrow would end it all.

Cervianus couldn't work out in that moment of decision whether he was proud of himself, or whether he hated what he had become.

The tribune let out a gasp of shock as the medic's shoulder

hit him full in the chest and the pair hurtled from the artillery platform, leaving a wide, empty space through which the world-changing arrow passed harmlessly, landing in the dusty ground with a thud.

'Haroeris, what have I done?'

It had been a strange hour. After an initial barrage of insults and threats from Vitalis for being apparently physically assaulted, the tribune had been made aware of the arrow shot and the fact that the capsarius at whom he had been screaming had, in fact, saved his life. Vitalis had fallen silent, speechless, and turned away and since that moment he had not spoken a word of thanks to Cervianus or even acknowledged his existence, turning his attention instead to the construction of mobile screens.

In a way, Cervianus was glad of the man's angry explosion. It made it easier to dislike him and, despite having in that split second made a choice to defy his true feelings and save the man, he knew in his heart that he should have let Vitalis die to save the rest of the army. Perhaps there would be another opportunity yet... it would not be totally unbelievable to suggest someone might slip a knife between his ribs during the attack. Certainly his own staff watched him with barely concealed loathing when his back was turned.

Their commander seemed to have changed since landing in Aegyptus. His vying for position with the other two legions and their commanders seemed to be bringing out a side of him that did not promise good things for the Twenty Second. Cervianus wished, not for the first time, that their legate could have stayed in command when the legion was assigned to Aegypt, rather than opening the way for Vitalis.

As Cervianus and Ulyxes, along with half a dozen other legionaries, finished constructing the platform and put together a few reed screens, gradually more and more boats docked on the island, delivering cohort after cohort of legionaries, all tense and apprehensive, eyeing the walls ahead. The arrows from the Kushites had tailed off to an occasional pot shot, and even *they* seemed half-hearted.

Now, almost an hour after Vitalis' narrow escape, the entire Twenty Second milled about behind the shelter of the stockade while the flotilla docked for the last time, carrying the rest of the Cretan archers and twenty of the legion's scorpions with their ammunition.

Secondary mounds had been thrown up, not as stable or large as the artillery platforms, to enable the auxiliary bowmen to shoot over the palisade, and the mail-clad Cretans in their dun-coloured tunics took position, crouched ready behind the timber defences, testing the tension of their bowstrings and jamming arrows point first into the timber in front of them for quick retrieval.

The feeling of tense expectancy was tangible and nerve-jangling, with the legionaries waiting for the order to fall into ranks, the archers in position, and the scorpions being borne aloft by their crews, across the ground from the jetties to the platforms, the legionaries grunting and sweating with their burdens.

The senior officers, including the prefect of the auxiliary archers, stood in a small group in the centre of the compound, quietly discussing the situation, though Vitalis, his expression sour, occasionally flicked a glance toward the capsarius.

Cervianus sighed and leaned against the palisade, watching four men struggling to carry the torsion weapon up the slope and onto their platform. He turned to Ulyxes and opened his mouth to speak, but stopped as there was a sudden roar.

Leaning close to the timber, he put an eye to one of the tiny cracks between the planks and drew back in surprise. The gate in the island's walls above them had swung open and a huge force of the enemy were issuing from it.

The capsarius had not been the only man to turn at the sudden noise and shouts of alarm arose in the bridgehead. The artillerists struggled as fast as they could to lift the scorpions into place while the auxiliary prefect ran back to his archers where the centurions were already shouting commands, their men nocking arrows to their bows. The legionary officers began to bellow orders, cornua sounding loudly, and the roar of the advancing enemy over it all. Cacophony and bedlam ruled the island.

As Draco shouted the order to fall in, echoed by the optio and the century's musician, Ulyxes grasped his shield and sword and moved back from the wall. Cervianus took one last, lingering look at this enemy they had never yet seen before turning away to join his comrades.

The Kushites were clearly different from the Aegyptians, even in their basic physical make-up. Their skin was a great deal darker and their faces wider and flatter; their hair was trimmed and beaded into a gleaming black bowl-shape on their crown, some with a white cloth wrapped around their brow to keep the fringe back from their eyes. Their only concession to armour appeared to be the hides of animals, including the spots of large cats, black and white stripes of some unknown creature, cow hides in monochrome splotches and others in varied plain colours. Some also carried shields coated with similar hides.

Their weapons were as varied as their attire, some armed with spears both long and short, others with axes on handles of equally varying length. Their swords were straight, reminiscent of the gladius. Their attack was a mad rush, such as the Gallic peoples used to employ: a screaming, roaring tide of humanity, bristling with weapons, designed to strike fear into their enemy.

The time for such warfare had passed, however, with the coming of Rome. The deafening rush merely charged the waiting legion with the fierce urge to fight back.

Loping away from the palisade, Cervianus shook his head as he fell in beside Ulyxes among the Roman ranks. What could the Kushites hope to achieve with this?

But the answer was clear to him as he thought deeper. There was nowhere for them to run now, with Rome gradually tightening its grip on Abu and Syene. They could hole up and make the legion pay heavily for every step, but that would not change their inevitable end. Shenti and the local garrison officer had said of them that they were bloodthirsty, without mercy or compassion, and so they were coming for blood. They were charging because there was nowhere else to go, because they had to try to destroy the invader before the artillery could start its work, and because their thirst for blood was too strong to stay confined and wait.

As the legion fell into formation, everything went strangely quiet in the camp, the only sounds the artillerists finalising their weapons and the rumble and roar of the enemy only a few paces now from the defences.

"Loose!" called the prefect and the Cretan archers, five

hundred strong, released their missiles in a seething mass, the angle high and short. A cloud of hissing death rose, seeming to hang for a moment at the apex, and then plunged down to earth once more on the far side of the palisade.

The Kushite roar ended abruptly, becoming a cacophony of screams, squeals, shouts of alarm and cries of rage. As if in answer to the volley, the enemy suddenly hit the wooden wall, the timbers shaking alarmingly. One of the junior tribunes below Vitalis stepped out in front of the legion as the archers nocked a second arrow and drew back, ready to loose. The scorpion crews were taking position, their ammunition now in place.

"First and Second centuries of each cohort, grab your pila and get to the wall. Anywhere there's a gap or a danger of breaking through, put a couple of feet of steel through the bastards."

Vitalis glared at the man, feeling his authority undercut by his junior officers, but said nothing as the centurions and their men rushed to the wall, filing between the archers and settling into defensive positions behind the wall and at the forward edge of the firing platforms. As Cervianus hefted his pilum over his shoulder, ready to thrust into or through the bound-plank wall as required, the archers behind released their second volley with a deafening hiss, just as the enemy were regrouping from the first hail.

Above, the scorpions began to loose at will, heavy iron bolts plunging into the crowd of warriors beyond the wall and causing devastation. The wall buckled suddenly under the pressing weight of the enemy. Despite the hundreds that had already been killed by missiles, many more threw themselves with fury onto the Roman defences, climbing over their own dead and hacking at the timbers with blades, thrusting with spears.

Cervianus leaned back in alarm as the timbers gave a good few inches toward him under the weight. The palisade had been a work of excellence, given the timescale and conditions in which it was raised, but it was flimsy, put up to save them from missile attack, not to hold back a mass of infantry. Along to the right there was a crack as one of the planks broke, spears stabbing through the hole and killing two legionaries before the defenders could get their weapons to the gap and begin fighting them back.

Again, the wall lurched toward Cervianus with a groan, rope fraying at the top. A narrow gap opened between two timbers and he thrust his pilum blindly into the hole. Whether he struck home or not he couldn't initially tell with the general noise and confusion, but as he drew the javelin back the tip was coated with glistening crimson.

Somewhere off to his left there was a resounding crash and a cry of alarm in Latin, followed by the sound of desperate combat. An order was bellowed and, though Cervianus couldn't spare the time to look around, jabbing repeatedly at the gap in the boards, he heard the rushing feet of reinforcements being sent forward from the lines to help hold the wall where it had caved.

Above, the scorpions continued their brutal work, twenty of the heavy weapons firing at will, joined by the hiss of a third volley of arrows from the Cretans. Ulyxes, to the capsarius's right, yelled a warning and leaned away as a wide-bladed spear thrust through the gap in the timber. Cervianus drew a sharp breath as the weapon neared his shoulder, and then smashed his shield against it, shattering the shaft so that the head fell to the ground inside the defences. While he readied his weapon again, Ulyxes took the opportunity to shove his own pilum back through the hole, biting home into flesh.

There was an ominous creak from the palisade and a crack from somewhere at the base. The earth that had been piled behind as a small embankment was being pushed inward as the weight gradually buckled the defences.

"This whole bloody wall's going to come down on top of us in a moment," Ulyxes shouted.

"We need more men here to hold it," Cervianus agreed, shouting over the din. "If it goes, they'll be among the archers and artillery!"

On the capsarius's far side, a cry of pain drew his attention. A gap almost six inches wide had opened in the wooden planks and two sword blades were jabbing and scything through, one of which had gouged a long rent in the next legionary's arm, causing him to fall back in pain.

Cervianus eyed the gap near him suspiciously and then risked a quick glance along the defences. The situation was the same all the way along: small holes had opened up in many places and whole chunks of the palisade were buckling inwards. Their optio was standing on their own well-built platform, watching the situation beyond the wall. Cervianus took a deep breath.

"Sir? Shouldn't we call for reinforcements to hold the wall?"

The officer looked down, frowning, though whether at the situation or the question, Cervianus couldn't tell.

"No. No reinforcements. They're close to breaking now. Another volley or two should see them running and then we have them easy."

Cervianus nodded and returned his attention to the

dangerously bowing palisade. A blade suddenly burst through the defence, driving another hole between the planks. Once again, still hefting his pilum, Cervianus used his huge, heavy and somewhat battered shield to slam the blade from the side, snapping the brittle iron near the hilt.

Things were starting to look desperate, but they should be able to hold a little longer at least. Another swish of arrows rose from the archers at their prefect's signal, peppering the enemy beyond the wall and raising cries of pain and alarm.

The optio would be right, of course. Along with Draco, for all their strictness, the two officers of their century were both experienced veterans and clever strategists, as was expected of officers that rose to command in the prestigious First cohort.

Indeed, as if to support the optio's statement, as the latest hail of arrows claimed their Kushite victims, there was a notable lessening of pressure on the palisade.

"He's right." The capsarius grinned at Ulyxes. "They're about to break!"

The shorter, stockier man grinned back and thrust his pilum through the gap again.

Behind them, the legion's cornu sounded a familiar but entirely unexpected call.

The pair looked round in surprise, along with many of the other defenders, and then, realising that the startling call for withdrawal was being confirmed by the cohort and century musicians, Cervianus looked up to their optio for further confirmation. The officer wore the same surprised look as he stared back at the commanders.

"What in the name of Jupiter's balls?"

But soldiers were already abandoning the creaking defences

and running back to their units. The archers, utterly confused, were replacing arrows in their quivers and turning to leave. The artillerists on the platforms looked stunned, unsure whether to abandon their weapons and run or keep on loosing as their comrades left them alone.

As Cervianus turned, reluctantly leaving that gap with the blades poking through it, he saw Draco storming out of the crowd of withdrawing soldiers and marching purposefully toward the commanders. As he did, he turned and shouted loud enough to be heard across the camp.

"Back to the wall… all of you!"

Chaos ensued once more as soldiers milled about, variously obeying the calls of the musicians or the authoritative voice of the legion's second most senior centurion.

Ulyxes and Cervianus stood still and watched. Vitalis had stepped out from the small group of staff officers, his face turning a shade of purple.

"Sir!" Draco yelled. "We *have* to hold the wall. They're about to *break*."

"You *dare* disobey my orders?" the tribune screeched. The other senior officers backed away nervously from the confrontation, but Nasica, the legion's feared and respected chief centurion appeared from the crowd and strode up to stand at Draco's shoulder.

"He's right, sir. We have to hold. A hundred heartbeats and we can break them where they stand. We can win the day here, without taking the walls."

Vitalis' face had darkened even further.

"Get your men into position. We are abandoning the walls and preparing to move in. I want this legion pushing them back into their own gates and all the way up to that temple in short order. Do you understand me?" His voice had gone dangerously quiet, but the entire compound had fallen silent, barring the noise beyond the palisade and the occasional clatter of the scorpions firing, and the words carried well.

Draco shared a look with his senior centurion. The two men between them had more command experience and strategic knowledge than a dozen Vitalises.

"Sir, we can destroy them with missiles without endangering any more men. Every moment lost weakens our defence. You give them an edge now and then march us on that wall and we'll lose *hundreds* of men before we even enter the gate!"

Nasica nodded seriously.

Vitalis, his eyes glittering, lip curling unpleasantly, grasped the Second century's centurion by the shoulder and turned him with some difficulty, pointing at the wall.

"What glory is there in *this*?"

Draco was dumbfounded. "Sir?"

"Greek auxiliaries fighting our battle *for* us? We're legionaries! It's *our* honour to take the fortress. I'm not about to hand over *my* mural crown to a bunch of degenerate barbarians. I will have that crown award for myself and for our standard. Now have your men fall in for an attack."

Draco looked to Nasica for help, but the primus pilus simply shook his head sadly. Their centurion had played a dangerous game in defying Vitalis' orders – committing an offence for which some tribunes would demand the death penalty. Only the situation and their current need for all the senior experienced officers they could get seemed to have saved him. Even then, Draco's escape was not guaranteed. As he saluted and turned to relay the order to fall in, Vitalis fixed a stare of pure hatred on the man's back.

Cervianus swallowed nervously as the artillerists abandoned their weapons and ran down to take their place in the infantry ranks.

They had almost managed to take Abu with barely a fight, but Vitalis' pride and obtuse idiocy was going to cost them dearly now. The wave of bitter regret over pushing the tribune out of harm's way once more washed through the capsarius.

Realising the worst danger had inexplicably ceased, a roar of triumph and rage arose beyond the defences, and with fresh and renewed vigour, the Kushites overran the palisade.

There was simply no time.

Vitalis put out the order to form into a wedge in order to punch through the seething mass of Kushites but, with only twenty paces separating the two forces as the horde of snarling warriors poured over the flattened and broken posts of the palisade, there was clearly no room to manoeuvre. The scorpions stood silent and still as yelping warriors climbed up the platforms' slopes and began to hack the weapons to pieces in blind fury.

Ignoring the tribune's call for an impossible formation change, the veteran centurions bellowed the commands to their men to form a shield wall.

Braced, leaning into his large, rectangular shield, Cervianus felt the shields of Ulyxes and Fuscus slam into place on either side.

It was a disaster. Due to the sudden withdrawal order and the lack of time to reorganise, most of the soldiers still held a pilum, while a few that had pulled back from the wall or the artillery platforms were waiting with drawn swords.

No one knew what to do. There would certainly be no time to cast the javelins and some of the more enterprising men at the back threw theirs aside and drew their swords ready.

As the front row's shields fell into place, Cervianus risked a glance over the top, only to discover that time was up: the enemy were upon them. He ducked back down as a Kushite axe buried itself in the bronze edging of his shield, the tip glancing off the brim of his helmet with a metallic ring.

An instant later the force of the wild charge hit them. Cervianus felt himself pushed back two steps in quick succession and then a third when a second wave of brutality hit the shield wall.

Chaos reigned. Centurions shouted orders, relayed by optios, standard bearers and musicians, but the plain truth was that, with the onslaught upon them, no time to move or breathe, and precious little unity of direction among the commanders, many of the orders were conflicting, picked up by the wrong musicians, or simply lost in the din.

Cervianus, finding it extremely difficult in the press, raised his pilum in his right arm and tried to thrust down at the enemy, taking advantage of his extra height, but there was just not enough room. Finally, giving up even trying, he threw the weapon over into the enemy, hoping it might do some damage, rocked back on his heel as something hit his shield with a massive thump, and drew his gladius with difficulty in the cramped conditions.

Other men around him were having the same trouble. Still armed with a pilum that was proving useless in the press, they cast them as best they could into the enemy mass and settled for their swords.

Over the roar of battle, Draco's voice bellowed, finally loud enough to cut through and be heard.

"First rank: advance slowly!"

Off to the other side, the primus pilus, Nasica, took up the call and ordered the advance for the whole cohort, a shout echoed finally in unison by all the officers within earshot.

Advance? thought the capsarius in disbelief, as a notched blade crashed into the top of his shield and scraped along the damaged edging, raising sparks as it went. Shifting weight slightly, he opened a gap just over an inch wide between the shields and thrust his gladius through, feeling the telltale change in pressure as the blade flashed through clear air and then buried itself in flesh, pushing through into softer organs.

Ripping it back, he felt it grate off bone and something slopped onto his foot. Paying no heed to the grisly effects of his blow, he pulled the sword back and closed the shield gap again.

Sure enough, despite the almost insurmountable difficulty of moving forward into the seething mass of shouting, dark-skinned warriors, legion discipline and the effect of Draco's commanding tone made the impossible possible.

Ulyxes and Fuscus braced and took a step forward, Cervianus slightly behind but leaning in to catch up. The line, heaving on their shields and putting their backs into physically driving back the riot with their sheer strength, managed a full pace forward, and then another.

To their right a clamour announced trouble. Here and there the Kushites were managing to land blows past the shields all along the front, but a crisis had opened up at the end of the Second century's lines, where several of the roaring, spittle-covered enemy warriors had used axes hooked over the top of shields to topple three of them forward, falling on the suddenly exposed legionaries in the gap and chopping them to pieces. Other Kushites joined them, stabbing and slicing with swords, screams of pain and cries of rage mingling in the melee. Slowly, as more legionaries went down under the flurry of blows, the third row managed to push forward and plug the gap.

The cohort took another step forward, and that extra pace finally made it easier. The Kushites had been thrown by the unexpected advance of their beleaguered enemy and the front lines, heaved into their own mass, began to lose their footing. The pressure of the bellowing crowd lessened and the First cohort moved forward purposefully another four steps.

Despite a failure at the top level of the staff, the centurions of the legion with their experience and discipline had managed to turn the tide of the fight and what had, a moment ago, been a roaring charge of blood-hungry warriors was now turning into a confused and milling mass of men trying desperately to fight back or get out of the way of this sudden brutal advance.

Off to the sides, the men of the First cohort kept the formation tight, only a narrow gap between them and the other cohorts. Seeing the success of Nasica's men, the other cohorts' centurions began shouting out orders, emulating the action, and gradually the entire legion began to move inexorably forward into the crowd of pelt-attired barbarians.

Draco's voice, however, still carried over the other centurions, with its deep, clear authority.

"Use your swords, not just your shields!"

In response, the centuries of the First cohort began to angle their shields as the opportunity presented itself and lash out with their swords. Behind, the advancing legionaries, finally, as the press of men opened up, finding that they had the room, cast their pila overhead and into the mass of confused and angry enemies, drawing their swords in preparation.

Another step forward and Cervianus opened the shield gap once more, stabbing forward with his sticky, glistening blade. It was impossible to miss, given the press of the enemy, and as he withdrew it and closed the gap in the shields it dripped with heavy gobbets of blood.

A desperate warrior somewhere in front managed, despite the confusion, to strike a heavy, overhand blow with a particularly long sword, and the tip punched through Cervianus' shield, the edge slicing deep into the wood. The capsarius grunted as he heaved the shield forward and the sword disappeared with the falling man.

All across the line, cries of pain rang out along with expletives and curses in both Latin and the strange tongue of the Kushites.

And suddenly the press of men before them faltered, broke and scattered.

The enemy force had turned and was running for the gates. The men of the Twenty Second heaved a sigh of relief and halted their advance, clambering over the bodies of fallen colleagues and enemies alike, a few last blows struck out at the backs of the fleeing Kushites.

The primus pilus, however, took several steps forward, out of the line. Cervianus, peering over the top of his shield, watched the officer. Nasica, a man of frightening appearance at the best of times, was coated in a slick of blood, his own shield battered and rent, his transverse crest missing a chunk of white horsehair. He held a sword high.

"Triple time! Secure the gates before they close!"

With a roar, the First cohort surged forward, their chief centurion falling back into the ranks as they ran, leaping over the bodies, shield wall tactics entirely abandoned. The tribune's cornicen blew out the order to advance at triple time, somewhat redundantly since the entire force was already moving forward under the orders of their centurions before the first note sounded. The men made for the gate eagerly and with purpose. Things would be bad enough taking the island without having to besiege the gate first.

The enemy were in full retreat, fleeing back into the island's defences, their charge having failed to drive the steel-clad invaders back to the boats, and the Twenty Second raced up the gentle slope toward them, bellowing violently.

For long moments, all detail of the attack escaped Cervianus, aware as he was only of his immediate surroundings, his chest heaving in laboured gasps as he ran alongside Ulyxes and Fuscus, jumping over corpses peppered with shafts, trying to keep his shield up and not lose his footing.

Behind them, the auxiliary unit followed up more slowly, bows on their shoulders as they gripped swords in their free hand and paused to dispatch any mobile wounded enemy in the lee of the main attack. Vitalis and the staff officers were somewhere behind the force now, largely forgotten – certainly unheard over the battle.

The first Cervianus knew of their proximity to the walls was a shout from Draco.

The First and Second centuries had pulled out ahead of the rest of the army, urged on by their stalwart officers, the best in the legion. So far ahead had they run, in fact, that they were almost upon the enemy. Some semblance of order seemed to have returned to the Kushites and a small, brave section of the retreating army had stopped before the gate and turned to face the pursuing Romans, presenting a solid front in order to give their comrades time to close the gate.

Draco, however, had other ideas.

"Don't stop. Run 'em down!"

The First cohort, their blood coursing, that strange euphoria that enveloped legionaries during battle pounding through their veins, gave a deafening roar and, far from falling into a combat-ready formation as the enemy would expect from a Roman force, hit the Kushites individually and hard as a rolling boulder.

Cervianus launched himself from the ground, putting every ounce of strength into the shoulder behind his shield as he hit a wide-eyed Kushite warrior square in the chest.

It would have been a magnificent sight from higher ground, the green-garbed mass of legionaries hitting the wall of hide-clad defenders like the crest of a wave on a violent sea crashing over a high reef. Along the line legionaries managed to barge through, or even vault over, the defending warriors, landing at a run and racing on toward the closing gate and the suddenly panicked men there. Other soldiers fell foul of the waiting blades of the warriors, impaled and falling, tumbling to the ground with their killers, to be overrun by yet more bellowing legionaries.

Wave after wave of roaring soldiers swarmed over the line of defenders, some pausing en-route to dispatch the desperately flailing warriors. The charge had been unconventional to say the least, and costly on the attackers, with dozens of green-garbed figures lying dead or thrashing around amid the enemy bodies, but the manoeuvre had gained them the time they needed, and the men of the Twenty Second closed with the gate even as desperate Kushites tried to close it on their own fleeing men.

The legionaries fell on the panicked crowd of Kushites like lions, stabbing and shield-barging, pommel-bashing and headbutting. Once again there was little time to view the larger situation or to even think beyond the next blow; every available man was hacking wildly at any non-Roman flesh that presented itself in an effort to push through the gate. Briefly, and with some sadness, Cervianus noted that Fuscus was no longer next to him and found himself hoping, despite the distance that had ever existed between him and his contubernium, that his fellow legionary had merely fallen behind in the rush.

Something metallic smashed into his cheek piece and Cervianus found himself staring at the nicked blade of a sword, less than an inch from his eye as it grated across the bronze. His heart lurching, he wrenched his head to the right to avoid the agonising contact that would come when the tip passed the metal and slid into his face. The sword whipped through open air as he pulled away and bit into Ulyxes' shield at the far side. The capsarius grunted and thrust his gladius into the bare chest of the sword's wielder and heaved him over, pulling it back out with an unpleasant noise as he pushed on forward.

The front ranks of the legion were now in the great square portal of the fortress gate, the doors half closed, and pushing inwards, smashing the resistance with Roman steel. The world here, in the press of men within the narrow entrance, was reduced to a flurry of blows and clashes, shouts of pain and warning, the spray of blood and a slick of slippery, sticky viscera coating the ground.

The legion had taken the gate.

Once again, the pressure was suddenly relieved. As the legionaries grasped the great timber gates and pushed them back wide, running inside, the enemy melted away before them. This time, however, it was no mass flight in a panic. In the blink of an eye, the defenders were simply gone, scattered into the fortress's interior.

The legionaries burst into the open, forum-like area behind the gate as the Kushites fell away, and paused for breath as their enemy disappeared. The fortress was more than a mere line of defences. Buildings of mud-brick filled the interior as it marched up the slope toward the far end of the island, forming a small town of its own with winding, narrow, vertiginous streets, four of which led off uphill from this square alone.

Instinctively, the men of the First cohort fell into a defensive formation as the other cohorts began to move in through the gate. Nasica, with Draco close behind, ran through the lines to the front, signifers struggling with their heavy standards following them, alongside musicians with their cornua. Both centurions were heavily bloodstained.

"First cohort split up. Centuries One, Three and Five to follow me up this road." He gestured to the most central thoroughfare. "The others are with Draco up there." With another pointing finger, he indicated the road to their right. "We meet at the top!"

The men under his command gave a shout and split off into the two groups, the centuries forming around their officers as they moved off. The other cohorts piled into the courtyard and a senior centurion divided his troops among the other two roads, while further soldiers secured the gate itself and began to move along its walls, gaining control of the fortress's perimeter.

As the men of the Second century ran into the narrow, winding, stepped street, Cervianus and Ulyxes found themselves toward the front of the unit again, only a few paces behind Draco and the optio.

"Looks like we might win out *despite* the tribune, eh sir?" the second in command noted with a wry smile.

Draco nodded as he ran. "Arsehole. He's going to lead this legion right into the latrine. Get to the back and keep the men running; things could get nasty in here."

Ulyxes turned to Cervianus and winked. "Some loyal fella ought to do away with Vitalis. Then Nasica could take over. Shit, we'd be in Kush in two days under *him*!"

Although Cervianus winced again at his friend's fearless outspokenness, clearly the sentiments were echoed by their centurion. Draco part-turned at the comment, but nodded slightly and returned his attention ahead.

They had run perhaps seven or eight hundred paces up the curved street, the sounds of the rest of the assault now drowned out by distance and intervening buildings, the curvature of the narrow way hiding anything behind them from sight.

"Halt!" Draco shouted as he came to a dead stop. Cervianus and Ulyxes, along with a number of their fellow legionaries, almost fell into him as they stopped running.

"What is…?" Ulyxes began, but Draco was pointing ahead.

The second line of ramparts crossed the road here, a single gateway in the thick walls standing open with half a dozen men in the gloomy shadowed passage beneath the flat-roofed portal.

"What in Hades?"

Draco suddenly shook his head in realisation.

"Cover!"

At his sharp command, the men of the centuries with him dived to the sides of the road, raising their shields, just as the Kushite archers appeared on the roofs to either side and began to shoot rapidly down. Despite the centurion's warning, there simply *was* no cover here, and shields would not be enough.

"Shit!"

Cervianus looked round to see that Vibius, their flatulent comrade, had now joined them, only to receive an arrow in the thigh.

"Can you move?"

"From *here*? Piss, yes!"

There were fortunately only a few archers above them, but their trap was well laid out, with no cover, and for every shot they took that thudded into an eagle-emblazoned shield, another found flesh.

A rumble from behind suddenly drew their attention and Cervianus glanced back in time to see a tall mud-brick wall from the side of the narrow street topple onto the legionaries in front of it. Screams announced the premature burial of a dozen men as the street became clogged with rubble and filled with blinding dust.

"Forward!" Draco bellowed, holding his shield over his head and coming up from a crouch into a run for the gateway, where the doors were slowly closing on them. Four black shafts protruded from the centurion's shield as he ran. Behind him, the men of the cohort followed suit. The way back was difficult, and becoming increasingly so as another wall came down, deliberately felled on top of the attackers by some unseen hand. Staying here while the archers used them for target practice was also not an option. Twenty legionaries remained in the street ahead of the blockage and they ran for the gateway with a surge of desperate energy.

The six men in the shadow of the gate started suddenly, surprised to see the Roman force still on the move, and the two who were slowly closing the gates redoubled their efforts. Four of them were dressed and armed in much the same fashion as the force that had attacked the beachhead. A fifth man, however, wore a shirt of interlinked bronze plates and a circlet, while his nearest companion bore a mail shirt and small, pot-like helmet. Both were armed with spears.

"Come here," Draco bellowed as he ran into the shade of the gate, the legionaries following him. Two more of the Roman force disappeared in a hail of arrows and a screech of pain at the rear of the attack but in a moment, in the cool shade, they fell on the enemy before the gates could fully close.

Draco had already carved a second grisly mouth in the throat of one of them with a swing of his gladius before his men managed to join him. Ulyxes leapt to his side and drove the bronze boss of his shield into the face of the man with the mail shirt, smashing his teeth and throwing him back against the wall, his spear clattering away to the ground. With a quick thrust of his gladius, he dispatched the man.

The centurion made straight for the warrior in the circlet as the legionaries behind him engaged the remaining three, taking them easily.

"Yield, you piece of shit," Draco snarled as he raised his gladius ready for a downward blow.

The man, presumably an officer or nobleman of the Kushites, straightened proudly and, grasping his spear, thrust it toward Draco. The centurion deftly stepped to the side, grasped the shaft as it swished past his ear, and wrenched it from the Kushite's hand.

"Fine," he said flatly, and delivered a punch to the side of the man's head that drove the consciousness from him before he even hit the ground.

Ulyxes grinned. "You ever considered taking up boxing, sir? You could make a *fortune* at the games!"

Draco turned a glare on him, but it was lacking the usual malice, and even a hint of a smile played at the corner of the officer's lips. "Careful, or I might practise on you. Pick this piece of shit up and let's get to the top of the town. I think this is about over."

Nodding, Ulyxes and Cervianus grasped the unconscious nobleman by the ankles and shoulders, swung him onto a shield and lifted him between them to carry.

"You think this is their leader, sir?"

Draco glanced over his shoulder at them as he walked. "Could be. Let's just hope they're all as tactically dumb as this one if the tribune's insistent on chasing the queen down. I hear she's a *real* bitch."

Draco and his remaining ten soldiers burst out of the narrow street and into the wide space at the highest point of the island. Their selected route had been tortuously winding and slow since the ambush that had separated them from the rest of their century.

The three Kushite warriors who had had the misfortune to round a corner halfway up the slope and bump into the invaders now raced ahead of them, heaving ragged breaths in an effort to stay out of the clutches of the roaring Romans.

The expression on Draco's face as he pursued them would have made Hades himself think twice about intervening, but Ulyxes and Cervianus merely looked exhausted, running along at the back of the unit, carrying aloft a shield bearing the unconscious form of the Kushite noble.

The three enemy warriors, wild-eyed and desperate, pelted out into the centre of the wide-open square and only stopped when they realised what they'd run into. The huge plaza was paved and enclosed by various important-looking buildings, including temples and high-walled official structures. Statues of crown-clad pharaohs and small ram-sphinxes stood in seemingly random positions. A huge temple of impressive dimensions and exquisite colour stood at the highest point, towering majestically over the square.

None of this was, of course, what brought the fleeing warriors up sharply.

The square was also filled with the glittering, green tunic'd forms of the Twenty Second legion. Nasica's journey up the central street had clearly been quicker and more successful than Draco's, and his legionaries were already falling into lines.

A group of dejected-looking Kushites, unarmed and stripped bare, stood before them in the centre. Draco grinned nastily as the three men turned to look at him, and slowed to a purposeful, malicious stride. The fugitives ran over to the relative safety of their captive compatriots.

"Draco? Where are the rest of your men?" Nasica's voice rang out. The primus pilus gestured to the small ragtag group following the centurion from the side street.

"They'll be working their way back round, sir," Draco replied. "We were ambushed and the street was blocked."

"Very well." Nasica nodded. "Looks like things are about done here. The other cohorts are on their way up the streets and along the walls. They have prisoners here and there, but it seems that the bulk of the enemy fled into that."

He pointed at a long, square building, reminiscent of a traditional Aegyptian temple, but considerably smaller. Walls uninterrupted by windows and doors showed no carving or paint.

"What is it, sir?"

"One of the prisoners who has the good fortune to know a little Latin tells me it was a government building at one point. Recently it's been their war-leader's headquarters. I don't want to waste men storming it, so when the tribune gets here I'm going to give them terms."

Draco nodded. "This might help." He indicated the capsarius and his friend, who plodded past their officer and laid the shield with its burden on the ground. "I think this might be their leader."

Nasica nodded thoughtfully. "Might be, but we've found two others with some sort of crown too. This one's certainly a man of import, though. Vitalis will want to see him."

"See who?"

As the legionaries all around came sharply to attention, the two senior centurions turned, covered in sand, dust and blood, to regard the pristine, shining figure of the senior tribune striding into the square, his musicians, standard bearers and junior tribunes in a cluster behind him. Cervianus saw Nasica mouth something to Draco and, although he didn't catch what was said, he saw the smile fighting for control of the centurion's face.

"We have a number of prisoners, sir." The primus pilus

clasped his hands behind his back and addressed the commander as he approached. "There are just over a hundred in the square here, my men report another couple of hundred being herded up here by the Fifth cohort, there are maybe a thousand crammed in that building over there, and we have three men that are clearly nobles and one could be the island's commander."

Vitalis nodded. "Good work, centurion. Very well done. I would have preferred you allowed *me* to lead the attack without running off ahead against orders, of course."

There was a dangerous glint in the tribune's eye, and Nasica straightened.

"No insult or insubordination intended, sir. In the tumult down there we just had to do whatever we could with the resources we had."

Vitalis studied him with flaring nostrils, weighing him up, trying to decide whether that was a sincere apology or, more likely, a thinly disguised attempt at further insubordination.

The primus pilus made several gestures and the three well-appointed captives were brought forward, two sullen and glaring angrily, the other lifted and held up by Cervianus and Ulyxes. An enormous purple and black mark was developing on the side of his face. Vitalis looked at Cervianus with a hint of recognition and noted the bag at his side.

"Wake him up."

"Sir? If I do that it could cause him considerable damage. We don't know—"

"I don't care *what* state he's in when we crucify him. I just want him awake to experience it. Now rouse him."

Cervianus swallowed nervously and nodded, reaching into his bag and withdrawing a small jar of white powder marked

Hammonicus sal. Opening the jar, he wafted it half a dozen times beneath the nostrils of the unconscious nobleman. Both Vitalis and Nasica's noses wrinkled in distaste and the tribune took a small step back. With a start, the Kushite came round, wide-eyed and confused.

"Good." Vitalis nodded approvingly. "Now take these three and have them crucified on the walls in the same places they nailed up our local garrison."

Cervianus shuddered involuntarily. Torture and execution sat badly with him at a deep level, given the teachings of Hippocrates. Grateful that he would have other duties and it would not be him roping, nailing and raising the enemy leaders on the T-shaped execution frames, he watched as fellow legionaries grabbed the three men roughly, saluted to the tribune, and dragged them away from the square. The noblemen, incapable of understanding even basic Latin, had no idea what horrible fate awaited them, and shuffled away despondently.

As he fell back into position, Cervianus noted how the victorious legionaries had, accommodatingly, gathered the healthy Kushite prisoners in one place and their badly wounded in another. Those disfigured and bleeding men leaned against the wall of the building or lay before it, perhaps fifty or sixty of them considered too badly injured to join the mobile captives.

The capsarius saluted to the officers and cleared his throat.

"If I may, sirs? I should be tending to the injured."

Draco nodded and pointed to the shady quarter of the square. "Set up there. The medicus should be here soon. It seems the support staff and the other commanders are all ashore now. I'll have the wounded gathered and sent to you. In the meantime, you can separate the salvageable prisoners and deal with them."

"Unnecessary," cut in the tribune.

"Sir?"

Vitalis pursed his lips.

"Gather all the enemy survivors and deliver them to their friends in that building."

"Sir?"

"For execution."

"But slaves, sir?" Nasica frowned. "The profit from the campaign?"

"No time to take slaves. We're heading south into Kush and we can't take prisoners with us. Send them to their friends and then wall the building up tight."

Cervianus blinked and opened his mouth to object, but Ulyxes subtly gripped his wrist and pressed so hard that the nails dug into flesh, causing him to draw a sharp breath. The smaller, stocky legionary mouthed the words "shut up" to him.

Nasica and Draco approached the tribune together.

"Sir? Even if we march on, we can leave them in a stockade under the guard of a small garrison unit. We'll have to leave men here anyway, including the local auxiliaries. We could pick them up on the way back to Nicopolis?"

Vitalis directed his flinty gaze at the second-most senior centurion. "I have had my orders questioned, ignored and countermanded all day. The next man who does so is looking for disciplinary measures. How would it look if I had to have a senior officer scourged in front of the army?"

The two centurions stared at him. To even suggest such a thing in front of the assembled legionaries was unheard of; it would undermine the authority of the entire centurionate. *Normally, it would*, Cervianus thought to himself, though. In the current circumstances the men were much more likely to feel their respect for these men deepen than fade with such a confrontation. Certainly *he* was seeing the two officers in a new light: the light of reason.

Nasica was the first to straighten, his face carefully neutral. "Very well, sir." Draco looked at his senior just once and followed suit. The primus pilus turned to him. "Centurion Draco? Have a detail force these men into the prisoners' refuge and seal it shut permanently."

Draco, his face pale with rage, saluted and turned, striding back to his unit to give the orders. Everything in the square had gone deathly quiet. Cervianus and Ulyxes stayed rigid where they were, not daring to move in the thick, dangerous atmosphere. Vitalis and Nasica still locked one another's gaze in a silent battle of wills.

The tense spell was suddenly broken by a bright voice from the edge of the square.

"Nice job, tribune Vitalis!"

The two men glared at one another for a moment longer and then wrenched their gaze away to see a group of senior officers in red tunics striding up from one of the streets. At the head were the chief centurions of the Third and the Twelfth legions.

"We watched the charge from the bank. Magnificent. Your centurions are to be commended."

Vitalis twitched slightly at a perceived insult, but nodded. "Syene is secured. I am having the survivors walled up and left. I want to be ready to move south by the end of the day."

The primus pilus of the Third frowned. "You're leaving the prisoners to die? What of slave booty? We've gathered our captives in the forum and roped them ready to move out."

"Frankly, I don't care what you do with your prisoners, but I cannot spare men to guard them as we move on."

The Third's temporary commander shook his head. "I have no intention of taking the men of the Third south of Syene, tribune. At the second cataract Rome's authority ends. We're not an invasion force; we're here to punish the Kushites and retake our lands. I'd say we've done that."

Vitalis began to shake again and pointed an angry finger at the centurion. "These *filth* took prisoners and loot from our lands and then went home with them. This is not over until their land swims in their own blood and we have every last coin and man back."

"That was not in the prefect's orders," the centurion said calmly, shaking his head. "He gave us the task of reclaiming our lands and driving out the Kushites and we've done that."

Again, the tribune shook his finger. "A push south was *implicit* in the orders. He told us to *punish* the Kushites, and that is what we will do. Their queen did this and she is now back in Kush. To punish them, we have to punish *her*."

The senior centurion of the Twelfth cleared his throat quietly. "Gentlemen, the entire army is listening to you. Perhaps we can retire to a more private place?"

His companion from the Third simply shook his head. "Not necessary. The Third will be gathering our prisoners and heading back to Thebes in the morning, leaving a few men to help the local garrison re-establish order."

Vitalis had gone white with anger. "I don't care *what* legion you are from, you are a centurion, while I am a tribune – one of the equites, appointed by the senate. You will take your orders from *me*!"

The senior centurion of the Twelfth fell in next to his

counterpart and both men glared at Vitalis. "The Twelfth will also be marching north, back to Nicopolis, where I intend to lodge a formal complaint over your handling of this entire campaign. I suspect the prefect will want your head, empty as it appears to be, if it ever returns from Kush!"

As Vitalis mouthed hollow words, so enraged he could hardly find his voice, the centurions of the two accompanying legions turned, without a salute, and strode from the square, their escorts following them.

Vitalis watched them go, vibrating slightly. The only sounds in the wide square were the cries of the vultures circling above and the moans of the wounded. After a long pause, while Cervianus and Ulyxes stood rigid, wondering whether they could slip away from the scene, Vitalis turned to his own officers. Nasica and Draco wore expressions of shock and disapproval, but the tribune's face had returned to a more normal colour. He took a deep breath, forcing himself to calm down.

"See to our wounded, wall up the prisoners, compile the usual figures, and begin ferrying men back across. I want to be out of Syene and five miles south before we make camp for the night."

As Vitalis stormed off toward his signifers and musicians and the sycophantic comfort of his junior tribunes, Cervianus turned to Ulyxes.

"He's leading us into trouble."

"That's obvious."

"No. I'm more than just sure. I think the gods have marked him somehow. Once we're encamped tonight, I need to speak to you and Shenti. I need to ask your opinions on a few things."

As Ulyxes frowned at him, shrugged, and wandered off to

the rest of the unit who had made their way around the long route and finally reached the square, Cervianus looked up at the birds above and shuddered, his mind reaching back to those images painted on the ceiling of the temple at Ambo.

The vultures were beginning to circle already.

IX

THE CATARACT

Sentries chatted quietly on the camp's ramparts some eight miles south of Syene. Despite the general stifling warmth that filled the Nile valley even during the hours of darkness, watch fires burned by the gates, and torches guttered intermittently along the palisade.

Cervianus appeared between two rows of tents, his head turning nervously this way and that. They were doing nothing wrong, of course, and even Draco would find no reason to punish them for meeting in the darkness in a deserted corner of the camp, but the whole situation was clandestine and seemed somehow wrong.

Shenti sat on the freshly cut and raised turf embankment, his white garb discarded in favour of a more miscellaneous brown that blended better with the landscape. Ulyxes was strolling along the intervallum walkway with his hands tucked into his belt, whistling: the very picture of a suspicious individual trying to look innocent. Cervianus rolled his eyes.

A quick dash across the walkway and the capsarius dropped to the turf next to Shenti. The cavalryman had an amused grin.

"Perhaps I should have dressed in black and covered my face against recognition?"

"There's no need for that."

The Aegyptian officer laughed quietly. "Then why do the pair of you creep around like children stealing sweetmeats from their mother's kitchen?"

Cervianus shuffled around uncomfortably and gave him a sheepish smile. "It's just that I don't want anyone else hearing about this yet; not at least until we've discussed it, and probably not even after."

"I am still not remotely sure what it is you wished to discuss. Your message was hopelessly cryptic."

Ulyxes strode up and dropped to the ground next to them, hauling a wine sack from his tunic and offering it to them. As they declined the beverage, he shrugged and took a deep pull, sighing with contentment.

"So what is it you wanted to say, Titus?"

Cervianus sat back and pursed his lips, unsure of how to begin without sounding like a superstitious fool. "This might sound stupid, but I was told by the gods to stop the army at Syene." He bit his lip. Superstitious fool it was, then.

"What?"

"At the temple at Ambo. The priest of Haroeris came to find me. He told me that we had to stop the campaign at Syene; that if we went beyond the second cataract we would suffer and die. There was a lot of embellishment in the usual priest-like way, but that was the upshot."

Ulyxes narrowed his eyes. "Why in Hades would a priest tell *you*? I mean it's not unknown for priests to see portents and warn of great dangers and all that crap, but usually they warn someone important. What did he expect *you* to do?"

Cervianus raised an eyebrow and fixed Ulyxes with a piercing gaze. "But I *did* have a chance to stop it, didn't I?"

The shorter legionary frowned in thought and he turned to the capsarius with a sharp look. "You mean Vitalis?"

"Of *course* I mean Vitalis. He's taking us exactly where the priest told me we shouldn't go. Even the commanders of the Third and Twelfth wouldn't go with us. I should have let Vitalis die, but I didn't. Problem is: what to do now? Do I even have cause to believe the priest?"

Shenti nodded. "You *do* believe him though, don't you? If you did not believe, we would not be having this conversation."

Cervianus shivered despite the warmth and the three of them fell silent as a legionary strode past on the rampart above, patrolling the wall. Once he was safely out of earshot, Cervianus leaned forward.

"What's special about the second cataract?"

Ulyxes spread his hands. "More importantly, what's a cataract?"

Shenti laughed lightly again. "The cataracts are places where the great river becomes shallow and rocky, with islands and white water, such as at the southern edge of Syene. They are the reason boats go no further than Syene these days. Long ago, ships used to ply the waters between the cataracts, but the difficulties passing these barriers make it less worthwhile these days. The first cataract is at Syene itself. The third through to the sixth are in Kush, but the second is at the border. It is where the lands of pharaoh end; where Rome's rule ends."

Cervianus nodded. "Then he's telling us not to leave Roman territory. It sounds like good advice."

"The second cataract is also the site of Buhen." Shenti's voice carried a hushed tone.

"Buhen?"

"The great border fortress; the most powerful fortress ever

built in the land of Kemet. The pharaohs used to garrison Buhen, but the lands around it have long been abandoned and Rome considered it unimportant enough to withdraw the southernmost troops to Syene. For certain the Kushites will have left a force in control of Buhen."

Cervianus nodded thoughtfully. "Perhaps there will be another opportunity to turn back there? The priest told me we should stop at Syene, but he also said we should go no further than the second cataract. Perhaps we're safe yet?"

Ulyxes shook his head. "So long as Vitalis is in command, he won't stop. He'll drag us into the jaws of Cerberus if need be to make a name for himself. You know what that means? What we have to do?"

The capsarius regarded his friend suspiciously. "Are you suggesting some sort of insurrection?"

Ulyxes shook his head, but Cervianus noted the look in his eye and the fact that his eyes shot momentarily, guardedly, toward Shenti. "No. Not insurrection. But if some *accident* were to befall Vitalis, we could just turn round and go home. Even the senior centurions like Draco and Nasica are aware of how much of a liability the man is. I'm not sure they'd even stick around long enough to bury him. Need I remind you of Syene?"

Cervianus shuddered, his mind involuntarily raising images of the Kushite nobles groaning as they hung there, nailed to the walls of the Abu fortress, the air in the background filled with the hollow, hopeless wailing of the other survivors as they watched their shelter become their tomb, with legionaries very efficiently and very thoroughly sealing it shut. Draco and Nasica had watched their commander with open loathing throughout the afternoon.

"No. But he's still the tribune in command of the legion. To even talk about... what you're talking about is a death sentence."

Ulyxes shrugged. "Then we'll have to take our chances south of the border, despite what your priest says. The gods are clearly against Vitalis, and if he drags us into Kush the gods will turn against us too, but obviously you'd rather defy the gods than a raving lunatic."

Shenti shrugged. "There is always personal choice. You can choose not to go. Simply leave your legion and travel north. I can provide you with supplies, and the way is not hard to ascertain. The river can be your guide."

"You mean *desert*?" Cervianus blinked. "The ultimate dishonour for a legionary?"

Ulyxes nodded slowly. "Better dishonoured than dead, I suspect, but that's an option for the future. For now we'd best go along with things and see what happens at this second cataract."

The three men fell silent, contemplating the coming troubles, and finally Shenti stood.

"Time for me to leave. I suggest you get a good night's sleep. The journey to Buhen will take more than a week, and the terrain becomes hotter and dryer from here."

The other two nodded.

"We'd best go check on Fuscus, anyway."

Their companion, feared lost during the assault on Abu, had been found among the corpses before the gate, concussed from a heavy blow to the head and missing a finger, a fine stripe across his knuckles showing how close he had come to losing the rest. Cervianus and Ulyxes rose slowly and plodded off in the direction of the medical section.

"You think your Aegyptian friend's trying to scare us, with his stories of the heat and the powerful fortress?"

Cervianus shook his head. "He might be exaggerating the conditions a little, but Shenti's one of us."

Despite Cervianus' scepticism at Shenti's description of the southern lands, the following ten days, spent tramping slowly and wearily through the yellow-brown sands, restricted to the maximum speed of the ox-drawn artillery and support carts, proved him to be correct in every way.

The legion had become more or less accustomed to the dry heat and parched landscape of Aegyptus in the weeks since landing at Alexandria. South of Syene, however, the landscape changed. It was almost like walking into another world. Gone were the fertile tended fields that crowded in on the silt-thick soil of the Nile valley. Here, the flood had a different effect, never settling quite the same. Above the first cataract, the river was narrower and less fertile, the lands to either side dusty and golden with just a narrow curtain of reeds and plants. The small areas of vegetation were few and far between.

There were occasional signs that this land had once been cultivated, though. A sharp eye could make out the criss-crossed lines of long-dry irrigation channels here and there, unused for so long that they were now mere grooves in the dry ground. There were no permanent settlements like the scattered villages they had seen on their journey to Syene; merely tracks and meeting places where the nomad occupants of the desert regions periodically came together. On occasion, though, Cervianus spotted what had once been a small settlement; now a collection of low mounds and piles of mud bricks. Some even appeared to have long-abandoned jetties. The lands beyond the first cataract had clearly been abandoned many decades ago.

By the fourth day, the legion had become sullen and surly. Ignorant of the warnings Cervianus had received, they had left Syene in generally good spirits, looking forward to chastising the Kushite queen and looting her kingdom. But four days of the lands to the south of the first cataract had parched and sapped the enthusiasm from even the most optimistic of men.

The marching songs had ceased and the nights were filled with tired, thirsty and bored men huddling in their tents. Roasted by day, chilled by night, the legion marched toward the unknown, spirits gradually descending as they moved south.

In response, Vitalis had shuffled the chief priest of the Twenty Second out front each morning to wax lyrical about how the gods favoured the legion's march into Kush and how so many signs were positive and the shape of some rock or other visible in front of the rising sun said that Kush would bring glory to Rome and so forth.

Unfortunately, that same priest had, on the first night, confided in one of his friends how poor the omens truly were; in particular the carrion feeders that followed and kept pace with the army, by both paw and wing. That friend had then disseminated the truth through the legion. From the second day the worried priest had let nothing further slip, but the damage had already been done.

The truth of the matter was nothing more than simple confirmation of the legion's suspicions, of course. Watching vultures circling as they marched through endless tracts of sand and hearing the howls and hisses of the predators at night was enough for most men, and the legion was rapidly forming the opinion that this entire campaign was a foolish waste of time and effort.

Now, as the tenth day neared its close, weary and sunburned, the Twenty Second legion with its accompanying auxiliary units caught their first sight of Buhen. There was a collective intake of breath and the sound of five thousand hearts sinking. Buhen was simply massive.

The landscape, here largely flat, with endless rolling waves of brown grit marching off to the horizon, beautifully accentuated the sheer scale of the monstrous fortress. Positioned by the edge of the Nile, a rocky slope separating it from the slow, ponderous flow, Buhen stood impregnable. The walls rose what seemed like a hundred feet, though in reality was probably thirty or forty, thick and powerful, buttressed against artillery and punctuated with towers designed for enfilade missiles. Beneath them a deep ditch provided an extra hazard. Even the engineers were whistling through their teeth and scratching their heads.

As the sun continued its descent toward the russet sands of the west, a call went out and the senior officers and scouts gathered at the front of the column and off to one side, close enough that Cervianus could see the disbelief on most of their faces and hear their hushed tones.

"Sir, how in Jupiter's name are we supposed to take that?"

"Efficiently and without complaint," Vitalis snapped at the junior tribune, silencing him.

The group waited, tense, as the Aegyptian scouts rode up to the commanders.

"Tell me about this place," the commander demanded with no preamble.

LEGION XXII – THE CAPSARIUS

The chief of the scouts, a man with passable Latin, who hailed from Syene and was familiar with the southern lands, sat easily on his horse and smiled, revealing several rotten teeth.

"Buhen in old time hold thousand men. Not now... when owned by pharaoh. Now: small number. This: outer wall. Inside is small fortress with same wall and ditch and small wall."

The tribune swung down from his horse and gestured for the others to join him. With a boot he swept a patch of dirt flat and pointed to it. "Show me."

Without comment, the scout master crouched and used his fingers to draw a rough plan of the fortress. Cervianus craned his neck to get a better view. Closer than most men, he could just make out the shapes, without much of the interior detail. The scout had drawn what looked like a rectangle with a smaller square attached to the interior of one of the longer sides. He finished the makeshift map with a set of wavy lines representing the river.

Vitalis frowned. "Weaknesses?"

The man cocked his head to one side as he ran the unfamiliar word through his head. Frowning, he hazarded, "You want easy way? No easy way. Big walls. Many men. Hard fight."

Once again, tense silence reigned over the group of officers.

"*Two* walls, sir," a junior tribune said nervously. "Two like that. We'll lose hundreds at the least just getting into the outer compound. *Twenty* men could hold that place."

As Vitalis threw the man an angry glance, Ulyxes nudged Cervianus. "Piss all chance of getting in there without losing a third of the men. It makes that fortress at Abu look like a child's toy."

Cervianus nodded thoughtfully.

A child's toy. Children played with many things, but one of the most popular was always... a boat. Sailing boats along streams and gutters; makeshift toys carved from wood or even folded leaves.

Boats.

The optio was so surprised when Cervianus wheeled around to face him, falling out of formation, that he skipped his usual sarcasm and frowned.

"What?"

"Sir? I think there's a way in."

The optio narrowed his eyes but said nothing.

"Sir, you've got to speak to the tribune before they commit to an assault. There's an easier way."

"So, not content with being a know-it-all prick, you're professing to be a tactician now?" the optio said darkly.

The capsarius shook his head. "I'm right, sir. I'm sure I am. It's the river, you see."

The officer's eyes flickered briefly to the Nile as it flowed past. "What about it?"

"Well sir, in the old days, when this was pharaoh's land, they used to trade up and down here in ships, as far as the first cataract at Syene. My friend told me all about it a few days ago when I asked him. There are deserted settlements with broken jetties all the way down."

"Make sense, Cervianus, and get to the point."

"Well sir, this place is right next to the river and the second cataract makes this the southernmost navigable reach of this part of the Nile. It's got to have had jetties and a water-side gate from those days. And if what I can see of that ground-plan over there is right, a water entrance would lead right into the main inner fortress itself."

"So…?"

Cervianus smiled. The optio was interested now.

"Well they clearly haven't had active shipping on this stretch in maybe a hundred years. Is it a fair bet that the river gates are poorly defended and badly kept? They'll not have been used in a century."

The optio shook his head and Cervianus felt the initiative draining away. He was losing the officer's attention.

"I know what you're thinking: that a riverward assault would be much harder than a landward one and they'd just redeploy the defence to there to stop us."

The officer nodded, his eyes narrowing again.

"But if the bulk of the army kept them occupied from the land side with a big show siege, a few centuries might be able to breach the walls at the river gate. Once they're in, the rest should be easy."

"It's unlike *you* to volunteer for special duties, Cervianus."

"Volunteer?" the capsarius said with a start. "No. I—"

His words were brushed aside with a waved hand as the optio strode past him toward Draco. Cervianus stood, watching nervously as the two officers of his century briefly discussed the situation. His attention was drawn rudely by a surreptitious kick on the ankle.

"Ow!"

"Shut up," Ulyxes hissed. "What in the name of Juno's tits are you doing?"

"Trying to find a way in that won't decimate the legion, or worse."

"You prat. You know you've just volunteered our century, and probably the First as well, to a stupid, dangerous river assault?"

"I'd still rather that than be one of the poor devils that Vitalis throws against the outer wall."

The pair fell silent and stood nervous along with the rest of the legion while tactics were discussed. Several moments passed before the optio returned.

"Cervianus: fall out of line and follow me."

With a nervous glance back at Ulyxes, the capsarius arranged the yoke on his shoulder and gripped his shield.

"Leave them."

Nodding, he leaned the pole and his two pila against the heavy shield that stood firm in the sand, and followed the optio. At the head of their century, Draco stood out to the side, arms folded, watching them. As they reached the centurion, Cervianus saluted crisply. Draco barely seemed to notice.

"Come with me, the pair of you."

Scurrying along with the two officers, Cervianus kept his head down as they approached the knot of officers. The scouts had now been dismissed from the huddle, their information given, and they stood with their horses perhaps seven or eight paces away. The legion's tribunes gathered around the dusty map, alongside Nasica, the camp prefect and the chief engineer and artillerist.

"Pardon the interruption, sirs?"

The officers looked up in surprise, but Nasica nodded immediately at his second centurion. "What is it, Draco?"

The centurion straightened. "Respectfully, sir, this legionary may have given us an alternative way in."

Vitalis frowned. "Explain," he said, quietly but sharply.

"Go on, lad," encouraged the centurion. Cervianus blinked at Draco's prompting, but he was nodding while the senior officers waited expectantly.

"Well, sirs, this stretch of the Nile used to be plied by ships, and this was the southern end of the route, so there'll be a water gate on the river side. If that map's accurate, the gate should open straight into the main inner fortress."

He paused, expecting to be gainsaid, but the officers merely waited, their eyes flicking back and forth between him and the map.

"Well, it's been maybe a century since the last ship ever sailed here. My feeling is that the gate won't even have been used since then. The whole fortress was abandoned for decades until the Kushites occupied it, so I suspect that the riverward entrance is badly kept."

"And probably not heavily guarded," Nasica finished for him. "You have some useful native sources, clearly. I'd like to speak to them at some point." The primus pilus turned to the legion's commander. "It's worth serious consideration, sir. We could save a lot of men."

Vitalis frowned, nodding his head slowly. "If a large-scale assault were to be launched in the morning, we could draw the bulk of their forces to the landward walls. A couple of centuries of men might be able to make their way along the river in the darkness beforehand and be ready to take the back door quickly and by surprise at the same time."

Draco cleared his throat.

Nasica spoke up at this prompt. "There might be an even better way, sir. Give me an hour and I think I can deliver you a plan to take the place without a siege, building on the lad's observations."

Vitalis stood for a while as the officers waited with bated breath.

"Very well, Nasica. For now we'll make camp and as soon

as everything's set up I want all officers at my tent for a full strategy meeting."

Cervianus chewed on his lip and looked up nervously at the circling vultures. This was it: they were at the first cataract.

"What if we find a crocodile?"

The optio stopped, his feet sloshing in the shallows, and turned to the man behind him, his face pale and unimpressed in the moonlight. A dozen soldiers bumped into one another in an effort to stop suddenly.

"Then, legionary Ulyxes," the optio said with quiet menace, "if you have not shut up complaining, I shall make every effort to feed you to the bloody thing!"

Ulyxes grinned. "I reckon they're too frightened of the centurions to come near us anyway."

Behind him, Cervianus rolled his eyes despairingly and then returned quickly to watching for the dangerous beasts. Crocodiles seemed to be considerably rarer here above the cataract, likely due to the absence of farmed land and the subsequent lack of prey, but the telltale V-shapes in the water had betrayed their presence at times during the journey, so they were still around somewhere.

The two centuries had had their ranks replenished by transfers from the other cohorts following the losses at Syene. Nasica had deemed it critical, given their task, that the two centuries be full, drafting in the required thirty-five extra men. Now, one hundred and sixty-four soldiers crept along the reed-knotted banks, clinking and sloshing despite their efforts.

Ahead, the bulk of Buhen rose like a mountain beside the Nile, a dizzying and heart-stopping prospect. Cervianus' assessment, based on the knowledge of Shenti and the guides, had proved to be accurate so far.

The side of the complex that rose above the great river was every bit as tall and heavily fortified as the inland face, but with several notable differences. Here, the slope between the reed-choked bank and the walls had been sealed off to land forces by an extra jutting wall and tower at each end, effectively creating a private dock area for the fortress. However, the century or so since it had been used for such purposes had seen the bank silt up heavily and reed beds expand, from an occasional nuisance that the defenders would have to remove, into an almost solid mass that blurred the division between land and water.

Two huge stone jetties projected out into the river, solidly constructed and still in good condition despite the decades of neglect, though the silted bank of the river now rendered them landlocked for over half their length. At the landward end of each jetty the buttressed fortress wall was punctured by a gate flanked by enormous square towers.

It was a terrifying prospect for an assault, with one redeeming point:

The lack of defenders.

During the daylight there had been some doubt and debate still about whether the Kushites would evenly distribute their defence force or concentrate them to face the bulk of the Roman threat inland.

Since nightfall, however, as the braziers and torches were lit along the wall tops, it had become clear that attention was mostly being paid to the landward side, where the blazing beacons on the walls lit the open ground around the fortress like a mockery of the hot sun.

Here, however, four fires were all that could be seen along the defences. One brazier burned on each end tower where the walls met the river, and two more flamed above the gates. No other flickering lights. The ghostly moonlight gave the walls a strange bluish tint.

"Aww, shit. I think I trod in something!"

Sniggers rippled through the century at the comment and the optio stopped again.

"Next man who makes a sound gets to dig the shit trenches for the whole camp alone tomorrow night."

Silence fell over the century at the officer's tone. Like Draco, he was not a man noted for his sense of humour. He had been allowing a certain leeway among his men so far tonight, knowing what the legion was asking of them, but as they closed on the fortress, secrecy was the prime factor and even a cough could change the whole course of the assault.

"That's better. We're getting too close now for piss-taking. Everyone keep an eye on me and watch for signals."

The men nodded silently, professionalism taking over.

Once the camp's fortifications had been put in place as the sun sank into the western sands, the men had gone about the business of erecting tents, digging latrines and preparing a meal, and the officers had met in the command tent and hammered out the basic structure of a strategy based on Draco's new plan. This had then been relayed via the centurions and their optios to the men later in the evening.

The plan was daring to say the least. Draco had told them that the strategy had been mostly devised by the tribune and agreed by all officers present, though Cervianus was sure that was not the case. The scheme had all the hallmarks of Nasica and Draco about it, placing a small number of units in a ridiculously dangerous position in order to safeguard the lives of the bulk of the army.

And thus, rather than getting a night's rest and setting off a few hours before dawn to fall into position, here they were only two hours after dark, traipsing through the murk by the Nile. The First and Second centuries bore the lightest possible kit, with only sword and armour; no pila, given the task ahead of them. Even the shields might be a problem, but they had been brought along anyway. Each century had been split into two units of forty men, commanded by a centurion or optio.

Cervianus, his unit being the last of the four in the line, peered over the heads of the others to see that the front of the silent, narrow column sloshing through the reeds had almost reached the corner tower. Locking his eyes on the top of the fortifications, he could just make out the silhouettes of several figures moving back and forth past the flames.

He estimated perhaps four or five men were active up there. If the same held true for the other towers they would have maybe a score of men to deal with, giving them generous odds, even taking into account the difficulties of access.

The native auxiliary officers and scouts had generally agreed that the Kushite garrison of the fortress would not likely number more than four hundred. Even in the days of its power, Buhen had held at most a thousand men at any one time, the crack troops of the pharaoh living in the central fortress while hired mercenaries and desert nomads lived within the outer enclosure.

Four hundred men was a pittance and would hardly make a legion commander blink were it not for the scale of the defences they manned, which more than doubled their effective strength.

Not *this* way, though.

The silence was broken by a splash and a curse ahead, followed by a great deal of hushing and the sound of a quiet blow with a vine stick. The unit commanded by Draco had dropped their ladder into the water. The entire column held its breath and came to a complete stop, trying to melt into the landscape. The river burbled and splashed on by, the voice of nature helping to disguise the noise of the Roman force.

No cry of alarm went up on the tower and after fifty thundering heartbeats the men of the assault force heaved sighs of relief and began to creep forward through the reeds, their care and silence even more absolute.

Grateful that he hadn't been one of the men carrying the enormous siege ladder, Cervianus flexed his knuckles and patted the hilt of the gladius at his side. Once more, for the third time since they had slipped down the bank and into the reeds, the entire column paused as Nasica, leading the front unit, encountered a place where the solidity of the ground beneath the reeds became questionable, the sloping bank giving way to sucking mud or deeper water.

Gradually, they worked a way around the troublesome spot and the column moved on again, following the trail the heavy, studded boots of those in front had left along the shore.

There was a tap on his shoulder and, his attention fixed on the approaching tower and its occupants, Cervianus nearly leapt out of his skin and had to fight to stop himself yelping. Turning angrily, he saw Ulyxes holding out the length of rope he'd been carrying and mouthing "your turn".

Grumbling silently and making an angry face at his friend, the capsarius snatched the rope and slung it over his shoulder, turning and stomping onwards.

As the last unit approached the corner defence tower, the front was nearing the far jetty and beginning to mass in position. Cervianus examined the defences as they came closer and closer. The tower had clearly been constructed as part of a complex system including the jetties, gates and a low outer defensive wall. Originally the huge tower had risen straight from the depths of the Nile, with the fortress's occupants no doubt dredging the side of the river annually to remove the silt build-up left by the inundation.

Failure to deal with the flood's effects for decades, however, had left the tower fully landlocked with enough of a silted bank around it to drive a wagon train across without getting wet. The Roman unit had simply walked around the defence among the reeds on the silty ground. Equally, the low wall had fallen into a state of almost hopeless disrepair, parts of it having gone entirely. Even those sections that almost reached the original height of ten feet were of no defensive value, the silt having largely submerged them and turned them into a low-banked dune that ran along the length of the fortress.

Despite their direct proximity to the fortress, the assault force was in increasingly better concealment, with the light from the tower unable to penetrate the shadowy area at the base of the walls. Slowly and with infinite care, the soldiers of the two centuries began to assemble in the area of ground between the enormous gatehouse and the piers. Each man stood tense, awaiting at any moment the cry of discovery from the top of the towers. The First century stood at the far pier, a huge scaling ladder still held by twenty men. The Second century, every bit the mirror of the First and with its own ladder, waited for the signal.

Over on the far pier the figure of Nasica, barely visible in the shadows even with his bright transverse crest, made a number of signals that were immediately picked up by Draco and his optio. Prepared beforehand with prior knowledge of both the plan and the various signals, the men of the Twenty Second legion began to move into position.

The water gates of the fortress were guarded by heavy, square towers that reached the same height as the main walls, and which opened onto a wide walkway above the gate itself. Access to any point above the gate would mean access to the entire wall system.

The door itself was heavy timber, apparently banded with bronze. Despite the ravages of time, the portal seemed to have lasted well and would be too strong to effect a simple entrance that way, but the ropes and ladders were clear evidence that Draco's plan had not been to slip in unnoticed through a door.

In the silence the men could hear, over the burble and stutter of the water, the low murmur of conversation from the defenders on the lit tower. Hearts pounded as the century's shields were stacked ready to be sent up at the end, the ladder manoeuvred out ready, and the six long ropes knotted together to create two enormous lengths.

As Cervianus tied the remaining two ropes together with the aid of Ulyxes, he nodded to his friend, testing the strength by hauling on it with satisfactory results. The stocky legionary grinned and let go of his end, stepping back. With a start, Cervianus realised that the other men who had been working on this rope had also let go and withdrawn.

Whipping his head this way and that, Cervianus tried to identify who had originally been carrying the first length of rope with the attached grapple. The man was nowhere to be seen.

"Well volunteered," Ulyxes mouthed at him, smiling wickedly. The capsarius felt his heart lurch and let go of the rope, dropping it to the dirt.

A voice, little more than a susurration next to his ear, said, "Pick the bloody thing up and get ready."

Cervianus turned to see the optio glaring at him. Flashing a look of anger and indignation at Ulyxes, he crouched and gathered the entire forty-foot length of rope, coiling it and hanging it on his shoulder, where it pressed down with the weight of a small cart horse, while the iron grapple scraped and bashed irritatingly on his mail shirt.

"Cheating bastard," he mouthed back at Ulyxes. The other men around his friend were also grinning at the capsarius and he realised he had been singled out by his companions in return for volunteering them for the dangerous duty.

With a sigh, he turned and watched as the optio moved among the unit, finding the other rope bearer and directing him into position. Draco's men were now gripping the ladder between them, eighty hands grasping the sides, ready to raise it as swiftly and quietly as possible. At the optio's signal, Cervianus carried his rope forward and fell in at the wall end of the ladder, opposite the other rope bearer. His heart sank a little further as the optio used his fingers to flash a "II" at the other man and a "I" at him. First over the wall. Not even a corona muralis, that prized military decoration, would make this worthwhile.

His blood rushing and pounding, Cervianus watched for more signals. Every passing moment felt like an hour of anticipation until at last some gesture that he couldn't see was given on the far pier and relayed by Draco and the optio.

With just the creak of wood and the sound of dozens of men

breathing heavily, the huge scaling ladder began to rise from where it lay perpendicular to the tower. The men at the far end, back along the pier, let go with gratitude as the top of the ladder rose above their heads. The grunting of the men at the wall end near Cervianus spoke volumes to the sheer strength and sweat involved in raising a ladder more than thirty feet in length and sturdy enough to carry the weight of half a dozen armoured men.

Slowly, almost ponderously, the ladder rose, more and more men letting go further back as it left their grasp, the strain falling ever more on the few men at the front. Cervianus could have felt sympathy for them, had he not been in a considerably worse position himself.

For a muscle-tearing moment, the optio gave them the signal to pause and the men held the ladder at a little over forty-five degrees while the one at the other gate, controlled by Nasica's men, caught up. Then at a further gesture, the two ladders continued to rise at an even rate.

Cervianus found himself holding his breath as it neared the vertical. This was the crucial moment. The engineers could so easily have miscalculated their estimate of the walls' height, resulting in a ladder so long it would stand proud, clear and rather obvious, above the battlements, or so short that a man could not reach the parapet from the top. Moreover, it only took one defender that happened to be alert and looking in the right direction to foil the whole plan.

However, the top of the ladder, controlled expertly by the men below, lowered to the stonework with hardly a sound and in perfect position. The entire force moved instantly to directions gestured by the officers. No time could be spared now.

Gritting his teeth and wishing he'd been alert enough to be the first to drop the rope and leave this "honour" in the hands of its originally intended recipient, Cervianus set his foot on the bottom rung and began to climb at a steady pace, sacrificing a little speed for the security of not slipping, dropping the rope, or making excess noise. Slowly he rose, his left hand gripping the side rail and his boots finding easy purchase on the well-constructed rungs. The huge coil of rope swung as he climbed, causing him to pause here and there and adjust it. Below him, he could see the other rope bearer perhaps ten rungs behind. The man seemed to be having a little trouble. As he climbed, Cervianus took the opportunity to peer down between his own knees at the legionary.

A soldier from another contubernium whom he recognised vaguely at best, the man was staring fixedly at the rungs as he climbed and his face had taken on a pale and waxy sheen. The capsarius shook his head in disbelief. Had the man not explained to the officers about his fear of heights before all this started? More likely he had done just that and the centurion had blithely ignored it anyway. Nothing could be done about it now but, had *he* been in control, he'd have sent that man up last.

Slowly, Cervianus approached the top of the ladder. The voices on the gatehouse became clearer and louder as he neared the crest. Obviously someone had made a joke, judging by the hoarse, deep belly laughs. The language was strange. He'd only heard the native Aegyptian tongue spoken in overheard conversation a few times, and it had seemed exotic and difficult. This language, though, made Shenti's mother tongue sound positively bland and northern.

Trying not to pay too much attention to the oddities and

interesting facets of the Kushites, Cervianus returned his attention to the task at hand. The top of the ladder, planned perfectly as always by the engineers and raised under the expert supervision of the optio, had touched down against the mud-brick walls just two feet below the parapet.

Taking a deep breath and holding it, Cervianus pulled himself up so that he was only a couple of feet below the edge, with the light and heat from the fire and the strange mixed scent of sweat and some sort of spice drifting out from the top. Pausing for only a second, the capsarius took another deep breath and, closing his eyes for a moment with sheer nerves, leaned out to his right with the grapple, the rest of the rope still coiled on his shoulder, his left hand gripping the ladder so tightly that his knuckles went white.

There was a horrible moment when he felt his foot move, the hobnails of his boot sliding along a rung as the tremendous weight of the rope threatened to pull him from the ladder while he leaned over thirty feet of space, flailing with the grapple.

Then, suddenly, and a cause of great relief, the iron prongs bit into the mud-brick crenel. Swiftly now, aware that discovery was inevitable at any moment, Cervianus released the rope into the air, reached down and grasped the other rope being held up by the ashen-faced man below. Repeating the procedure with his other hand, Cervianus hooked the second grapple over the far crenel and let the rope unfold down to the ground.

Clenching his teeth and holding as tight as he could, Cervianus reached down and slid his gladius from its scabbard. Now he would just—

A cry of alarm went up from the second gate, some fifty paces upriver, and was swiftly picked up by the men above. Desperately, aware now that speed was crucial, Cervianus struggled up the last few rungs and thrust himself up over the top of the battlements, lunging forward and rolling onto the flat walkway.

The five men on the tower top had just begun to react to the alarm call from their allies further along the wall, drawing their weapons and rushing to that side of the fire to try and identify what was happening without the dancing flames ruining their night vision. It was a poor move as it turned out, giving Cervianus plenty of space to roll out across the surface and come up, sword in hand.

The five men, weapons out and ready, had not yet noticed him. Sparing a quick glance over the edge, he was pleased to see legionaries already climbing both ropes as well as swarming up the ladder. A flickering light to one side caught his eye and he noted with satisfaction that a warrior had left a burnished bronze shield, perhaps two and a half feet across, leaning against the parapet. Good. His own shield would not be hauled up until the whole unit had arrived. Quickly, he stooped to grasp the bronze disc and slid the shield onto his arm.

Finally, as four of the men bellowed urgent questions at their friends, the fifth turned and saw Cervianus, shouting another warning.

"Come on!" the capsarius bellowed to the man on the ladder behind him. He could see the legionary's hands hooked over the brick of the parapet, gripping for dear life, but the man appeared to have stopped there.

"Shit!"

The tower's defenders had split up, two of them circling around one side of the fire, the other three at the far side. Any moment now he was going to be fighting five men on his own, largely because of a case of acrophobia that had left the second man clinging onto the wall's edge, unable to take that last desperate step and haul himself over to the relative safety of the tower top. The man was blocking the ladder and shouts of anger and consternation were now ringing out from below, from the men who should even now be pouring out onto the top to help take the tower. At this rate, the rope-climbers would get here before anyone reached the top of the ladder, by which time Cervianus would be long dead.

The five Kushites continued to close on him around the fire. There was nothing he could do. Once they had him between them, he was as good as dead. Taking yet another deep breath and throwing a quick prayer into the ether for any god that happened to be listening, he took a running jump and leapt across the fire that roared away in a low, circular iron grate at the tower's centre.

Feeling the tortuous heat as he passed through the flickering flames, he came down at the far side and went straight into a roll in case his clothes had caught. The mail shirt protected him from the worst jarring as he hit the floor and he came up breathless but uninjured.

The capsarius allowed himself a moment to take stock of the situation. Three of the men had changed direction and were now bearing down on him again. The soldiers on the unaffected towers around the fortress had become aware of the trouble and Kushite warriors were pouring along the walls on their way toward the water gates. The remaining two men on this tower bore down on the ladder-bound panicked legionary, transfixed by his fears. With a sneer, a warrior kicked the man's knuckles hard, breaking fingers and causing the soldier to lose his grip.

With a scream that pierced the night, the terrified legionary plunged back into the air, tumbling the thirty-some feet to land below among the Romans. The Kushite and his companion leaned forward to push the ladder away from the wall, but retreated in surprise as the grinning face of Ulyxes appeared over the lip and the tip of the legionary's sword burst through the back of the first ebony warrior.

In a feat of what seemed like superhuman strength, Ulyxes heaved the two men, one already dying as he clutched at the blade in his chest, back from the wall and stepped out onto the surface. Cervianus didn't have time to pay any further attention, however, as the other three men were on him. Unable to think of another way out, he found himself backed up against the parapet on the inner side of the gatehouse.

As the first man swung a heavy axe, the capsarius raised the shield to block the blow, his blade coming up to parry the sword of the second. Weight of numbers would decide this fight, though. Having successfully fought off the first two blows, there was nothing left to help against the third, and the spear thrust glanced off his armour at the collar bone, smashing into the mail shirt, carving a chunk out of the top of his shoulder and sending loose metal links scattering this way and that.

Wincing at the pain, Cervianus did his best to ignore it. The swordsman came in for another swing and, having to make an impossible choice, the capsarius left himself open to the axe man, slamming his shield in the way of the sword blow while stabbing out at its author with his gladius. The Kushite gasped as the sword entered his gut, and Cervianus made sure he wrenched sideways and up with the blade as he withdrew it, delivering the most painful and terminal wounds he could in order to remove the man from the fight.

So much attention had he invested in the swordsman that he barely had time to react as the axe came round for a second swing and he ducked at the last moment, feeling the blow smash off his helmet at the forehead, slicing the crest holder from the top and leaving the perfect bowl hopelessly misshapen.

His ears rang and hissed with the deafening sound caused within by the heavy axe head striking his bronze helmet, and his eyes crossed and defocused. It was blind luck really that he saw the second spear thrust coming. Desperately, fighting for his life, he dipped to the side and the spear plunged through the air where he had been standing a heartbeat before. Thrusting his leg out wildly, Cervianus caught the spearman as he leaned in to the failed blow. The momentum caused the Kushite to trip and sail out over the parapet, wild-eyed and shrieking as he plummeted down to the ground below.

Cervianus tried to focus and his eyesight began to return just as the axe's shaft, held in two hands, thrust up against his throat, pressing into his Adam's apple. The Kushite leaned forward against him, his hot, stinking breath inches from Cervianus' face as the capsarius fought to regain his senses following the blow to the head.

Desperately, as the man began to squeeze his windpipe with the shaft, Cervianus tried to bring his gladius round for a blow but the big Kushite simply delivered him a painful knee in the wrist, smashing his arm against the parapet, the sword falling 'away, useless.'

Speckles and lights began to dance in front of the legionary's eyes as the lack of breath began to deal real damage. The Kushite's rotten teeth grinned at him and those black-upon-pure-white eyes poured their rage down on him.

Desperate. No air. Cervianus felt the shield fall from his weakening arm.

And suddenly he was staring at the tip of a gladius that emerged from the man's neck. The spurt of warm blood soaked and blinded Cervianus, spraying across his face as the shocked Kushite staggered back from Ulyxes' blow, releasing the pressure as he dropped the axe.

"Don't fall asleep, you prat. There's loads more coming."

Cervianus' ears were still ringing but his sight had returned, much as he'd rather it hadn't right now. He had taken advantage of the free moments after Ulyxes had saved him from being choked to death to adjust his gear. His mail shirt hung ragged, a patch of links gone from the shoulder where it was soaked red, the shoulder flap detached by the blow and hanging uselessly down the back. Damaged, but still serviceable for the moment.

His helmet, on the other hand, had become more of a hindrance than a help. The axe blow that had sheared off the crest holder had also left such a massive dent in it that the metal pressed deeply into Cervianus' head just above the hairline. After a cursory glance, he discarded the helm, rubbing the tender spot on his head.

That had been all the time they could spare, however. There were clearly more than the predicted four hundred Kushites in the fortress. At a rough guess there was almost that number already on the walls or mounting the stairs just visible further along, rushing to repel this incursion, never mind the reinforcements that continually appeared from doorways.

The Roman forces had taken control of both water gates

and the section of wall between them was now secured, while the first bundle of shields arrived and was distributed among the men.

Both Nasica and Draco had assigned legionaries to control the stairwells that rose from the depths of the gatehouses and opened onto the top. The heavy wooden trap doors had been slammed shut and four men kept each closed, piling Kushite bodies on top to help prevent access.

Now the men serving under Cervianus' optio fell into formation on the wall top. Even at their narrowest, the massive walls of Buhen were wide enough for five men to stand abreast. Given the need for manoeuvring room, the optio had formed his legionaries into a column four men wide and ten deep, a solid wall presented at the front, the forward ranks of the column having now been re-equipped with the huge eagle-emblazoned shields.

Screaming, dark-skinned warriors in animal pelts were racing around the wall system toward them while more poured up a staircase that fed the walls from the inner fortress a little ahead.

Cervianus had settled into the third row of the column, grateful not to be at the front, given his lack of protective headgear. The unit moved forward slowly and deliberately, its objective to secure the walls. Draco's theory had been sound, of course. Four hundred defenders could easily be overcome by two centuries if the Romans maintained control of the walls. Then no slow and deadly assault on the outer walls would be necessary. Odds of three to one against meant nothing when legionaries had the advantage.

But the odds were gradually changing. Risking a glance over the edge, Cervianus could see yet more Kushite warriors pouring out of the buildings within the inner fortress. More like eight hundred. Almost a full garrison.

In front, someone shouted "Brace!", and the half-century came to a halt, feet planted firmly on the mud-brick wall walk, shields forward and swords ready to begin the brutal butchery.

Behind the unit, the last of the men arrived on the wall top, clambering up the ladder and falling in at Draco's commands. The remaining bundles of shields were drawn up on the ropes and distributed. Leaving four men in control of the tower, the centurion brought the other half of the century along the walls, following the optio's unit.

Suddenly, the world two rows in front of Cervianus exploded. A screaming mass of warriors, visible as strange, almost animal-like figures in the sporadic flickering firelight, threw themselves against the four-man shield wall at the front, yelling things in their strange language and bringing axes and swords down in overhand blows, trying to find a way around the solid shield defence, while men behind them thrust blindly with spears.

The initial pressure as the charging barbarians fell against the wall of steel was soon relieved as the Roman swords began to lance out between the shields in carefully opened gaps, biting into flesh again and again like some grisly machine. Warriors were stabbed and knocked aside to fall, screaming, into the compound below or collapse, half-draped over the crenels of the battlements.

Cervianus, with a clearer view than most, his height advantage increased by his lack of a restricting helmet, was forced to continually duck his head this way and that to avoid the random desperate spear points that found their way back past the first line of men.

Hot liquid sprayed across the capsarius's face, forcing him to squeeze his eyes shut for a moment. As he felt it stop, he opened them again to see the men surrounding him soaked in blood, a legionary on the front line lolling to one side and missing most of his head as a blood-soaked axe was withdrawn for a second swing.

Ignoring the gore, the man in front of Cervianus lifted his shield and barged the body out of the way. The dead legionary, still standing in the press, unable to collapse due to the close mass of bodies, was thrown to one side as the replacement legionary stepped forward to take his place. Cervianus moved into the gap, taking his new position in the second row and blinking as blood and other matter ran down his face.

The unit took a step forward at the optio's bellowed command, good footing a difficult proposition among the bodies. A scream announced the second Roman casualty. The man at the inner side of the wall had succumbed to a blow from that same axe, blocking it with his shield just in time, but the momentum causing him to lose his balance and tumble over the precipice into the fortress itself. Once more the lines shuffled forward to fill the gap.

The fighting began to thicken now, more and more groans or shrieks coming back from the front line. Barely had Cervianus time to count to five before another man disappeared to a well-aimed sword blow or a lucky spear thrust; the lines shuffled forward almost continually.

This was not what he had envisaged. Cervianus' original thought, before it had been taken from him by the officers and turned into some brutal and heroic assault, had been a sneaky incursion to get the gates open.

He could *understand* Nasica and Draco, of course, wanting

to try and take the entire fortification without committing to a hugely costly frontal assault, but it was hard to appreciate the manpower-saving tactic when you were standing soaked with blood and brains as your companions were carved away around you. Of course, some blame had to fall on the scouts for so seriously underestimating the defending numbers, almost halving them in fact.

His inner monologue of recriminations was rudely interrupted as the man in front crumpled under an axe blow that managed to reach over his shield, biting deep into his shoulder. His arm all but severed, the legionary disappeared, screaming, under the press, leaving Cervianus desperately pushing his shield up into a defensive position. He was now at the front.

The unit had moved perhaps twenty steps from the edge of the tower. Ahead, the stairs up from the ground level were still feeding men into the fight, but the press was beginning to even out and each step forward was becoming easier.

A warrior smashed into Cervianus' shield and the shock made him yelp as his wounded shoulder, raw and pink, took the worst of the blow.

"All good fun, eh?"

Cervianus blinked as he stabbed out with his gladius, sliding the blade into the chest cavity of the warrior before him. Unable to afford time to turn his head, he mentally rolled his eyes at Ulyxes' idiotic comment. The two friends now formed the centre of the front row and it was with some gratitude that Cervianus remembered just how vicious and bloodthirsty the shorter man could be when he got the taste for a fight. Frantic sword slashes and axe blows rained down on their shields and the four men at the front rhythmically stabbed out with their gladii, feeling the blades strike home every time in the tight press.

To Cervianus' left, the man at the flank succumbed to a lucky spear strike that smashed into his face and thrust through until it struck the back of his helmet. Dead instantly, the legionary slumped without even time to cry out, and the man behind unceremoniously knocked him from the wall and took his place.

"Fancy meeting you two ponces here!" Vibius, the ruddy-faced soldier who shared their tent, fell in alongside them and began to help carve out a path.

"Maybe you could fart and blow them off the wall," Ulyxes bellowed helpfully.

"This is pissing ridiculous. We're losing too many men!"

Cervianus nodded his agreement with Vibius' assessment as he struck again and again, his head lurching to one side to avoid an errant spear.

The optio at the column's rear repeated the order for slow advance, and the men took another laboured, difficult step forward.

"So what can we do?" Cervianus asked, an intentionally rhetorical question. There was nothing that could be done but push slowly forward, fighting like lions, until either they died or the enemy thinned out enough for them to give in.

"Screw it. Let's charge the bastards!"

Despite the clear need to keep his close attention on the dangerous mass in front, Cervianus found himself turning to stare in disbelief at Ulyxes. A sword swipe that came close enough for him to feel the current in the air as it whistled past drew his attention back forward.

"*What*?"

"Let's break 'em."

Vibius laughed to his other side. "Might give us an edge!" he agreed.

The legionary to the far side of Ulyxes, a man Cervianus didn't recognise, cleared his throat. "Are you lot frigging mad?"

"Come on."

Cervianus found himself bracing his left leg ready, despite his misgivings. Ulyxes took a deep breath and shouted over his shoulder to the supporting lines. "We're going to charge the whoresons! Ready?"

There was a rousing cheer behind him that almost drowned out the optio's voice snapping orders at the rear.

"Charge!" Ulyxes bellowed.

Launching forward from their braced left feet, the four front men put all their weight behind their shields, the use of swords all but forgotten. The second, third and fourth rows behind added their weight and strength to the push and the Kushites, taken by surprise by this sudden reversal of the action, found themselves being barged back among their own advancing mass. Men all along the wall, unable to keep their footing as the wave of warriors crumpled backwards, found themselves thrust into open air over the edge of the wall, plummeting to their deaths.

The optio at the back, a man who knew an advantage when he saw it, had stopped calling out the slow advance and had picked up the cry to charge that was already being bellowed by most of his men.

The very first push had broken the advance of the Kushites and they found themselves now being driven back along the wall. The arrival of reinforcements up the staircase halted; more and more warriors found themselves pushed and squeezed out over the edge of the precipice, grasping on to their friends to arrest their fall and invariably pulling those men to their doom alongside them.

Cervianus laughed at the absurdity of it. Forty men had not only fought off and pushed back a force of perhaps two hundred, but they had now managed to put them to flight. And such was apparently the case. The Kushites were retreating along the walls toward the tower at the corner of the inner fort, where they would have the choice of rushing inland along the inner defences, or continuing along the riverbank walls of the outer compound.

The optio called the command to halt, reining in his men before they overextended their insane charge. A man of great experience, the officer could see beyond the euphoria of the moment. The enemy still outnumbered them by more than two to one at the very best estimate and as soon as their panic died down they would regroup for a second attempt to repulse the Romans.

Ahead, the mass of fleeing men had passed the stairway that led on to the wall; a few warriors appeared up from it, staring wildly at the blood-spattered gleaming Romans, and running back along the wall to join their retreating companions.

"Move forward at a steady pace and secure the stairs!"

Settling back into a shield wall, the remaining thirty men of the optio's command marched along the wall, stepping over the bodies until they had fully cleared the site of the brutal combat and entered the open wall top that the enemy had fled and left clear. On they stepped until the rear of the small column passed the stairway, now devoid of men, the reinforcements who had been using it having withdrawn, finding other, safer, ways up to help their friends.

Behind the optio's unit, Draco's half-century set guards on the stairway and then moved up to join them again. The two officers conferred for a moment, their voices carrying in the sudden silence left by the absence of fighting.

"Take your men along the outer wall. Try and get to the main gate and open it. Then the tribune can come in as he wishes. I'll take the rest and push along the wall of the inner fort until we can open that gate too; lay the whole place bare."

The optio saluted. "Be careful, sir. They fight like trapped animals and they're getting ready for a second push."

Draco nodded and waved him away. The optio turned back to his men.

"Alright. I expect you all heard that. We go to the next tower and then straight on and leave the left-hand wall to the centurion and his men. Soon as we get to that tower they might start to fight back hard, so hit 'em with everything you have. Ulyxes? That was some nice work back there, but you pull a stunt like that again without consulting me and I'll have you turned inside out and nailed to the supply carts. Am I clear?"

Ulyxes snapped out a surly affirmative as the unit prepared to move again.

"Right. Double speed to the tower and form a shield wall as soon as we begin to close."

The unit moved off at a fast trot along the walls. Down below, in the inner fortress, groups of warriors could be seen moving between the buildings, making for the inner gatehouse. Draco would certainly have his work cut out when he got there.

Ahead, the fleeing Kushites had gathered on the tower and were being redeployed by a noble or commander of some sort. The warriors were clearly less than happy about the situation as they turned and set themselves ready for the mass of shining steel and green shields that was descending on them with violent purpose.

This time, however, the clash was different. The enemy, already demoralised after their failure to hold the Roman attackers at the gates, broke easily and split, some of them retreating along the inner fortress wall, the rest falling back along the river-front walls toward the outer gate. There was a roar of triumph from the Roman column and only the optio's bellowed commands and threats prevented them from breaking into a run after the cowardly Kushites.

The optio's men flooded onto the tower, their eyes locked on the wall straight ahead, beside the river. As the unit carried on, bearing down on the rabble, and Draco's party split off behind them and moved in to secure the inner walls, Cervianus felt a sudden chill. Something was dreadfully wrong here. These could not be the Kushites that Shenti spoke of? The warriors that the auxiliary commander at Syene had described? Bloodthirsty maniacs, who quailed at rallying for a second push? They had run too easily. They still outnumbered the Romans considerably, and they knew it, so why break and run when they had marshalled their strength?

Visions of the trap Draco and his men had found themselves in among the narrow streets of Abu Island came unbidden to his mind. These men were *not* cowards, but they *were* devious. The optio's unit marched out along the outer perimeter wall, jeering after the retreating Kushites.

But they were no longer retreating.

Now others began to sense that something was wrong; something had changed. The Kushites had *not* been fleeing the Roman column after a second attempt had broken. They had been drawing their Roman enemy along the walls, leading them on. Ahead, the retreating warriors had gathered once more and turned to face their pursuers ready for a fight.

Behind, the optio bellowed out the command for shield wall.

Something drew Cervianus' attention. There was a deep, mass groaning noise from the fortress's outer compound and his gaze fell over the edge of the wall into the dark area below, spotted by flickering lights.

Each light was a camp fire, bright, but barely illuminating the black tents that covered the ground like hundreds of glistening cockroaches.

And between the tents hundreds upon hundreds of figures stood, wrapped in black, almost invisible, wraith-like in the shadows, the gleaming heads of half a thousand arrows nocked and pointed up at the wall.

Cervianus' eyes widened even as the air filled with the sound of hundreds of bow strings twanging and the hiss of myriad deadly missiles.

"Shields!" he managed to bellow as the trap sprang shut.

X

BUHEN

The cloud of black hissing death rose from the ground, iron points gleaming in the moonlight, ebony shafts and black fletching blending into the darkness. The men of the Second century, forewarned by Cervianus' sharp eyes and quick call to action, managed to raise their shields in time to catch the volley and only four struck home, the men plummeting from the wall with a screech as the missiles punched through their legs or caught them in the neck.

The optio began to yell the order for a testudo formation at the back and men tried to shuffle into position to fill the gaps formed by dying legionaries. The second volley of arrows, coming only moments after the first and while the Romans were still reeling from the shock, took another seven men.

"Get to the gate!" the optio yelled. "We've got to let the tribune's men in!"

Trying to maintain their semi-testudo formation, shields raised to protect from the volleys of deadly missiles, the Second century pushed on, picking up the pace, the survival of them all resting now on getting that gate open so the rest of the legion could join the fray.

How could things have gone so wrong so quickly? Of course, Cervianus knew the practical answer to that: the scouts had seriously underestimated the defensive garrison, which seemed to be around four times the initial figure including these strange figures in black. Yet he still couldn't shake the feeling that this was another sign that the gods were turning against them as they moved south.

Make Syene your end.

The Second century was down to around two-thirds of their number already, fighting along the walls, and the remaining distance to the gate seemed so immense that the chances of any man reaching it alive looked unfeasible. The Kushites had formed up further along the wall, ready to halt the Roman force in their tracks. It was the first mistake they had made, and Cervianus was pleased to see it.

"Run," he bellowed, and the men around him redoubled their speed as they bore down on the waiting warriors, each man aware of what the close combat would mean: the arrows would stop for fear of striking their own men. The casualty rate would slow drastically in hand-to-hand fighting as opposed to their simply being picked off a half-dozen at a time by the volleys of missiles.

The Kushites readied themselves. There were perhaps a dozen or so here, while others had run along the inside wall where they were now being pursued by Draco and his men. More still had run on ahead, presumably to secure the gate. A dozen was a manageable number.

With a cry of frustrated rage, the men of the Twenty Second legion fell upon the enemy, desperation driving them on like madmen. Eschewing the traditional disciplined approach of the legions, the soldiers threw their weight behind their shields, swords drawn back and ready to stab, all thought of a cooperative shield wall forgotten. Speed was everything, now.

On the far side of the outer corner tower another flight of stairs led down to the tent-filled enclosure and black figures were starting to move up it with a spine-tingling motion reminiscent of spiders scuttling. The archers released one last volley, aiming for the rear of the unit to avoid hitting the Kushite warriors. Two more squawks confirmed their success. The optio was shouting something about securing the stairs, but the men at the front had precious little spare attention to pay him.

The legionaries piled into the ebony-skinned, pelt-wearing warriors, shouting curses and the names of any god that might still look favourably on them. Shields smashed into Kushite bodies; swords began rhythmically stabbing into flesh and drawing back, blood splashing onto the mud-brick surface, spattering legs and arms and faces, coating shields. Howls of pain and cries of rage mingled.

Cervianus felt the second wound of the night with only passing interest as a nicked blade scythed the bronze edging strip from his shield and carved a neat line along his upper arm in the process. Three stitches would easily solve that.

A shout from the right announced the death of the man next to Ulyxes, a sword having managed to find the gap between shield and helmet and biting deep into the side of his neck. As the man collapsed over the embrasure in the outer wall, a replacement from the second line arrived, bellowing cries of defiance, to fill the gap.

The Kushite warriors were fighting like demons, painful blows managing to find their targets despite the huge shields that protected the Romans. One had to admire them in a way:

hardly a shield or a scrap of armour among them, and yet they were managing to hold their own and pick off the century at a surprising rate.

Finally the dozen or so defenders gave way, the last two falling to well-placed gladius blows, and the scene beyond became clear. The remaining Kushites on this wall had retreated to the gatehouse and were drawing up there to prevent the critical position falling to the invaders. The corner tower was clear, but black-clad figures were leaping up the stairway two steps at a time, moving lightly and with incredible dexterity, and were beginning to reach the tower top.

The archers down below had dropped their bows, the use of missiles now impossible given the press of both sides, and were drawing shining blades and moving toward stairs and both inner and outer gatehouses.

Cervianus swallowed. There was something very eerie about these black figures. They were no better armed or armoured than the Kushites, yet they frightened him for some reason. With a shiver, he realised what it was. The Kushites who garrisoned Buhen, like their counterparts at Syene, were warriors born and bred, in a similar mould to the Celts that lay at the Galatian root of the Twenty Second's national pride. They ran into battle, heedless of the danger, baying for blood, and were not afeared of fighting a superior enemy against the odds, bellowing defiance as they went.

Not so these new figures. Not a single word had issued from them. Indeed, the only noise they seemed to have made at all since the Romans had arrived on the outer walls and fallen into their trap was the hiss of arrow volleys.

They moved soundlessly and with grace and speed. They were black upon black, their skin the same colour as the garb that almost hid them from sight. Even their arrows had been ebony. Only the gleam of iron and steel betrayed their existence once among the shadows. They moved like the lemures, dark spirits of the dead come back to prey upon the waking world.

"What the shit *are* they?" Ulyxes asked, seemingly reading Cervianus' mind.

Before he could find voice to reply, the optio called out again.

"Once we've taken the tower, we split up. Right two columns will keep going round the walls and make for the gatehouse and the left two secure the stairs and head straight through the tents for the gate at ground level."

The mind-boggling danger of trying to fight their way down a staircase from the wall's side and then running through the enemy camp struck Cervianus, but already he was raising his shield again as he moved, ignoring the pains in the shoulder and upper arm.

The front line of the Roman advance reached the tower at the same time as the first black-clad figures from the staircase, and the legionaries began to spread out, the tower top allowing for more manoeuvring room despite the large brazier in the centre. The four-man front became eight, the rear ranks pushing up to join them. Because of the central fire, however, no shield wall was possible and the Romans and their foe separated into two groups, closing on either side of the orange flames.

Cervianus set his weight behind his huge shield and took a couple of steps toward one of the black-upon-black figures moving toward them, preparing to run the man down with a shield-barge.

The man, wrapped in black cloth, only his eyes visible in the strange garb, wore no armour and held no shield. In each hand he held a straight-edged blade just over a foot long. Cervianus eyed his opposition, planting his feet hard ready to launch himself forward.

The black-clad man's eyes narrowed and his hand began to move, the blades blurring and spinning with a fascinating speed and dexterity. Clenching his teeth, Cervianus pushed forward and ran at the warrior, raising the shield as he moved, aiming the heavy bronze boss straight for his enemy's chest in an attempt to knock him flat, following which he could be dispatched with alacrity.

The warrior, however, simply stepped a wide pace back and made a strange, complicated move with his arms, the blades in his hands carving chunks from Cervianus' shield.

The capsarius stopped abruptly, staring down in astonishment as a piece of his shield almost two square feet in size simply fell away to the floor, drastically reducing his coverage. Leaping forward, he thrust efficiently with his gladius, only to find the man deftly stepped to one side, his straight blade deflecting the blow while the other hand carved another corner from the shield.

A tiniest move of Cervianus' head allowed him to see that the other Romans were having similar problems. The black-clad men were simply breathtaking. Cervianus gritted his teeth. Another lunge with his sword, feinting and at the last moment changing the direction of his thrust, almost caught the man out. The warrior's deft change of footing allowed him to dance out of the way of the blow but only just. The capsarius's gladius had slipped through the cloth of the man's garb beneath his armpit.

A retaliation blow, however, struck the shield with either an astoundingly calculated or unbelievably lucky blow. The blade plunged through the wood and leather at the edge of the boss, miraculously severing one end of the grip on the inside. Cervianus struggled to hold the battered and carved remains of his shield and at the last moment decided that caution was getting him nowhere.

Giving up the hope of his shield, he simply threw the useless article at the black figure before him. Unprepared for the move, the man failed to duck out of the way fast enough and the large, heavy shield smashed into him flat on, sending him staggering back and to the floor.

Caution thrown entirely to the wind, Cervianus threw himself into the air and landed on top of the flailing, black-clad man. Stabbing repeatedly with his gladius, he left the man no time to recover, punching holes in his chest again and again. Finally, after what felt like hours of repeated attacks, he rose to his feet and stepped back, covered in blood.

He turned to take in the chaos around him. The rest of the Roman force was now pouring onto the tower top and dealing with the black figures. A legionary pushed past his right-hand side, close to the flames, and made for another black-clad figure, but it was to his left, at the tower's inner edge, that Cervianus found his gaze being inexorably drawn.

Vibius had fared less well than him. The flatulent soldier had shared their tent for the past two years, was instrumental in the shunning of the capsarius and equally at the heart of his miraculous reacceptance following the crocodile incident. Vibius, the stinky, raucous, absolutely model legionary, lay dead on the surface a foot or so from the parapet.

The black-clad figure that had apparently easily dispatched him had, ridiculously, taken time from fighting his enemies to crouch by Vibius' body and begin sawing through the neck with his blade. Cervianus watched for a moment, feeling sick to his stomach. His eyes strayed and he realised this was happening all across the walls. Heedless of the danger posed by the remaining legionaries, any soldier that had fallen to one of the black assailants was having his head removed. Judging by the screams, not all of them were dead at the time.

Anger and bile rose in Cervianus and he turned, stamping over to the black-clad man as he delivered the final slash, pulling away Vibius' head with a bone-chilling tearing noise. The warrior began to rise, his prize in his left hand, and was turning when Cervianus hit him full in the torso, knocking him backwards out over the parapet and into the empty air.

Breathing heavily, the scent of blood filling his nostrils and obliterating thoughts of anything else, the capsarius turned, his foot splashing in the pool of blood still pouring from Vibius' neck.

Despite the violence of the black-clad figures, the Romans were managing to push them back and take control of the tower. Their curious and horrifying apparent need to take the heads of their targets meant that each defending black warrior was leaving the scene whenever he managed to grab a grisly trophy. Three of the warriors were already pushing back down the stairs past their fellows, carrying heads, still silent and other-worldly.

Ulyxes, his shield gone, gripping his sword in one hand while fresh blood ran down the other and dripped from his fingertips, stopped and stared at his friend.

"Juno, what happened to you?"

Cervianus stared in incomprehension. His mind seemed to have shut down at the sight of the man tearing away Vibius' head. His emotions had settled somewhere deep inside him and a cold fire burned in his mind. He ignored Ulyxes' comment, unaware that hardly an inch of him showed from beneath the coating of blood that soaked his clothes and armour.

Turning, he began to walk off toward the far side of the tower where the fighting was now raging. Ulyxes, shouting something that went entirely unheard, ran after him and was suddenly by his side.

A figure in black stepped out from the stairway and on to the tower. The blade in his hand turned and whipped this way and that with amazing agility. The warrior's eyes settled on the gladius in Cervianus' hand and he went into a defensive crouch.

The capsarius stormed toward him, his pace increasing. He was shouting something and was not entirely sure what it was, as the blade cut him twice, once on the wrist and once on the jaw; light wounds for certain, but painful. Paying as little heed to the shocking pain as he was to the friend at his side, Cervianus reached out and grasped the warrior by the throat. The move was so sudden, forceful and surprising that the black figure, trying to back away, instead lost his footing and was only prevented from toppling back down the stairway by the choking hold that this crazed Roman had on his windpipe.

Still shouting something over the chaos, Cervianus closed his grip and felt muscle, cartilage and bone crunch as the black-clad man died in agony, his body spasming and shaking.

"What?" He suddenly shook his head as though waking from a dream. Staring at the shaking thing in his hand, Cervianus blinked twice.

"I said what the shit is *up* with you?" Ulyxes yelled again.

"I don't... I don't know. They're taking *heads*, Ulyxes!"

"Yes, I can see that, but you—"

"I can't have them doing that, Ulyxes. Taking Vibius' head like that. I can't let them, Ulyxes. I just can't."

A shout of rage came from the busy stairway ahead. Blinking and looking around, Cervianus realised that the Roman force had taken the tower. A dozen men ran on toward the gate, a long stretch of open wall ahead of them. The optio came to a halt beside them.

"What's up with him?"

Ulyxes shook his head. "I think he's pissed off."

"So am I. Get down those stairs. I want that gate open before we're all torn to pieces."

Cervianus turned, still confused, to look at the optio. The officer was clutching his upper arm, a great deal of blood flowing from a wound beneath his fingers. Everywhere was blood. He himself was covered in it. It flowed freely from all his companions as he looked at them. The floor of the tower was slick with it, making footing dangerous and difficult. All he could smell was blood.

But all he could see as he closed his eyes was Vibius' head coming away with that tearing sound. He shuddered. The weight in his hand was suddenly relieved as the optio took the dead warrior from him. With a grin, ignoring the sudden increase of blood, the officer let go of his wound, lifted the body in both arms and cast it toward the stairs.

The effect was impressive. Legionaries at the wall top were fighting to stop the black-clad figures gaining a foothold again but suddenly their efforts were pointless, as the body hit the remaining warriors on the stairs, knocking them back into their companions and beginning a chain reaction that could have been humorous in other circumstances as men fell into one another all down the thirty-foot staircase, surprised warriors falling from the edge into the press below.

Suddenly the staircase was almost clear and the legionaries who had been fighting at the top were beginning to descend, their target the main gate that lay at the far side, some two hundred paces away, through the very centre of the nightmare force's encampment.

The optio took one look at Ulyxes and Cervianus and shook his head before turning and descending with the rest of the legionaries. Ulyxes grinned nervously. "We'd best get going with them. Careful on those stairs, though. You look strange. You alright?"

"I feel… I don't know. I just lost it, I think."

"What were you shouting back there?"

"I don't know."

"It was Greek. Sounded like…" Ulyxes paused and closed his eyes, concentrating, before repeating back syllables, retained despite their unfamiliarity by his perfect recall.

Cervianus stared at him.

"Don't know Greek," the shorter man shrugged, "but I know what I heard."

The capsarius shook his head. "It *is* Greek – from Herodotus. 'My gods, Mardonius… what sort of men have you brought me to fight against?'"

Ulyxes furrowed his eyebrows. "You are really *weird*, you know that? Most people settle for simple cursing."

Cervianus shook his head again in confusion as the pair began to make their way carefully onto the steps. Here the going became easier, away from the slick of blood that coated the tower.

At the base of the stairs, the first men of the Twenty Second legion were forming a shield wall against the press of the black-clad men while the rest of the dozen-strong group rushed down to join them.

"Testudo and double speed!"

The optio's plan was simple: form up as defensively as possible and run to the gate, ignoring anything in their way. It was insane, clearly, but was also probably the only option. With a quick glance upwards, Cervianus spotted the Roman forces closing on the gate along the wall top, and stepped from the stairway with his friend, falling into the small testudo. As soon as he reached the rest, Cervianus found himself pulled into the centre. Lacking a shield he was precious little use on the periphery.

As soon as the shields closed around them with a thump, the unit began to move.

Initially, the going was tough. The black-clad warriors pounded on the shields' exterior with a variety of exotic weapons, occasional slivers being sliced off them or the points stabbing through into the inside, sometimes drawing blood. Quickly, though, as they moved away from the stairs, the going became easier. Peering out over the shields, they could see something was clearly happening in the outer compound of Buhen. The number of black-clad figures seemed to be thinning out for no obvious reason.

With a shriek, the legionary to Cervianus' right succumbed to a lucky or horribly accurate blow as a blade scythed out beneath the shields and bit into his Achilles tendon, felling him instantly. As he dropped, Cervianus desperately grasped his shield and wrenched it from his hand. Though it sickened him to take it and leave the man to his fate, there really was no other option. Dropping the shield back into position and taking the soldier's place, he tried not to listen to the screams as the prone man became another dangling trophy carried off by the head-takers.

Ulyxes, just behind him, panting as they ran, leaned forward next to his ear. "What are you muttering?"

"Prayer to Sobek. Seemed like a good time."

On they ran, the optio at the front guiding the armoured formation as they ran between the tents. Despite the occasional blow on the shields, there was clearly something happening. The area in front of them had opened up, black-clad figures now few and far between rather than crowding in to get to them.

"What in Hades is going on?" the optio wondered as they ran.

By the time they were thirty paces from the gate, even the occasional blows had stopped. The optio bellowed the command to break formation and the testudo split up, the eleven soldiers and their officer glancing around nervously.

Not a single black-garbed warrior could be seen among the tents.

"This is putting the shits up me," Ulyxes said quietly. "Where have they gone?"

Cervianus nodded. Ahead, the figures of the Twenty Second's legionaries now held the top of the gatehouse. Behind the advancing unit, Draco and his men had gained control of the inner gate. Despite everything, they seemed to be winning. The legionaries bore down on the gatehouse, peering apprehensively into the shadows where the moonlight could not penetrate. No figures seemed to be visible in the recess and the unit moved in, shields raised ready, swords gripped tight.

The scene inside the gatehouse was that of nightmares.

Perhaps twenty Kushite warriors had been here, holding the gate itself against the Roman attackers. Their bodies lay scattered around the gatehouse floor, glistening in the lake of blood, not a head to be seen anywhere.

"What in the name of Dis?" The optio shook his head as he took in the scene. "Looks like these animals turned on their masters as soon as we started winning. But where did they go?"

Ulyxes shrugged. "Frankly, sir, I don't give a shit *where* they are right now, so long as they're not here."

There was a chorus of affirmative noises and even the optio was nodding.

"Let's get this gate open and let the legion in before we come across any other nasty surprises."

"Agh!"

Cervianus bit his lip against the pain and glared up accusingly at Ulyxes. "I can't believe you can really be this clumsy by nature. Are you doing this on purpose?"

The stocky legionary grinned at him.

The pair sat in the lee of the great outer walls of Buhen, in the shade, sheltering from the already searing heat of the mid-morning sun. Around them, the aftermath of the fight went on. Ulyxes tugged the stitch, causing his patient to yelp again.

"For gods' sake, will you try and be a bit gentler? It's like being stitched by a blind camel."

"If you don't like it, you could always piss off and get the medical staff to do this?" Ulyxes grinned. "You know... the way they're *supposed* to?"

Cervianus glowered at him. "You may have the light touch

of a ballista operator, but I'd still take your hand over the medicus and his trained monkeys any day. Just concentrate. Now, you need to tie it off, preferably without tugging so hard that my arm stays puckered for the rest of my life."

Ulyxes gave a small, wicked tug on the thread and then tied it as carefully as he could, grinning at the look on the capsarius's face.

"When you've finished with me I'll sort out your arm and then get on to the others."

"You needn't think I'm letting you near me after I've had the chance to play with your wounds, Titus. Don't be daft!"

Cervianus grumbled again. The small cut on his jaw would heal of its own accord and he could apply the salves himself. The egg-shaped lump on his head would be there a week or more before it subsided, and the headache would probably last as long as the constant whining in his ear from the bell-like helmet blow. The neat line on his wrist hardly warranted a stitch. Thus the cut on his upper arm was the only wound, despite everything he had suffered, that would require attention.

Apart possibly from his apparently declining mental state, that was. That was the most worrying aftermath of the fight: the knowledge that at some point in the scuffle on the wall top, he appeared to have almost entirely lost his mind and plunged into a killing frenzy, yelling quotes in Greek. Ulyxes had ribbed him about it mercilessly this morning but, despite the general humour the others seemed to find in the scene, he himself found it distinctly worrying. The Gauls back in the campaigns of Caesar were said to suffer from blind killing rages. Could it be that they ran in his race's blood? The Galatians and Caesar's erstwhile enemies did share a common ancestry, after all...

He shook his head irritably and looked down to see Ulyxes mopping the freshly stitched line.

"Now put some of the amaracinum oil on the wound and then bind it tight and seal it with the bee glue."

Ulyxes nodded and worked away, his tongue protruding from the corner of his mouth as he concentrated. Despite Cervianus' complaints, his friend was actually doing as good a job as any man could on a simple wound stitching. Given the incorrigible legionary's lack of medical knowledge, he was performing extremely well. The capsarius ignored the aching and let his gaze wander, along with his thoughts.

Once the remains of his century had managed to secure the gate, things had been over in less than a quarter of an hour. Draco's unit had met with Nasica's optio and his men at the inner gatehouse and secured the walls of the main fortress with little trouble. Nasica himself had arrived at the outer gatehouse with thirty men to bolster Cervianus' unit just as they had managed to open the great gates.

Outside, the tribune, aware from the shouts and the sudden explosion of activity that things had not gone entirely according to plan, had drawn up three cohorts of the legion. They had been about to begin besieging the outer wall when Roman infiltrators had appeared over the parapet, running for the gatehouse, confirming that the fortress had all but fallen and the main entrance should be accessible any moment.

As soon as the great wooden portal swung inwards, Vitalis had entered, safely surrounded by his personal guard, the three cohorts immediately sweeping into Buhen and searching out resistance.

Finding none.

In the strangest and most disturbing turn of events, they

located not a single enemy survivor. Probably two-thirds of the Kushite garrison lay dead on the walls or on the ground, their wounds labelling them victims of Nasica and Draco's assault. The remaining third littered the more secure spots, their headless bodies mute testament to the horrible and fickle nature of their black-clad allies.

And of those allies?

Not a single prisoner.

Not one black-garbed warrior had been found alive, despite a thorough search of the fortress. Where they had gone was the subject of hushed talk among the legion now. How had several hundred men vanished in the midst of a siege, apparently passing the invading army unseen? Even black-clad and in the dark, the feat was almost Herculean. Their dead remained, to prove that they had been there, but that was all. The legionaries of the Twenty Second were already calling them ghosts and demons and making fervent prayers to any familiar or friendly god they could name.

Vitalis had raged and ranted at the two senior centurions in the moonlit outer compound for half an hour, while the legion went about securing the fortress, piling up the enemy dead out in the desert for the carrion feeders and gathering the fallen legionaries, retrieving their useful equipment and preparing a mass pyre near the water's edge for them.

The tribune had been almost apoplectic in his anger at the result.

No words of reason from Nasica or Draco could persuade him of the monumental success they had pulled out of the abyss here. Fewer than eighty men dead to take the whole fortress was a record that would earn most officers awards and bonuses that would weigh them down like pack animals.

Instead, Vitalis strode back and forth in front of them, tearing strips off them for failing to adapt adequately to the situation, losing too many legionaries and, most importantly, allowing the worst of the enemy to escape the scene and leave behind no defenders to interrogate.

Unbelievably, and unprofessionally, the rant had taken place in such a public area that every man in the Twenty Second became uncomfortably aware of the growing rift between the commander and his senior officers. Draco and Nasica might be martinets in their own right, and occasionally made enemies among their men, but the sheer scale of their achievement and the lives they had saved had put every last soldier firmly in their camp during the dressing-down, the feeling of the men toward their senior commander beginning to turn unpleasant.

Finally, the tribune had left them with a hanging threat, telling the two senior centurions that they were lucky to have escaped this without a beating, before turning and stalking off out of the fortress to where his tent stood in the Roman camp, sweetmeats and watered wine waiting for him like a pampered senator while his men moved stinking corpses to be burned.

Cervianus shook his head. Things were clearly going from bad to worse. Vitalis was rapidly losing his grip on reality, as had been evidenced by the spittle on his lips as he raged. The two senior centurions had stood fast and taken the tirade with straight faces and stoic expressions though no passer-by could fail to notice the proud defiance that emanated from their very stance.

Since that exchange in the middle of the night, the tribune had returned to his camp, and its remaining six cohorts, and left the senior centurions to clean up the mess at the fortress. The

Roman wounded, mostly light cuts, breaks and dislocations, gathered in one corner of the compound, awaiting the attentions of the various capsarii and medical staff. Due to the nature of their foe last night, most of the wounds had either been light glancing blows or horribly fatal, leaving the medical unit with surprisingly little work.

Legionaries moved around the ground level removing the few things of value from the black tents and then collapsing them, gathering them into a pile in the centre where they would then be taken out and burned. The lack of even the slightest breeze caused the stench of crisping flesh from the Roman pyre outside the walls to saturate the whole area around Buhen and the smell of charring corpses filled every nostril and permeated every tent. And yet, despite everything that felt wrong or unpleasant about the assault, it was important to remember how truly successful it had been.

Cervianus nodded to himself as Ulyxes finished wrapping his arm and retrieved the bee glue from the battered leather bag.

"Here comes shit-brains again," Ulyxes noted.

The capsarius looked up in confusion at his friend's words and then turned his head to see Vitalis striding across the dusty ground from the gatehouse.

"Wonder what he's up to now?"

Ulyxes shrugged. "Probably come to finish a few of the wounded lads off. Mercy killings and all that."

Cervianus nodded at his friend's acerbic comment. It was no laughing matter really. Vitalis, with two junior tribunes and half a dozen cavalry guards at his back, strode across toward the wounded men.

"Perhaps he's going to hand out commendations?"

Ulyxes turned to Cervianus, shaking his head. "I don't think so. Not that prick."

The capsarius closed his eyes, wishing his friend's voice carried a little less. One or two of the wounded men nearby had turned to look at Ulyxes as he spoke. The tribune strode into the centre of the medical section. While Cervianus and Ulyxes sat on the periphery tending to one another, the medicus and his staff, along with three other capsarii, were working on the various other injuries. One of the orderlies tapped the medicus on the shoulder as he probed a leg wound.

"Don't touch me, you moron. I could have cut an artery then!"

"Sir? The tribune's here."

Cervianus felt the tiniest morsel of respect for the medicus as the man turned to face Vitalis, his front covered in blood, scalpel in hand and a sour, unappreciative look on his face.

"Can I help you, commander?"

Vitalis came to a halt not far from the medicus and looked around. "How many casualties?

"Twenty-seven, sir. Only three bad, miraculously. I'm looking at them now and then they can be loaded on the cart and sent back to Syene and Thebes. The rest will be able to march with the legion, though they'll have to be excused duties for a week or more and their packs stored with the wagons. All in all, a good result I'd say."

Vitalis, his face expressionless, scanned the men. "Unnecessary. There are plenty of supplies here. I want to leave a small garrison at Buhen. The twenty-seven men can form part of that garrison, along with a group of troublemakers and convalescents from the other cohorts. They can all stay here and rest until we return."

The medicus blinked. "Sir? Even the lightest wounded of those men will have to have occasional check-ups and treatment. If they get an infection or the humours go out of balance they could rot and die. If you leave men in that sort of circumstance without proper medical checks you're inviting *plague* to descend."

The tribune waved aside his objection. "If you feel it's that important, leave one of your orderlies with them. I'm not taking anyone with me that can't pull their weight, and I want Buhen in Roman hands. Make it happen."

Vitalis ignored the flapping, astonished mouth of the medicus and turned on his heel, marching away with his escort.

"Ouch!"

Ulyxes, his teeth grinding together, had exerted a little too much pressure on Cervianus' arm and blood oozed up through the dressing.

"Sorry. What a prick."

The comment was loud enough that one of the retreating cavalry guard turned and scanned the men, frowning and trying to identify the speaker. As the officers turned the corner into the gatehouse on their way to some other unknown and officious engagement, there was a collective release of tension and no few grumbles of misery.

"You've *got* to watch your mouth," Cervianus said to his friend. "One of those bastards heard you. If *Vitalis* hears you call him names, you'll be dangling from a crucifix by sundown."

"Prick, prick, pricking, pricketty-pricking PRICK!" shouted the shorter man after the retreating officers, causing a burst of grins and laughs to rise from the wounded across the way. The medicus turned and frowned at them, though his face betrayed his true feelings and he decided not to admonish them.

"It's about time that prick was sent back to Alexandria strapped to a mule. At least the mule will have more sense."

More grins erupted at Ulyxes' comment.

"I'd love to catch the posh bastard on his own in the latrines," one of the others said. "I'd soon teach him a thing or two."

"Oh, aye? You been hanging around with the Greeks again?" another man laughed.

The group burst into a low cacophony of humorous comments, a standard defence mechanism when faced with unpleasant truths.

"You can make jokes about it," Ulyxes said quietly, his voice low and yet carrying enough weight that it cut through the general humour. "It's all very funny, I know, but there's a real problem here. Vitalis is walking us into the jaws of Cerberus and I for one am not ready to be the demon dog's snack."

The murmur died away. Some of the wounded were nodding sagely, while others looked increasingly worried.

"The time is coming when those of us in the legion with an ounce of sense are going to have to decide between Vitalis and saving our own skins."

"Shut up," hissed Cervianus. "Don't start this again."

"You all know I'm right. Draco and Nasica are still following him, bound by their oaths, but how long do you think even *they* are going to follow the prick after this morning's shit storm?"

Again there were murmurs of agreement and nods.

"Anyway, you lot are alright. You'll get to stay here. There's going to be enough stores in Buhen to let you live like kings until Vitalis pushes Nasica too far. Once the man's face down in a ditch with a gladius in his back, we can turn round and come back for you."

This time even the medicus glared at Ulyxes and made motions for him to be quiet.

"Pah!" He finished sealing off the dressing and sat back on his haunches. "I'm only saying what most of you are thinking. You listen carefully when you're among the others. I've not heard so much talk of rebellion since the days of Pompey, when we were still a Galatian army. The men will only follow Vitalis as long as Nasica and Draco do; you know that. And the pair of them are reaching the end of their tether."

The entire medical corner fell into quiet contemplation. For all his outspoken nature, courting danger, Ulyxes was absolutely correct and everyone knew it. The spell was broken by a groan from the man on the table with the gash in his leg. The medicus took a deep breath.

"Right. That's enough idle chatter. Seems to me like you lot have some deciding to do. Are you fit enough to make the rest of the campaign on full duties and with full kit, or would you prefer to take your chances here? I'll leave an orderly who's capable of handling dressings, bleedings and minor infections, so I'm hoping you'll be alright until the legion returns from the south."

The men began to discuss the situation earnestly while Cervianus tried hard not to consider the possibility that the frightening men in black might return to Buhen as soon as the legion moved on. There was the very real chance that remaining in the fortress was a simple route to decapitation. He locked eyes with Ulyxes.

"I think we'll head on south, eh?"

The stocky legionary nodded, clearly preferring the uncertain dangers surrounding Vitalis' campaign to the possibility of waiting in a plague-ridden fortress for the deadly black-clad maniacs to return.

"Come on. I'll stitch and bind your arm and then you can head back and start putting our things together while I help patch this lot up. You'll want to lay claim to some of Vibius' gear too before it's taken away by the quartermaster. Get me his helmet, will you? Mine's gone. Don't go near his tunic though. He's probably burned a hole in the arse over the years."

Ulyxes nodded, ignoring the humorous comment, and settled in as the capsarius opened his medical bag. Glancing round, he rolled his eyes. "Here comes your friend. Wonder if he's learned to count yet?"

Cervianus frowned in incomprehension and then turned to see Shenti tying up his horse at one of the iron rings in the wall and then strolling toward them.

"Learned to count?"

"Well, to estimate numbers, anyway."

Cervianus shook his head. "Hardly *his* doing. That was the scouts. Be nice."

The short, wiry officer, clad in his white linen tunic and mail shirt, removed the scarf from his head and wiped his face with it as he approached them. His face was serious and bore a slightly hunted look.

"I trust the two of you are not seriously harmed?"

The capsarius shook his head. "A few minor cuts and bruises is all. You been busy?"

Shenti nodded as he stopped and dropped into a crouch. "All the mounted auxiliaries and scout units have been scouring the desert for ten miles in every direction. The tribune desires that we bring him the survivors of Buhen. He will be disappointed, I fear."

"You found no trace?" Ulyxes frowned. "Surely they must have left tracks?"

Shenti shook his head. "They move very lightly and use bound brush and sticks to wipe clear their trail. If they do not wish to be found, we will not find them. By now they will be out in the deepest dunes of the desert, following trails known only to them and seeking out hidden supplies of water. If we are lucky we have seen the last of them."

"Who are they?" Cervianus asked as he cleaned Ulyxes' wound expertly with hardly a glance.

"They have many names. They dwell in the deserts to either side of the Nile south of Buhen and north of the Kushite lands. It is said that they have magnificent oasis fortresses, decked in silver and peppered with precious stones. I think this is a lie. They are a people that value food, water, privacy and the taking of trophies. Jewels would not interest them, I think."

"I've never seen anyone like them."

"They are nomads. They have no cities, but they build only fortresses and temples to use as they move around. We know little about them, really, just rumour and fable. Pharaohs at times have used them as mercenaries. It would seem that now the Kushites are following the same principle."

Cervianus shivered. "I'd think twice before hiring them. As soon as the battle turned against the Kushites, these bastards turned on their masters, took their heads and ran off into the desert."

Shenti nodded absently. Something was clearly still worrying him.

"Anything on your mind?"

"That the desert dwellers are fighting with the Kandake

of Kush bodes badly for any trek to the south. From here we will be travelling through the heart of their lands. Between here and the edge of the kingdom of Kush, the only safe route for an army is along the Nile, while this enemy can move about the desert quickly and by paths unknown to even me. If they decide to do so, the nomads could very well whittle down the legion to nothing by the time we reach the fourth cataract."

Cervianus and Ulyxes shared a look.

Overhead, a lone vulture cried out its hoarse call.

"What's this about, then? The move south?" Cervianus hazarded, risking familiarity with a man who theoretically outranked him. The artillery and engineering chiefs were notorious for their down-to-earth attitude, though, and, true to form, the optio simply shrugged and glanced over his shoulder as they walked.

"Bollocksed if I know. Everyone with position in the legion's here though. Look."

Cervianus followed the ageing engineer's pointing finger.

Vitalis stood on a raised rocky platform to one side of the flat ground, his junior tribunes standing around him looking pristine and unreal in their resplendent green cloaks.

The dusty locale, reminiscent of a parade ground, and presumably chosen for that very reason, was filled with men of influence and power in the army. Centurions flooded the area, apparently *all* of them, many having left their optios in charge of the soldiers back at the camp and the fortress.

In addition to the senior officers and centurions, the entire medical staff was present, including all ten capsarii, the officers of engineers and artillery, the camp prefect, the quartermaster and even the pack and wagon masters.

A veritable panoply of power.

Cervianus fell into position somewhere off to one side, a comfortable distance away from the medicus and his men and just in sight of Nasica and Draco, who stood at the front, viewing their commander with professionally blank expressions.

The capsarius swept his gaze around the gathering while the last of the attendees arrived, trying to ascertain a reason for the whole affair and failing dismally. The stragglers were almost entirely engineers, scruffy and late as was almost expected of them, so wrapped up were they in their own affairs as a matter of habit.

When the last were in position, Vitalis paused for a moment on the rock, allowing the tiniest breeze to ruffle his cloak in what he presumably believed was an impressive and oratorical fashion. Finally, he stepped to the fore and cleared his throat.

"You represent the command of the Twenty Second legion: my right arm." He narrowed his eyes. "I feel I may need to remind you all of a few things. In the manner of all Rome's legions, the praetor gives us our remit. In this case, the praetor is Prefect Petronius in Alexandria. When the remit is given, the legion's commander makes the decision on how to accomplish the praetor's goals. *I* am that commander."

He paused, allowing the assembled officers to take in this clear statement of autonomy. "When I decide how to accomplish those goals, I pass on my decisions to you, my officers. You find ways to achieve what I require and in turn pass that on to your men, who follow the orders and achieve those goals. This is the way of the army. This is how things are done in Rome."

There was a menacing tone to the end of this flat statement. The assembly shifted slightly in anticipation.

"I am neither deaf nor stupid," the tribune said quietly, his voice carrying regardless in the uncomfortable silence. "There are mutterings of dissatisfaction among the men. Whispers, I might add, that I have heard echoed even among the lower officers. I hear my name spoken with vitriol. I hear fear and cowardice, treachery, rebellion and downright stupidity."

A few of the men near Cervianus looked away guiltily. He hadn't realised just how far this rot had spread and how much Ulyxes was, in fact, just voicing the fears of the whole legion each time his mouth ran off in far too public a place.

"This will be an *end to it*," the tribune continued. "It is the duty of each of you and your optios to stamp out signs of disaffection and disobedience. You are required by both your position and your oath to punish such behaviour appropriately and I will break any man that I observe failing to perform this duty."

Again a pause to let this ominous threat sink in.

"I will brook *no* disobedience. Mark my words."

He straightened in the dangerous silence. "Very well. If that is all clear, we shall move on from such unprofessionalism, as makes me sick to my stomach, and consider what is to be done."

He gestured grandly to the great walls of Buhen some quarter of a mile from this meeting site, where the legion was finishing the job of clearing up. "We are currently at the border of Rome's governed lands. Buhen stands at the northern edge of the second cataract and south of here lie the lands claimed as the 'kingdom' of Kush. We have driven the invaders from our territory and reinstated our control, in spite of the Twelfth and Third legions."

The insult was appalling from a man who had so recently accused his officers of unprofessionalism. Cervianus could feel the thick air of disapproval rising from the men around him. While there had been an initial dislike between the legions, the soldiers of the Twenty Second's allies had accounted themselves well at Syene.

The tribune seemed not to have noticed the feel of the crowd, or at least he ignored it.

"However," he went on, "the remit given to us by the prefect contained an implicit instruction to revenge ourselves on Kush and their *queen*. As such, while we have now achieved with glorious efficiency the broad goals of the campaign, I intend, as I formerly stated, to carry this campaign into the heart of Kush and make them pay back what they owe us in both loot and blood."

A pause again. Perhaps the tribune had been expecting a rousing cheer at his words. Perhaps not. His face betrayed no emotion.

"Not only must they be punished, but they must be so thoroughly chastised that they never again dream of crossing Rome. I intend to march the Twenty Second on their capital of Meroe, taking and razing any and all settlements of import on the way. When the eagle of Rome is planted atop the Kandake's palace in Meroe we will have achieved our full goal, and we will claim Kush and its resources for the Princeps and the republic."

Cervianus felt his heart lurch. Not only did Vitalis intend

to march them into the unknown world of Kush, but a new motive had suddenly emerged. This was not just a campaign of revenge to the tribune, but of conquest. Just as Caesar had taken Gaul beyond the remit given him by the senate, and like Pompey's claims in Anatolia, Vitalis would be a new conqueror in the mould of Rome's most famous sons.

But Vitalis was no Caesar or Pompey. His was a barely tenable command held together only by the two most senior centurions clinging to their oath in spite of everything. And the gods had turned their backs on him. Cervianus shuddered as the tribune resumed.

"Thus far we have treated this campaign as any other: marched as a standard legion on campaign. Now, though, the terrain changes. To Buhen we have been in Roman territory, familiar to our guides and scouts and, nominally at least, supporting the republic."

He pointed upriver, past the fortress that stood brooding in the afternoon sun. "From here to the south, the terrain is less familiar even to our scouts. We will be moving into Kushite territory that could hide garrisoned forts and way-stations; we could fall foul of traps or surprise attacks at any time."

Cervianus found himself nodding, though in the recesses of his mind it was not forts garrisoned by screaming Kushite warriors that formed the great danger ahead, but the very real presence of the eerie, black-garbed nomads who inhabited the lands of the border regions. The thought of traps sprung by them made his flesh grow cold. Silent masses of killers in black waiting in the dark to decimate the Twenty Second.

"Thus," Vitalis continued in a resonant tone, "we must travel light and fast and be prepared for any eventuality. I intend to more than double the army's marching speed – triple it if possible. To that end, we will be leaving the wagons at Buhen."

A murmur of astonishment and disapproval rose from the crowd, but Vitalis raised his voice and spoke over the top of it.

"The artillery, siege machines, supply wagons and even the water wagons will be staying here. We will not rely on anything that uses wheels or more than two legs as they dictate a dangerously slow pace. We have been covering fifteen miles a day at best with the supply train. Without it and with the men carrying everything we need as is their duty and privilege, we can achieve forty miles a day. More, if I know the mettle of the Galatian soldier. This will give us the speed and flexibility to deal with the land's harsh conditions and the unknown nature of our foe."

He waited, watching, with a twitch in his eye as the officers of his legion grumbled. After a long moment, he turned and muttered something to one of the other tribunes. Nasica, the primus pilus of the legion, turned and looked over his shoulder at the assembled officers.

"Quiet!" he bellowed.

The hubbub died away instantly. Far from thanking Nasica, the tribune merely gave him a disdainful look and then drew breath to continue.

"The supply wagons will be stripped of anything that is necessary and can be carried. The wagon master and the quartermaster will supervise both this and the distribution of those supplies among the men. Despite the fact that we will not be taking artillery and siege weapons, we will be taking a core group of those trained officers and men with us, enabling us to construct siege equipment on site as needed. If feasible, we will also transport some of the small scorpion weapons, utilising the spare cavalry horses without the carts."

The engineers, typical of their breed, simply shrugged, accepting the situation, and began to quietly discuss how to go about transporting the scorpions and what equipment would be needed along with them for construction. Cervianus shook his head at the professional one-track madness inherent in the minds of a legion's engineers. There was even a twinkle in the eye of a number of them as they began to relish the challenge of constructing great engines from nothing in testing circumstances.

Lunatics.

The tribune continued, folding his arms. "The medical staff is here for two reasons."

Cervianus looked up, paying close attention.

"Firstly, only those who are capable of marching at full pace and in full kit will be joining us. The wounded will be staying here with the supply carts. That includes the wagon for the non-walking wounded. I'm sure you all know what that means?"

Though carefully quiet, the atmosphere in the gathering plunged even deeper into dark dismay. The lack of a wagon for the wounded meant that any man incapable of marching with them would have no method of transport. A man who could not keep up with his unit was effectively dead, left behind for predators. It was a measure taken by legion commanders only in times of dire crisis or panicked retreat. It was not an approved method to carry out a campaign of conquest.

"I see that you all understand. Also, I need the medical corps to spend the rest of the afternoon formulating a plan to enable units to cross long tracts of open desert."

The whole assembly suddenly became very still. Was the man mad?

"My native scouts tell me that the northernmost of the Kushites' major settlements that we are making for is their holy city of Napata. Following the Nile along its great curve, the legion will have to march approximately four hundred miles to reach Napata. As we do so, we will undoubtedly pass outposts of the Kushites, who will fall back or send word and prepare Napata against us."

The tribune's face hardened. "The scouts also inform me of the existence of a nomad trail that runs almost directly from this cataract to Napata across the desert. That track, though hard and forbidding, is a little over half the distance of the river route. Thus we will send a smaller force along that trail to arrive at Napata considerably ahead of the army and hopefully also ahead of any warning. They should be able to take the city by surprise, holding it as a staging post ready for the rest of the army when it arrives."

A general murmur broke out again, leading to a darkening of the tribune's expression and causing his eye twitch to return. Nasica turned and bellowed for silence again. The medicus, two of his more senior orderlies at his shoulders, shuffled out to the front.

"With respect, sir, such a route would be extraordinarily dangerous. Quite apart from the perils posed by wildlife, the nomads who made the trail, and myriad other things I could mention, one must also remember the gruelling conditions in the deep desert. Even the hardiest of men will succumb to the heat, the cold, the lack of water and food. And if they should lose their bearings the desert will swallow them."

Cervianus found himself nodding, agreeing with the .

medicus, despite their differences. At least the man had spoken up. The trail the tribune was speaking of would be one of the paths of those very same ebony nightmares that had inhabited Buhen's outer compound.

The tribune glared down at his chief medicus, a challenge in his eyes. "Are you saying that it is impossible?"

The medicus blinked and stepped back. "Of course not, sir. It's far from *impossible*, just excessively dangerous."

Cervianus groaned. *The idiot. How could he be so stupid?*

"So you agree," the tribune continued, "that it is possible for a unit of soldiers to cross such an area of desert?"

"Well, yes, sir? I would advise against it with all my heart, but I couldn't say it's *impossible*."

The tribune nodded. "I thought so. The First and Second cohorts will cross the desert route with the aid of two or three of the native scouts and take Napata upon arrival, preparing it for us to use as a base against Kush." He clasped his hands behind his back. "Do any of you have questions?"

There was a hint of challenge once again in his tone and, despite the misgivings of almost every man in the gathering, not a voice cut through the thick silence.

"Then get back to your units and begin organising. The army will move out in the morning. Dismissed!"

Ulyxes hovered with Shenti by a large boulder some distance from the gathering. The stocky, moustachioed legionary was leaning against the stone in a fairly relaxed pose until he spotted the transverse crests of the officers approaching.

Cervianus, still turning over all this insane new information in his head, hardly noticed the pair until he heard his friend shout his name. Veering out from the column of officers returning to camp, he left the company of the engineers as they plotted and planned their miracle-working in the face of adversity.

"How did you get away from duty?" he asked his friend.

Ulyxes grinned. "Our friends the cavalry of the Nome of Sapi-Res requested the optio release me to their unit for an hour or two. He grumbled a bit, but he agreed."

Shenti smiled encouragingly. "I needed the company. Now tell us what has been said, my friend."

Cervianus' expression became grave once more. "I'll do that, certainly, though you'll be hearing through channels imminently, anyway. The tribune—"

He stopped mid-sentence as a deep voice called his name from back in the column. Turning, he swallowed nervously as Draco stepped out of the line, Nasica close behind him. The three soldiers came to attention and saluted as the legion's two most senior centurions closed on them. Nasica returned the salute and Draco simply nodded in response.

"Stand at ease, lads."

"Can we help, sir? We were just heading back into camp."

Draco raised an eyebrow. "I might ask what this dangerously insolent soldier is doing *outside* of camp." He sighed. "But this isn't the time. Cervianus, we need to talk."

"Sir?"

Nasica gestured to the retreating column heading back to the fort. "Walk and talk."

Falling silent, he let his deputy take the reins of the conversation again as the five men strode back toward the rest of the officers, Ulyxes and Shenti keeping respectfully a few paces back from the centurions.

"I saw your face as medicus Albinus essentially justified the tribune's plan. You are less than convinced of the feasibility?"

Cervianus hesitated. The direction this conversation was taking was making him uneasy. "Yes, sir," he said finally. "There are so many problems with the tribune's plan, I wouldn't even know where to begin. The medicus mentioned only the tiniest fraction of them. I'm not sure he's..."

He paused again. To speak ill of a senior medicus could be a bad career move. He swallowed. "I'm not sure he's fully *aware* of all the dangers, sir. If he was, he would never have told the tribune the journey was possible."

Draco turned to Nasica and the three friends couldn't see his expression, but the primus pilus nodded in response and clapped a huge hand on Draco's shoulder before addressing Cervianus himself.

"Your centurion here tells me that you're an inventive and knowledgeable man. I gather you were behind the information that won us Buhen. A man with an analytical mind like yours is likely to look at every angle of a problem and anticipate any issues."

Cervianus shrugged. "I would hope so, sir. Missing things is a bad habit in a surgeon."

Nasica laughed out loud, his deep voice registering rare humour. "Good. We are unlikely to argue our way out of the task at hand and, despite the sentiments being bandied about among the men," a quick glance in the direction of Ulyxes, "we are soldiers of Rome and not about to gainsay our commander."

"Of course, sir."

"So the First and Second cohorts will be marching into the desert and assaulting Napata. However, we still have half a day and night before we must depart. I want you, as our cohort's capsarius, to start thinking of everything we'll have to watch out for and guard against and I want to take any extra stores or gear that might make the journey easier. Essentially, you've bought yourself a free afternoon. Just get yourself and the rest of the men as prepared and armed against the journey as you can."

Cervianus saluted quickly. "Yessir!"

Draco turned again as they fell into line with the column, and regarded Shenti and Ulyxes. "Take your disobedient friend to help you, too."

Ulyxes grinned and the centurion's eyes narrowed in contemplation. A slow smile broke out across Draco's face as he turned back to his superior.

"Did you hear any mention of replacing our lost men or the disposition of troops, sir?"

Nasica shook his head, frowning.

"Then could I submit, sir, that you might want to arrange the transfers of the hardiest and strongest men from around the legion to fill the losses in our centuries? We should have a full complement if we're to try this and stronger backs and constitutions will be very helpful in the coming week."

His smile spread to the primus pilus.

"Good idea, Draco. If the tribune's sending us into Hades, let's make sure we're ready for it."

Cervianus turned, swallowing nervously, his eyes straying to the endless stretches of golden brown on the horizon. Without even contemplating the many things living in the desert that bit or stung, or simply ate, the unwary, just the sun, the sand and the air could kill a man in mere days. Only a true fool would willingly leave a life-giving river and march out into the unforgiving desert.

'All hail the legion of fools,' sighed the capsarius as he squared his shoulders and took a deep breath. 'Here we go…'

HISTORICAL NOTE

The history of the Twenty Second legion has always fascinated me. Galatia, of Biblical fame, was a once-independent land in the heart of Anatolia (modern Asian Turkey). The entire region had been contested for centuries between Greek and Persian cultures and yet in the third century BC, Gauls from modern France migrated east through the Balkans and managed to settle and create a Gallic-speaking state in the midst of this eastern region. The state of Galatia lasted more than two centuries, and by the mid-first century BC the last king of independent Galatia, Deiotarus, was a staunch ally of Rome. The great Pompey aided the king in levying a private royal Galatian army, organised and trained on the Roman model. In 25 BC, after the death of Deiotarus and brief rule by a son-in-law and then a grandson, the kingdom was peacefully assimilated into the Roman republic as a province, and its army became the Twenty Second legion, retaining the name of its founder as part of the unit name, 'Deiotariana'.

It is easy to imagine, in the years following their incorporation into Rome's military, how different they might still have been in comparison with the other legions. Their adherence to ancient custom, language, gods and such forth can easily be pictured and, like the auxilia raised from distant provinces, it seems highly likely that Roman officers had been foisted upon the Galatian legion. The soldiers would have spoken their native Galatian language, but with the prevalence of Greek-speaking states around them, that language, too, may well have been commonly spoken. Moreover, given the longstanding ties to Rome, and the fact that the legion had been formed and trained by Romans, Latin was likely quickly learned.

I have done what I deemed appropriate in the story to make the unit stand out as different. The subject of the colour of legionary uniforms is a matter of constant debate among experts. The only pictorial representations from the principate show red tunics, and this has long been taken to be the standard. However, such images may represent officers or specific units. Most likely the legions wore undyed wool and linen, for dyeing was expensive; so off-white would seem the natural, perhaps with centurions in red. I have taken the traditional line, portraying the other legions in red, and making the Twenty Second stand out in green. My own choice. Mea culpa.

Egypt was the province of a prefect. No one of senatorial rank could hold a command there, for the place was seen as a potential source of usurpers. Mark Antony had based himself there, and rumour has it that Caesar was also planning to do so at the time of his murder. The Third Cyrenaica was based at Thebes and later, after the time of this tale, moved first to Alexandria and was then reassigned to Syria in AD 106. The Twelfth Fulminata was assigned to Egypt in 30 BC, and may have been at Nicopolis, or possibly Babylon (Cairo), at this time. They would then move to Syria in AD 14. We do not know when the Twenty Second Deiotariana moved to Egypt, other than that they were in Galatia in 25 BC and in Nicopolis by 8 BC, where they would remain until at least AD 119. They may have been destroyed during the Bar Kokhba revolt of AD 132, for there is no mention of them after this time.

The ill-fated expedition of Gallus to Arabia Felix was one of the most appalling debacles in Roman military history and is described by Strabo, Pliny the Elder and Cassius Dio. I shall not dwell too long on it, for its merit to this tale is merely as background and an opening scene. Its importance, however, in leaving Egypt undefended and open to attack, cannot be overstated.

Another subject that fascinates me, and which also gave rise to this story, is that of Roman military medics. This is a massive subject in and of itself, and I have only peripherally dealt with the legion's medicus and his staff, since my main subject is the capsarius. This character, named for the *capsa*, or leather satchel in which he carried his equipment, was one of the most interesting figures in the army, and is not widely understood. Like several figures in the legion with specific jobs, the capsarius was 'excused duty', allowing him to concentrate on his role rather than fortifying camps and digging latrines. This put him at a slight rank advantage over the normal soldier, though with no authority over them. The capsarius was not part of the legion's medical team and was primarily a soldier, though in battle his duties would include field dressings and the removal of the wounded from the fighting.

In studying their skills, I am indebted to a work called *The Healing Hand* by Guido Majno, which goes into ancient medicine in much detail – including Roman and Greek medicine, as would have been practiced within the republic, but also including ancient-Egyptian medicine, which involved a deal more magic and mysticism and was clearly of import to this story. Every procedure I have described in the book has a solid basis in history. It is clear that, despite reliance upon the four humours and libations to healing gods, there was a great deal of accuracy and skill in Roman medicine, some of it even on a par with modern skill.

The journey up the Nile is something of a *Heart of Darkness* journey. Each site I have used is a historical site and, where possible, is based upon personal visits combined with archaeological investigations and modern reconstructions. One that clearly stands out is the double temple of Sobek and Haroeris at Ambo (now Kom Ombo.) Nowhere is the ancient-Egyptian veneration of the crocodile more keenly felt than there, where the visitor can even view mummified crocodiles from the site.

The first place where my imagination has had to take priority over research is Buhen. When the Aswan Dam was constructed in 1964 and the waters of Lake Nasser rose, the imposing fortress of Buhen was one of the many monuments sadly lost to history beneath the surface, along with the cataract a few miles away. However, enough investigation had already been carried out for a good plan and idea of Buhen to have survived, and there are even photographs of its massive ramparts. In labelling the border between Aegyptus and Kush here, I have somewhat simplified matters. The border seems to have been a lot more nebulous, and there were other fortresses manned against Kush. Interestingly, though, Buhen *was* a border fortress, and even now the location lies mid-lake but only five miles from the Egypt-Sudan border.

The desert journey is something of a composite in which I have attempted to portray all the many perils of such a trek.

Nothing here is entirely unrealistic. Indeed, in the sources, there is the following line: 'after passing through the sand-dunes, where the army of Cambyses was overwhelmed when a wind-storm struck them'. The bleakness of this journey is somewhat amplified by the mention of Cambyses II, an Achaemenid emperor who is noted as losing his army to the sands on an ill-advised invasion of Ethiopia.

Kush (modern Sudan) was a powerful state. Though it displayed a number of differences to Egypt, the two cultures were closely linked, and Egypt had been ruled by Kushite pharaohs for a time. The Meroitic period, during which this is set, is the last flowering of that culture, and is characterised in particular by a series of impressive warrior queens. They are shown in scattered representations, but the vast majority of what we know about them comes from Graeco-Roman sources. In particular, the Kandake of this story, Amanirenas, is mostly known from three Roman sources (Strabo, Pliny and Cassius Dio), all of which I have quoted at the end of this note for reference. It can therefore safely be said that the image painted is coloured by a healthy dose of fiction and xenophobia. Still, it is what we have to work with, and so I have built upon their image.

One primary source that is fascinating beyond those three is an image carved on the side of a pyramid wall at Barwa, which shows this Kandake and to some extent confirms the portrayal by the Roman writers. The images show the queen standing in violent pose with a sword in each hand, using her right to crush an army, believed to represent a Roman force, which is then being eaten by her lion.

The black-clad tribesmen that appear in the book are my own portrayal of the tribe known as the Blemmyes, which occupied the desert highlands east of the Nile, to the south of Egypt and the north of Kush. The Blemmyes are somewhat mysterious. All we know of them is from ancient writers, though they are now thought to be the ancestors of the nomadic Beja people. However, though they may have developed into a relatively peaceful tribe, there has to have been something frightening and martial in their past. Not only were they used as mercenaries by later Roman emperors (and they themselves invaded and occupied parts of Roman Egypt on at least two occasions), but they must have been a powerful military force in their own right, for there is a somewhat telling hint that they terrified their Roman enemies. Of them, Pliny writes, 'The Blemmyes, by report, have no heads, but mouths and eyes in their chests' (author's translation), and Pomponius Mela echoes this peculiar and worrying image. What, then, were these monsters? I have made them human, at least.

Therein I have explained all I feel is needed. I leave you with the three historical source texts that cover this campaign (as far as the end of *The Capsarius*, at least). Firstly, the work of Strabo's *Geography* (Book XVII.54, Loeb Edition 1932):

But the Aethiopians, emboldened by the fact that a part of the Roman force in Aegypt had been drawn away with aelius Gallus when he was carrying on war against the Arabians, attacked the Thebaïs and the garrison of the three cohorts at Syenê, and by an unexpected onset took Syenê and Elephantinê and Philae, and enslaved the inhabitants, and also pulled down the statues of Caesar. But Petronius, setting out with less than ten thousand infantry and eight hundred cavalry against thirty thousand men, first forced them to flee back to Pselchis, an Aethiopian city, and sent ambassadors to demand what they had taken, as also to ask the reasons why they had begun war; and when they said that they had been wronged by the Nomarchs, he replied that these were not rulers of the country, but Caesar; and when they had requested three days for deliberation, but did nothing they should have done, he made an attack and forced them to come forth to battle; and he quickly turned them to flight, since they were badly marshalled and badly armed; for they had large oblong shields, and those too made of raw ox-hide, and as weapons some had only axes, others pikes, and others swords. Now some were driven together into the city, others fled into the desert, and others found refuge on a neighbouring island, having waded into the channel, for on account of the current the crocodiles were not numerous there. Among these fugitive were the generals of Queen Candacê, who was ruler of the Aethiopians in my time — a masculine sort of woman, and blind in one eye. These, one and all, he captured alive, having sailed after them in both rafts and ships, and he sent them forthwith down to Alexandria; and he also attacked Pselchis and captured it; and if the multitude of those who fell in the battle be added to the number of the captives, those who escaped must have been altogether few in number.

And from Cassius Dio, *History* (Book LIV.5.4, Loeb Edition 1917):

About this time the Ethiopians, who dwell beyond Egypt, advanced as far as the city called Elephantine, with Candace as their leader, ravaging everything they encountered. At Elephantine, however, learning that Gaius Petronius, the governor of Egypt, was approaching, they hastily retreated before he arrived, hoping to make good their escape.

And finally from Pliny the Elder's *The Natural History* (Book VI.35, ed. Bostock & Riley 1857):

The Roman arms also penetrated into these regions in the time of the late Emperor Augustus, under the command of P. Petronius, a man of Equestrian rank, and prefect of Egypt. That general took the following cities, the only ones we now find mentioned there, in the following order; Pselcis, Primis, Abuncis, Phthuris, Cambusis, Atteva, and Stadasis, where the river Nile, as it thunders down the precipices, has quite deprived the inhabitants of the power of hearing.

ABOUT THE AUTHOR

SIMON TURNEY is from Yorkshire and, having spent much of his childhood visiting historic sites, fell in love with the Roman heritage of the region. His fascination with the ancient world snowballed from there with great interest in Rome, Egypt, Greece and Byzantium. His works include the Marius' Mules and Praetorian series, the Tales of the Empire and The Damned Emperor series, and the Rise of Emperors books with Gordon Doherty.

www.simonturney.com @SJATurney